Small Animal Theriogenology

Editor

BRUCE W. CHRISTENSEN

VETERINARY CLINICS OF NORTH AMERICA: SMALL ANIMAL PRACTICE

www.vetsmall.theclinics.com

September 2023 • Volume 53 • Number 5

ELSEVIER

1600 John F. Kennedy Boulevard • Suite 1800 • Philadelphia, Pennsylvania, 19103-2899
http://www.vetsmall.theclinics.com

VETERINARY CLINICS OF NORTH AMERICA: SMALL ANIMAL PRACTICE Volume 53, Number 5
September 2023 ISSN 0195-5616, ISBN-13: 978-0-443-18266-2

Editor: Stacy Eastman
Developmental Editor: Varun Gopal

Veterinary Clinics of North America: Small Animal Practice (ISSN 0195-5616) is published bimonthly by Elsevier Inc., 360 Park Avenue South, New York, NY 10010-1710. Months of issue are January, March, May, July, September, and November. Business and Editorial Offices: 1600 John F. Kennedy Blvd., Ste. 1800, Philadelphia, PA 19103-2899. Customer Service Office: 3251 Riverport Lane, Maryland Heights, MO 63043. Periodicals postage paid at New York, NY and additional mailing offices. Subscription prices are $387.00 per year (domestic individuals), $844.00 per year (domestic institutions), $100.00 per year (domestic students/residents), $488.00 per year (Canadian individuals), $1049.00 per year (Canadian institutions), $528.00 per year (international individuals), $1049.00 per year (international institutions), $100.00 per year (Canadian students/residents), and $220.00 per year (international students/residents). To receive student/resident rate, orders must be accompanied by name of affiliated institution, date of term, and the *signature* of program/residency coordinator on institution letterhead. Orders will be billed at individual rate until proof of status is received. Foreign air speed delivery is included in all *Clinics* subscription prices. All prices are subject to change without notice. **POSTMASTER:** Send address changes to *Veterinary Clinics of North America: Small Animal Practice*, Elsevier Health Sciences Division, Subscription Customer Service, 3251 Riverport Lane, Maryland Heights, MO 63043. Customer Service (orders, claims, online, change of address): Elsevier Periodicals Customer Service, Elsevier Health Sciences Division Subscription **Customer Service 3251 Riverport Lane Maryland Heights, MO 63043. Tel: 1-800-654-2452 (U.S. and Canada); 314-447-8871 (outside U.S. and Canada). Fax: 314-447-8029. E-mail: journalscustomerservice-usa@elsevier.com (for print support); journalsonlinesupport-usa@elsevier.com (for online support).**

Reprints. For copies of 100 or more of articles in this publication, please contact the Commercial Reprints Department, Elsevier Inc., 360 Park Avenue South, New York, NY 10010-1710. Tel.: 212-633-3874; Fax: 212-633-3820; E-mail: reprints@elsevier.com.

Veterinary Clinics of North America: Small Animal Practice is also published in Japanese by Inter Zoo Publishing Co., Ltd., Aoyama Crystal-Bldg 5F, 3-5-12 Kitaaoyama, Minato-ku, Tokyo 107-0061, Japan.

Veterinary Clinics of North America: Small Animal Practice is covered in *Current Contents/Agriculture, Biology and Environmental Sciences, Science Citation Index, ASCA, MEDLINE/PubMed (Index Medicus), Excerpta Medica,* and *BIOSIS.*

Contributors

EDITOR

BRUCE W. CHRISTENSEN, DVM, MS
Diplomate, American College of Theriogenologists; Chief Veterinarian, Assisted
Reproductive Services, Kokopelli Veterinary Center, Sacramento, California,
USA

AUTHORS

DALEN AGNEW, DVM, PhD
Diplomate, American College of Veterinary Pathologists; Professor and Department
Chairperson, Department of Pathobiology and Diagnostic Investigation, Michigan
State University College of Veterinary Medicine, East Lansing, Michigan,
USA

**MICHAEL AHERNE, MVB (Hons 1), Graduate Diploma of Veterinary Studies
(GradDipVetStud), MS**
Diplomate, American College of Veterinary Internal Medicine (Cardiology); Member,
Australian and New Zealand College of Veterinary Scientists (Small Animal Surgery),
Department of Small Animal Clinical Sciences, University of Florida College of Veterinary
Medicine, Gainesville, Florida, USA

SONIA KUHN ASIF, DVM
Diplomate, American College of Veterinary Ophthalmologists; Blue Pearl Veterinary Eye
Care, Bessemer, Alabama, USA

ORSOLYA BALOGH, DVM, PhD
Department of Small Animal Clinical Science, Virginia-Maryland College of Veterinary
Medicine, Blacksburg, Virginia, USA

BART J.G. BROECKX, MSc Vet Med, MSc Stat Data Analysis, PhD
Professor, Department of Veterinary and Biosciences, Laboratory of Animal Genetics,
Faculty of Veterinary Medicine, Ghent University, Merelbeke, Belgium

JANICE CAIN, DVM
Diplomate, American College of Veterinary Internal Medicine (Small Animal Internal
Medicine); Canine Reproduction Center at Ironhorse Vet Care, Dublin, California, USA

BRUCE W. CHRISTENSEN, DVM, MS
Diplomate, American College of Theriogenologists; Chief Veterinarian, Assisted
Reproductive Services, Kokopelli Veterinary Center, Sacramento, California, USA

ALAN J. CONLEY, BVSc, MS, PhD, FRCVS
Diplomate, American College of Theriogenologists (Honorary); Department of Population
Health and Reproduction, School of Veterinary Medicine, University of California, Davis,
Davis, California, USA

AUTUMN DAVIDSON, DVM, MS
Diplomate, American College of Theriogenologists (Honorary); Diplomate, American College of Veterinary Internal Medicine (Small Animal Internal Medicine); School of Veterinary Medicine, University of California, Davis, Davis, California, USA

KATHRYN A. DIEHL, MS, DVM
Diplomate, American College of Veterinary Ophthalmologists; Department of Small Animal Medicine and Surgery, University of Georgia College of Veterinary Medicine, Athens, Georgia, USA

HOLLIS N. ERB, DVM, MS, PhD
Department of Population Medicine and Diagnostic Sciences, Cornell University College of Veterinary Medicine, Ithaca, New York, USA

KRISTINE L. GONZALES, BS, DVM
Diplomate, American College of Theriogenologists; Guide Dogs for the Blind, California Campus, San Rafael, California, USA

SOPHIE A. GRUNDY BVSc (Hons)
MANZCVS (Small Animal Medicine), Diplomate American College of Veterinary Internal Medicine (Small Animal Internal Medicine); Veterinarian, Banfield Pet Hospital, Sacramento, California, USA

RAGNVI HAGMAN, DVM, PhD
Associate Professor, Department of Clinical Sciences, Swedish University of Agricultural Sciences, Uppsala, Sweden

BENJAMIN L. HART, DVM, PhD
Distinguished Professor Emeritus, School of Veterinary Medicine, University of California, Davis, Davis, California, USA

LYNETTE A. HART, MA, PhD
Professor, Department of Population Health and Reproduction, School of Veterinary Medicine, University of California, Davis, Davis, California, USA

JESSICA J. HAYWARD, PhD
Senior Research Associate, Department of Biomedical Sciences, College of Veterinary Medicine, Cornell University, Ithaca, New York, USA

LIN K. KAUFFMAN, DVM
Associate Veterinarian at Prairie View Animal Hospital, Grimes, Iowa, USA; Veterinarian/Owner of Enhanced Animal Reproduction Services, LLC, Ames, Iowa, USA

HYUN-TAE KIM, DVM, MS
Department of Clinical Sciences and Advanced Medicine, School of Veterinary Medicine, University of Pennsylvania, Philadelphia, Pennsylvania, USA

STUART J. MASON, BVSc (Hons)
MANZCVS, Diplomate, American College of Theriogenologists; Monash Veterinary Clinic, Victoria, Australia

ERICKA MENDEZ, DVM
Flagler Beach, Florida, USA

STUART MEYERS, DVM, PhD
School of Veterinary Medicine, University of California, Davis, Davis, California, USA

FREYA MOWAT, BVSc, PhD
MRCVS, Diplomate, European College of Veterinary Ophthalmologists; Diplomate, American College of Veterinary Ophthalmologists; Department of Surgical Sciences, School of Veterinary Medicine, University of Wisconsin-Madison, Department of Ophthalmology and Visual Sciences, School of Medicine and Public Health, Madison, Wisconsin, USA

MARY K. SEBZDA, DVM
Diplomate, American College of Theriogenologists; Associate Veterinarian at Newport Harbor Animal Hospital, Costa Mesa, California, USA; Clinical Assistant Professor of Veterinary Medicine at Western University of Health Sciences, Pomona, California, USA

JENNIFER SONES, DVM, PhD
Veterinary Clinical Sciences, Louisiana State University School of Veterinary Medicine, Baton Rouge, Louisiana, USA

ABIGAIL P. THIGPEN, BS
Associate Specialist, Department of Population Health and Reproduction, School of Veterinary Medicine, University of California, Davis, Davis, California, USA

RORY J. TODHUNTER, BVSc, MS, PhD
Diplomate, American College of Veterinary Surgeons; Professor of Surgery, Department of Clinical Sciences, College of Veterinary Medicine, Cornell University, Ithaca, New York, USA

JOSEPH J. WAKSHLAG, DVM, PhD
Diplomate, American College of Veterinary Internal Medicine (Nutrition); Diplomate, American College of Veterinary Sports Medicine and Rehabilitation; Department of Clinical Sciences, College of Veterinary Medicine, Cornell University, Ithaca, New York, USA

Contents

Advances in canine semen evaluation have progressed over time in fits and spurts, interspersed with long periods of relative inactivity. Despite exciting advances in the semen analysis, clinical canine theriogenology has been in a period of relative inactivity for a number of decades since initial advances in canine semen freezing in the mid 20th century. This review describes ways that the clinical practice of canine semen evaluation should improve, given the state of current knowledge.

Progesterone is a worthwhile addition to the clinical assessment of cycle stage for breeding, elective cesarian delivery, and reproductive management in the bitch if reliably measured. Clinical decisions based on systemic progesterone concentrations also require the rapid return of results. Most commercially accessible analyses capable of returning results within a day still rely primarily on immunoassays of one kind or another. Point-of-care instruments utilizing similar technology have been developed more recently to enable results to be generated in-house. Repeated monitoring of progesterone on whatever platform can be useful if consistent collection and analysis protocols ensure acceptable precision, accuracy, and repeatability.

Genetic tests are powerful tools that enable (1) a focus on genetic diversity as mating outcomes can be predicted and thus optimized to minimize or even avoid exclusion and (2) working toward breeding goals by improving a phenotype.

This article describes the history and infrastructure associated with canine breed-related eye screening and certification by Diplomates of the American College of Veterinary Ophthalmologists. Some of the common or otherwise particularly problematic specific inherited ophthalmic conditions are discussed.

acknowledged. This review will focus on new information that has been obtained since our last *B canis* article in 2018. Readers are encouraged to look to that article for information not presented within this update. Current *B canis* epidemiology along with a complete review of diagnostic testing options will be covered. Regulations for the international movement of dogs will be discussed in addition to concerns for increased zoonosis potential. Future goals would include better management of this disease including proposed screening of all imported dogs. Canine brucellosis prevention, owner and shelter/rescue education along with proposed therapies for the future will also be explored.

Infertility in the dog is a common reason for presentation of stud dogs for assessment with veterinarians. This article aims to discuss and outline some of the tests that can be done to try to ascertain the underlying cause of abnormalities found in a semen assessment. Topics discussed are semen alkaline phosphatase measurement, retrograde ejaculation assessment, ultrasound of the male reproductive tract, semen culture, human chorionic gonadotropin response testing, dietary assessment for phytoestrogens, environmental impacts on spermatogenesis, testicular biopsy, supplements to improve semen quality and quantity, and when to expect an improvement in semen quality after starting treatment.

Feeding during normal reproduction is often not thought of until there is a problem with conception or gestational losses. Energy demands of lactation and early puppy/kitten are of concern, particularly in large and giant breed dogs where mineral balance is crucial to normal development. There is a paucity of information around optimizing feeding during conception and gestation with many myths around ingredients which will be explored in this article along with supplements that may be able to support spermatogenesis and conception which primarily comes from the human literature and may have validity in times of difficult conception.

 Video content accompanies this article at http://www.vetsmall. theclinics.com.

Veterinary care of breeding dogs begins before a breeding takes place, during prebreeding consultations, through matings, gestation, and delivery of newborns.

Canine Cesarean Section (CS) is primarily performed to increase survival of newborns and less commonly to save the life or reproductive future of

some dog breeds when neutered at young ages. These risks are breed-, gender-, and body-size specific and related to neutering age. Current guidelines suggest making a personalized decision for each dog's neutering age. Recommendations are presented for 40 breeds and mixed-breed weight classes.

Ragnvi Hagman

 Video content accompanies this article at http://www.vetsmall. theclinics.com.

Pyometra is a common disease in intact bitches and queens and occurs, although less frequently, in most other female pets. In bitches and queens, the illness is generally diagnosed within 4 months after estrus, in middle-aged to older individuals. Complications such as peritonitis, endotoxemia, and systemic inflammatory response syndrome are not uncommon and associated with more severe illness. Ovary-sparing surgical options such as hysterectomy could be considered in individuals with high-risk for detrimental side effects of spaying or without infection of the uterus but has not yet been evaluated for safety in pyometra.

VETERINARY CLINICS OF NORTH AMERICA: SMALL ANIMAL PRACTICE

SERIES OF RELATED INTEREST

Veterinary Clinics: Exotic Animal Practice
https://www.vetexotic.theclinics.com/
Advances in Small Animal Care
https://www.advancesinsmallanimalcare.com/

THE CLINICS ARE NOW AVAILABLE ONLINE!
Access your subscription at:
www.theclinics.com

Preface

A Profession Dedicated to Healthy Breeding Programs

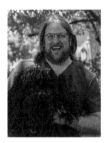

Bruce W. Christensen, DVM, MS
Editor

When I was interviewing for veterinary school admissions, I was asked to differentiate a job from a profession. There are undoubtedly a lot of appropriate ways to answer that question. My thoughts were along the lines that the motivation to do a job is mostly the payment, and when the required tasks are done, you go home; but a profession is a part of you, and you are a part of it, and so you don't just do the minimum required tasks, you also find ways to contribute and build it up. The professionals who present their contributions here received no compensation for their work, just the fulfillment of doing something worthwhile to add to the betterment of small animal theriogenology. I have no doubt that any member of our profession who reads the information here will discover many worthwhile things.

In putting together the 2023 issue of *Veterinary Clinics of North America: Small Animal Practice* dedicated to theriogenology, I evaluated previous issues published in 2001, 2012, and 2018 and tried to conscientiously choose topics that would flesh out and strengthen the canon. This led to the updated articles on semen processing, stud dog infertility, genetic testing, neonatal health, pregnancy, C-sections, brucellosis, and pyometra. While there were past articles on male and female reproductive lesions, we lacked one on neonatal lesions. I chose a couple of articles on current issues in clinical canine reproduction, namely the onslaught of in-house progesterone testing and when or how to spay and neuter. To fill out the rest of the issue, I focused on our responsibility as veterinarians to help create and support healthy canine breeding programs. This inspired articles on genetic screening, nutrition, obesity, puppy behavior, and Orthopedic Foundation for Animals testing in eyes, heart, and hips.

The resultant issue presented here is a robust and informative collection of articles written by talented and experienced veterinarians. I express my appreciation to each of

Vet Clin Small Anim 53 (2023) xiii–xiv
https://doi.org/10.1016/j.cvsm.2023.06.001
0195-5616/23/© 2023 Published by Elsevier Inc.

them for the significant time they took out of their lives to thoughtfully prepare material for the betterment of our profession.

Bruce W. Christensen, DVM, MS
Assisted Reproductive Services
Kokopelli Veterinary Center
1420 Fulton Avenue
Sacramento, CA 95825, USA

E-mail address:
drbruce@kokopellivet.net

Canine Semen Evaluation and Processing

Bruce W. Christensen, DVM, MS[a],*, Stuart Meyers, DVM, PhD[b]

KEYWORDS

- Semen • Cryopreservation • Sperm motility • Morphology • Fluoroscopy

KEY POINTS

- Basic semen evaluation should include objective measures of motility and concentration and subjective evaluation of morphology.
- Advanced semen evaluation should include viability analyses and kinematic parameters.
- Advances in sperm cryopreservation include new extender types and parameters to predict cryopreservation success.
- Clinics offering reproductive services should utilize objective diagnostics.
- Clinics specializing or having a special interest in theriogenology have opportunities to also increase and improve their diagnostic offerings by including evaluations of sperm function.

INTRODUCTION

Semen evaluation began in 1677 when Dutch scientist Anton van Leeuwenhoek and his student Johan Ham viewed a human ejaculate under a compound microscope Leeuwenhoek had constructed and observed sperm for the first time in history. With the publication of their findings in 1678, sperm biology was born.[1] They called the sperm "animalcules" (little animals), believing that each sperm was a tiny, preformed human.[2] This may seem silly from our twenty first century hindsight, but consider that the mammalian ovum was not discovered for another 150 years. For many years the scientific dialogue focused on the source of the embryo (from the male or the female?) and the purpose of sperm, which were argued to be complete embryos or, alternatively, parasites. Roughly 100 years after the discovery of sperm, the Italian priest Lazzar Spallanzani demonstrated with frogs that contact between eggs and sperm result in offspring. He incorrectly determined that the male contribution came from seminal fluid "vapor" that stimulated the eggs and that the sperm were incidental parasites. Spallanzani was, nevertheless, the first to successfully perform

[a] Kokopelli Veterinary Center, 1420 Fulton Avenue, Sacramento, CA 94825, USA; [b] School of Veterinary Medicine, University of California, One Shields Avenue, Davis, CA 95616, USA
* Corresponding author.
E-mail address: drbruce@kokopellivet.net

Vet Clin Small Anim 53 (2023) 921–930
https://doi.org/10.1016/j.cvsm.2023.05.006
0195-5616/23/© 2023 Elsevier Inc. All rights reserved.

artificial insemination (AI), and in 1776 the dog was the first mammal to successfully produce offspring after AI.[3]

Perhaps due to the focus of reproductive biologists on whether or not sperm played a direct role in fertility, it wasn't until the early 20th century that semen analysis parameters began to be established. Initial studies focused on concentration, subjective motility, and morphology, and it was not until the mid-20th century that studies investigating the processing and cryopreservation of sperm were conducted. This pattern of progression in fits and starts with long intervals of stasis has persisted. Despite advances in our ability to evaluate sperm functionality, most clinicians are still stuck in patterns and technology from decades ago: using densimeters for concentration, evaluating morphology on stained slides at 400x, and evaluating sperm motility in a subjective manner. This review will explore options for advanced semen analysis and processing for the shipping and cryopreservation of semen in dogs.

DISCUSSION
Sperm Motility Evaluation

During natural mating in the dog, sperm are deposited into the cranial vagina. Transport of the sperm from there to the oviductal ampulla, where oocytes are located after ovulation, is accomplished through a combination of prostatic fluid waves produced in the third ejaculatory fraction during the copulatory tie, contractions of the uterus, ciliary movement in the oviduct, and actual self-propulsion of the sperm (forward, progressive motility). The progressive motility of sperm has long been considered to be a strong, measurable marker of male fertility.[4] Most clinical evaluations of sperm motility are done subjectively by an observer looking through a microscope at 200x and giving a "best impression" of the percentage of sperm that are motile. Some clinicians go one step further and differentiate subjectively between all motile sperm and those moving in a relatively straightforward or progressive manner. Evidence in stallions indicates that total motility (and morphology) are better correlated to actual fertility than progressive motility.[5] In other species, progressive motility is thought to be a more accurate reflection on sperm function and fertility.[6]

It is hard to overstate the advantage of having a reliable, objective system for calculating motility and concentration. The current state of canine reproductive services in most clinics is embarrassingly archaic and inaccurate with the use of subjective measures for determining semen quality. Most of the time fresh/chilled semen is shipped with no documentation whatsoever, sometimes without even identifying the information of the stud dog, let alone estimations of the quantity or quality of the sperm. When those evaluations are performed, they are usually done subjectively, which is sometimes little better than guess work, or even aspirational hopes in some instances. Because of the variable precision inherent in subjective measures, little confidence can be placed in these estimations. Whether conscious or subconscious, there will be an intrinsic bias in the mind of the evaluator to overestimate the quality of the ejaculate, especially in cases where semen is being frozen with the accompanying hopes and expectations for maximal quality and number of insemination doses produced. This is further compounded by the fact that some practices charge by the dose, both to freeze the ejaculate and to store it. Using subjective measures to calculate sperm quality is not only less accurate but in these cases is a conflict of interest and is a disservice to clients. Using objective measures to calculate sperm motility and concentration is more accurate and more defensible from legal, ethical, and professional standpoints.

Objective measurements of sperm motility have been around since the 1990's[7] and are now readily available through numerous computer-assisted semen analysis

(CASA) platforms.[8–11] Until about 2017, CASA systems seemed prohibitively expensive (usually more than $20,000) for all but clinics with active, heavy reproductive caseloads. As with most technology, time allows for improvements in performance and reductions in cost; a reliable system may now be purchased for a few thousand dollars with reasonable accuracy to measure objective motility and concentration.[9] Clinicians should do their homework before purchasing a unit to be as sure as possible of the accuracy, precision, and limits of the systems they purchase.[11]

KINEMATICS

The advent of CASA systems for sperm motility analysis has allowed for precise evaluations into different aspects of sperm motility. These systems can determine parameters beyond simple total motility or progressive motility. Different kinematic parameters evaluated include the following.[6,12]

- Velocity of the curved line (VCL): analyzes the velocity of a sperm head on time-average basis along its actual curvilinear path (measured in 2 dimensions)
- Velocity of the straight line (VSL): measures the velocity of a sperm head on a time-average basis along the straight line between its first and last detected position
- Velocity of the average path (VAP): measures the velocity of a sperm head along its average path on a time-average basis; this path is computed by smoothing the actual path according to algorithms in the CASA instrument, these algorithms vary among instruments
- Linearity (LIN): estimates a curvilinear path reflecting the straightness of the sperm path (VSL/VCL $\times$ 100 [%])
- Straightness (STR): reflecting the righteousness of motion (VSL/VAP $\times$ 100 [%])
- Wobble (WOB): balancing, expressed as percentage; the degree of oscillation of the actual path of the sperm head in its relationship with VAP (VAP/VCL $\times$ 100 [%])
- Beat cross-frequency (BCF): the average rate at which the actual sperm trajectory crosses the VAP (a derivation of the true frequency of flagellar beat and frequency of rotation of the head)
- Amplitude of lateral head displacement (ALH): measures the magnitude of the lateral displacement of a sperm head about its average path; this can be expressed as the maximum or an average of such displacement; the amplitude of variations of the current path of the sperm head in its relationship with VAP

Studies have not directly correlated specific kinematic properties or ranges with fertility, although some ranges have been correlated with the ability of sperm to be cryopreserved successfully.[10] Establishing normal ranges for the different values will be a strong step towards more comparable, objective practice and a step forward from the current practice of simply estimating "vigor" on a subjective scale of 0-4. Of course, studies that objectively determine the value of any adjunctive motility parameters will be critical for clinical implementation to further our understanding of canine fertility.

MORPHOLOGY

The importance of normal sperm morphology in relation to fertility has been demonstrated in other species.[5,13] Evidence suggests that the female tract is able to differentiate fertile sperm based, in part, on morphological cues. Traditional morphological evaluation entails subjective, visual analysis of sperm either fixed on a slide (bright- or dark-field) or preserved in a droplet for phase or differential interference contrast evaluation. A recommended bright field stain is rose bengal and a recommended dark field stain is eosin/nigrosin. Analysis is typically done at 400x or (better) 1000x under immersion oil. This type of analysis is relatively quick and easy, and can pick up many types of morphological abnormalities, such as detached heads, cytoplasmic droplets, abnormally shaped midpieces, and bent or coiled tails or midpieces.

More subtle head or midpiece defects can be missed in these traditional morphological analyses. More detailed morphometry can be performed for objective sperm measurements. The process involves capturing images of what appear to be normal sperm using a phase contrast microscope at 1000x coupled with a specialized camera and software programs. Measurements are taken of length, width, area, and perimeter of the head; length, width, area, and perimeter of the midpiece; tail length and total length of the sperm. From the data obtained from the measurements of the sperm head, ellipticity, elongation, roughness and regularity of the sperm head can be calculated.[8] More data are needed to determine to what degree, if any, this increased sensitivity of morphology evaluation gives insight into sperm subfertility. Until this is known, it may be difficult to justify as a practical application for clinical practice. Further, new methods are emerging in which imaging flow cytometry can be used to capture bright-field images of sperm in a high-throughput system that can also detect fluorescence staining. In this way, reported thus far for stallions, thousands of sperm can be analyzed along with other morphologic fluorescence parameters that increases the precision and accuracy of semen analysis.[14] Although promising tools, equipment expense would prevent these methods from being adapted by clinicians in the near future. It is anticipated that with time these objective measures will become easier and less expensive to use and will eventually replace the subjective morphology measures currently used by most clinicians and researchers.

CONCENTRATION

The gold standard for concentration determination has been, and some consider it still to be, manual counts with a hemocytometer or Neubauer chamber. Certainly, this method should be a tool used at least on a periodic, but regular basis in clinical practice, alongside more sophisticated measures, to determine the accuracy of the quicker, more technical tools.

Densimeters and spectrophotometers have been used for decades to estimate concentration and are still in use in many practices. This optical density technology is centered on how much light travels through a sample. More light means a less concentrated sample. Obviously this method is nonspecific as any cells or other debris in the sample will cause an erroneously high concentration calculation.

Beyond their role in objective motility assessment, CASA systems also give concentration measurements of sperm cells detected in a chamber, usually 20 μm deep, while also calculating the motility.

The NucleoCounter SP-100 (Chemometec, Denmark) uses the binding of propidium iodide (PI) to sperm and then a fluorescence assay to count those cells. The method is highly specific for sperm and produces a very accurate estimation of concentration.

A study in 2006 compared a photometer, two types of CASA, and the Nucleo-Counter against the gold standard Neubauer hemocytometer.[15] That study determined that the best agreement was with one of the CASA systems (SpermVision, Minitube, Germany) in dilute semen and with the NuceloCounter in concentrated semen. In addition to improvements in technology for existing CASA systems, many newer CASA systems have been developed in recent years. Again, clinicians are recommended to do their homework and look closely at validating studies when deciding on a system to purchase.

VIABILITY

The sperm membrane is integral in capacitation, acrosome reaction, and binding of the sperm to the egg surface. Viability of sperm is often determined based on membrane integrity and a variety of stains and assays are used. One of the older methods is the dark field stain, eosin/nigrosin, mentioned earlier for morphology evaluation. Sperm sit mostly unstained on top of the dark, stained background (the nigrosin stain). Those with damaged membranes appear pink, having allowed the eosin portion of the stain to enter the cell. Those sperm with intact membranes exclude the eosin and appear white. As a modification on this method, bromophenol blue may be used with nigrosin to a similar effect.

The NucleoCounter SP-100 can also be used to detect non-viable sperm and calculate the number of viable sperm in the sample. It does this by coupling a cell membrane lysing agent to the PI assay.

The hypo-osmotic swelling (HOS) test is used to evaluate the functional integrity of the sperm plasma membrane by determining the ability of the membrane to maintain equilibrium between the sperm and its environment.[16] The basis for this test is that only sperm with an intact and functional cell membrane can maintain equilibrium between the intracellular and extracellular compartments and react to changes in the environment. Influx of the assay fluid due to hypo-osmotic stress causes the sperm tail to coil and balloon or "swell." A higher percentage of swollen sperm indicates the presence of sperm having functional and intact plasma membranes. The utility of the HOS test has been evaluated in dogs and found to correlate with motility and the acrosome reaction, indicating it has value in evaluating viability in canine sperm.[17,18] For dogs, it is recommended to use a 60 mOsm fructose solution incubated in a 37° C water bath for 45 minutes prior to evaluation.[19]

SEMEN EXTENDERS

Initially, canine semen was extended using a very basic skim milk-based extender. Later Tris-based extenders were developed, in which buffering action reduced fructose metabolism and thus preserved sperm motility. More recently, powdered coconut water has been used as an extender base, being composed of a mixture of proteins, salts, sugars, vitamins, amino acids, and growth factors.[20–22] Sperm morphology does not seem to degrade significantly through the freeze/thaw process, regardless of extender type used.[8]

For cryopreservation, extenders often include egg yolk as a support for the phospholipid cellular membrane of sperm. Different methods of processing egg yolk to create low-density lipoproteins (LDL) have yielded significantly better post-thaw motility in cryopreserved canine semen compared to control samples with egg yolk not subjected to the agitation needed to create the LDLs.[23]

Shipping fresh semen at chilled temperatures for short-term storage prior to insemination is a common practice in canine breeding management. Most of the time the ejaculate arrives at the intended location and is used to inseminate the bitch within 24- 48 hours. Many commercial and homemade extenders have been used successfully for this process and canine sperm seems to be relatively resilient to minor temperature fluctuations. Some extenders even allow for maintenance of motility over longer periods, up to 10 days, as long as the temperature remains low (4°–5° C) and the extender is changed out every few days.[24]

Recent research in canine semen extenders has focused on the reduction of oxidative stress experienced by sperm in the chilling and cryopreservation processes. Researchers have looked to various methods and additives to buffer and protect sperm, with variable success.[18,22,25–30]

Prediction of Sperm Cryopreservation Potential

A high percentage of motile sperm in fresh semen does not always correlate with good post-thaw motility in cryopreserved sperm.[31] Several assays may give better predictability for the success of cryopreservation of a particular ejaculate. Quantification of sperm volume has been suggested to be predictive of post-cryopreservation quality in canine sperm, since the ability of the cell to survive osmotic changes through shrinking and swelling is key to the cryopreservation process.[32] Evaluation of sperm membrane integrity should be a valuable predictor of post-thaw fertility and can be done through the use of fluorescent assays using SYBR-1, PI, and carboxyfluorescein diacetate succinimidyl ester (CFDA-SE) stains. Mitochondrial activity in the sperm midpiece is critical to the kinematic activity of the sperm. Assessment of mitochondrial membrane integrity can be done with the JC-1 probe, which can therefore be a good indicator of mitochondrial function and oxidative ATP production prior to cryopreservation. Evaluation of DNA integrity is key to knowing the ability of sperm to function, whether fresh or cryopreserved. Different fluorescent assays assess DNA damage, including COMET, TUNEL, and toluidine blue.[33] A Raman spectrometer has successfully evaluated the light-scattering patterns caused by the interaction of light protons with molecules and thus assess the DNA integrity of sperm.[34] Currently, most of these evaluation techniques have been limited to research laboratories.

We are at a point, however, where the adoption of some of these techniques may be practical in a clinical setting and raise the standard of canine sperm cryopreservation evaluations. Fresh sperm samples with PM < 83.1%, VCL < 161.3 m/s, STR < 0.83% and LIN < 0.48% will have a probability of 85.5% that the post-thaw sperm quality will be low.[10] It has been proposed that a combination of certain CASA kinematic markers (VCL, STR, LIN, and PM), coupled with staining with JC-1 and COMET or toluidine blue (all of which are relatively simple to perform) to predict the potential for a dog to be a "good freezer" could be useful in a clinical setting[33] as discussed above for imaging flow cytometry.

Miscellaneous Improvements in Semen Processing

Traditional semen cryopreservation protocols include only one semen collection per day and on-site semen freezing. Collecting two ejaculates the same day, one hour apart, and pooling the two ejaculates for one cryopreservation process has been shown to increase the number of total sperm by an average of 80% without a decrease in semen quality.[35] In addition, while freezing on-site immediately after semen collection is the gold standard, acceptable post-thaw motility can be obtained from the cryopreservation of chilled/shipped semen, opening up the opportunity for semen cryopreservation to dog breeders in areas that do not have a canine fertility clinic close to them.[36] The benefits and risks of inclusion of prostatic fluid in the canine ejaculate during cryopreservation is still in question and likely the answer varies with individual dogs.[37] Elements of the seminal plasma (which in the dog is solely prostatic fluid) have been shown to exert a protective effect on mitochondria.[38,39] Poor quality ejaculates or those from older males, however, may benefit from the removal of prostatic fluid. Removal of the seminal fluid, and efforts to target specific sperm concentrations, require centrifugation, which in and of itself increases DNA damage and decreases post-thaw fertility in some ejaculates.[40] Use of centrifugation cushion media may help mitigate the damage.

FUTURE DIRECTIONS

Fertility rates in humans have been dropping steadily over the past decades, which is a major concern and incentive for active research. Lessons learned and tools developed for human fertility evaluation and treatment may also eventually benefit canine breeding programs.[41] Active research is also well-funded in farm animal production, where higher fertility means better efficiency and therefore better profits. Techniques currently being investigated in these other species include ways of selecting the most fertile sperm for use in advanced reproductive techniques, such as intracytoplasmic sperm injection, in vitro maturation of embryos, and embryo transfer. Density gradient centrifugation can be used to select for motile sperm but cannot select for DNA fragmentation and other functional problems.[42,43] Microfluidics[44,45] and hyaluronic acid binding[46] seek to mimic attributes of the female reproductive tract to select for normally functioning sperm. Apoptotic markers are used to differentiate viable from degenerating sperm.[47] Sex-sorting of canine sperm to produce litters of all (or predominantly) males or females can, in theory, be done, but logistics of semen handling, breeding management, and cryopreservation still need to be worked out.[48–50] One study successfully produced male or female dominated litters (86.4% and 87.5%, respectively) from sex-sorted, frozen-thawed canine semen, but the insemination doses were very low (4×10^6 total sperm) and overall pregnancy rates were only 20% and 25%, respectively.[51] CASA systems are dramatically improving and include 3-D digital holography[52] and imaging flow cytometry.[14] Non-invasive methods are developing that do not require sacrificing sperm for evaluation.[34,53] Next-generation sequencing allows for more accurate chromosomal analysis.[54] Specific components in seminal plasma have been shown in certain species to be reliable markers of sperm freezability, but to date no marker has been identified in canine semen.[33] It has been demonstrated that seminal proteins differ markedly between breeds,[37] perhaps indicating a reason why some individuals or some breeds lend themselves to cryopreservation more than others.

CLINICS CARE POINTS

- Objective measurements of sperm motility and concentration are now the standard of care and should replace subjective measures in veterinary clinics offering semen services.
- Morphological evaluation should be done on every semen sample and can be done on a bright field, dark field, or phase contrast preparation.
- Kinematic parameters can be used to predict post-thaw viability (PM < 83.1%, VCL < 161.3 m/s, STR < 0.83%, and LIN < 0.48% will have a probability of 85.5% that the post-thaw sperm quality will be low).
- It is usually beneficial to collect semen from a male twice in a day, one hour apart, when freezing, and pool the two ejaculates, in order to increase the insemination doses obtained.

DISCLOSURE

The authors have no conflicts of interest to disclose.

REFERENCES

1. Andrade-Rocha FT. On the origins of the semen analysis: a close relationship with the history of the reproductive medicine. J Hum Reprod Sci 2017;10(4):242–55.

2. Leeuwenhoek A. De natis e semine genital animalculis. Philosophical Transactions 1678;12:1040–6.

3. Spallanzani L., Prodromo della nuova enciclopedia italiana. Siena: pazzini-carli and bindi, Fecondazione artificiale, 1779, Siena, 129–134.

4. Biologic Markers of Human Male Reproductive Health, Physiologic Damage. National Research Council. Biologic Markers in Reproductive Toxicology. Washington, DC: The National Academies Press; 1989. https://doi.org/10.17226/774.

5. Love CC. Relationship between sperm motility, morphology and the fertility of stallions. Theriogenology 2011;76(3):547–57.

6. Tanga BM, Qamar AY, Raza S, et al. Semen evaluation: methodological advancements in sperm quality-specific fertility assessment - A review. Anim Biosci 2021; 34(8):1253–70.

7. Ellington J, Scarlett J, Meyers-Wallen V, et al. Computer-assisted sperm analysis of canine spermatozoa motility measurements. Theriogenology 1993;40(4): 725–33.

8. Teixeira DO, Silva HVR, Brito BF, et al. Sperm quality and morphometry characterization of cryopreserved canine sperm in acp-106c or tris. Anim Reprod 2022;19(3):e20210069.

9. Bulkeley E, Collins C, Foutouhi A, et al. Assessment of an iPad-based sperm motility analyzer for determination of canine sperm motility. Transl Anim Sci 2021;5(2):txab066.

10. Schäfer-Somi S, Tichy A. Canine post-thaw sperm quality can be predicted by using CASA, and classification and regression tree (CART)-analysis. Pol J Vet Sci 2019;22(1):51–9.

11. Surmacz P, Niwinska A, Kautz E, et al. Comparison of two staining techniques on the manual and automated canine sperm morphology analysis. Reprod Domest Anim 2022;57(6):678–84.

12. Aghazarian A, Huf W, Pflüger H, et al. Standard semen parameters *vs.*Sperm kinematics to predict sperm DNA damage. World J Mens Health 2021;39(1): 116–22.

13. Garcia-Vazquez FA, Gadea J, Matas C, et al. Importance of sperm morphology during sperm transport and fertilization in mammals. Asian J Androl 2016; 18(6):844–50.

14. Bulkeley E, Santistevan AC, Varner D, et al. Imaging flow cytometry to characterize the relationship between abnormal sperm morphologies and reactive oxygen species in stallion sperm. Reprod Domest Anim 2023;58(1):10–9.

15. Hansen C, Vermeiden T, Vermeiden JP, et al. Comparison of FACSCount AF system, Improved Neubauer hemocytometer, Corning 254 photometer, SpermVision, UltiMate and NucleoCounter SP-100 for determination of sperm concentration of boar semen. Theriogenology 2006;66(9):2188–94.

16. Ramu S, Jeyendran RS. The hypo-osmotic swelling test for evaluation of sperm membrane integrity. Methods Mol Biol 2013;927:21–5.

17. Kumi-Diaka J, Badtram G. Effect of storage on sperm membrane integrity and other functional characteristics of canine spermatozoa: In vitro bioassay for canine semen. Theriogenology 1994;41(7):1355–66.

18. Michael AJ, Alexopoulos C, Pontiki EA, et al. Effect of antioxidant supplementation in semen extenders on semen quality and reactive oxygen species of chilled canine spermatozoa. Anim Reprod Sci 2009;112(1–2):119–35.
19. Kumi-Diaka J. Subjecting canine semen to the hypo-osmotic test. Theriogenology 1993;39(6):1279–89.
20. Cardoso Rde C, Silva AR, Uchoa DC, et al. Cryopreservation of canine semen using a coconut water extender with egg yolk and three different glycerol concentrations. Theriogenology 2003;59(3–4):743–51.
21. de Cássia Soares Cardoso R, Silva AR, da Silva LD. Comparison of two dilution rates on canine semen quality after cryopreservation in a coconut water extender. Anim Reprod Sci 2006;92(3–4):384–91.
22. Uchoa DC, Silva TF, Mota Filho AC, et al. Intravaginal artificial insemination in bitches using frozen/thawed semen after dilution in powdered coconut water (ACP-106c). Reprod Domest Anim 2012;47(Suppl 6):289–92.
23. Anastácio da Silva E, Corcini CD, de Assis Araújo Camelo Junior F, et al. Probe ultrasonification of egg yolk plasma forms low-density lipoprotein nanoparticles that efficiently protect canine semen during cryofreezing. J Biol Chem 2022;298(7):101975.
24. Goericke-Pesch S, Klaus D, Failing K, et al. Longevity of chilled canine semen comparing different extenders. Anim Reprod Sci 2012;135(1–4):97–105.
25. Divar MR, Azari M, Mogheiseh A, et al. Supplementation of melatonin to cooling and freezing extenders improves canine spermatozoa quality measures. BMC Vet Res 2022;18(1):86.
26. Bencharif D, Dordas-Perpinya M. Canine semen cryoconservation: Emerging data over the last 20 years. Reprod Domest Anim 2020;55(Suppl 2):61–5.
27. Bencharif D, Amirat-Briand L, Garand A, et al. Freezing canine sperm: comparison of semen extenders containing Equex and LDL (Low Density Lipoproteins). Anim Reprod Sci 2010;119(3–4):305–13.
28. Michael AJ, Alexopoulos C, Pontiki EA, et al. Effect of N-acetyl-L-cysteine supplementation in semen extenders on semen quality and reactive oxygen species of chilled canine spermatozoa. Reprod Domest Anim 2010;45(2):201–7.
29. Usuga A, Tejera I, Gómez J, et al. Cryoprotective effects of ergothioneine and isoespintanol on canine semen. Animals (Basel) 2021;11(10):2757.
30. Del Prete C, Calabria A, Longobardi V, et al. Effect of aqueous extract of maca addition to an extender for chilled canine semen. Animals (Basel) 2022;12(13):1638.
31. Nöthling JO, Gerstenberg C, Volkmann DH. Semen quality after thawing: correlation with fertility and fresh semen quality in dogs. J Reprod Fertil Suppl 1997;51:109–16.
32. Petrunkina AM, Gröpper B, Günzel-Apel AR, et al. Functional significance of the cell volume for detecting sperm membrane changes and predicting freezability in dog semen. Reproduction 2004;128(6):829–42.
33. Schäfer-Somi S, Colombo M, Luvoni GC. Canine Spermatozoa-Predictability of Cryotolerance. Animals (Basel) 2022;12(6):733.
34. Sánchez V, Redmann K, Wistuba J, et al. Oxidative DNA damage in human sperm can be detected by Raman microspectroscopy. Fertil Steril 2012 Nov;98(5):1124–9.
35. Lechner D, Aurich J, Schäfer-Somi S, et al. Combined cryopreservation of canine ejaculates collected at a one-hour interval increases semen doses for artificial insemination without negative effects on post-thaw sperm characteristics. Reprod Domest Anim 2021;56(9):1220–6.

36. Colombo M, Morselli MG, Franchi G, et al. Freezability of dog semen after collection in field conditions and cooled transport. Animals (Basel) 2022;12(7):816.

37. Araujo MS, de Oliveira Henriques Paulo OL, Scott C, et al. Insights into the influence of canine breed on proteomics of the spermatozoa and seminal plasma. J Proteomics 2022;257:104508.

38. Aquino-Cortez A, Pinheiro BQ, Lima DBC, et al. Proteomic characterization of canine seminal plasma. Theriogenology 2017;95:178–86.

39. Domoslawska A, Zdunczyk S, Franczyk M, et al. Total antioxidant capacity and protein peroxidation intensity in seminal plasma of infertile and fertile dogs. Reprod Domest Anim 2019;54(2):252–7.

40. Kim SH, Yu DH, Kim YJ. Effects of cryopreservation on phosphatidylserine translocation, intracellular hydrogen peroxide, and DNA integrity in canine sperm. Theriogenology 2010;73(3):282–92.

41. Dai C, Zhang Z, Shan G, et al. Advances in sperm analysis: techniques, discoveries and applications. Nat Rev Urol 2021;18(8):447–67.

42. Esteves SC, Roque M, Bedoschi G, et al. Intracytoplasmic sperm injection for male infertility and consequences for offspring. Nat Rev Urol 2018;15(9):535–62.

43. Domain G, Ali Hassan H, Wydooghe E, et al. Influence of Single Layer Centrifugation with Canicoll on Semen Freezability in Dogs. Animals (Basel) 2022; 12(6):714.

44. Eamer L, Vollmer M, Nosrati R, et al. Turning the corner in fertility: high DNA integrity of boundary-following sperm. Lab Chip 2016;16(13):2418–22.

45. Orsolini MF, Verstraete MH, van Heule M, et al. Characterization of sperm cell membrane charge and selection of high-quality sperm using microfluidics in stallions. Theriogenology 2022;192:1–8.

46. Parmegiani L. Physiologic ICSI: Hyaluronic acid (HA) favors selection of spermatozoa without DNA fragmentation ande with normal nucleus, resulting in improvement of embryo quality. Fertil Steril 2010;93:598–604.

47. Hoogendijk CF, Kruger TF, Bouic PJ, et al. A novel approach for the selection of human sperm using annexin V-binding and flow cytometry. Fertil Steril 2009; 91(4):1285–92.

48. Merlo B, Zambelli D, Cunto M, et al. Sex-sorted canine sperm cryopreservation: limits and procedural considerations. Theriogenology 2015;83(7):1121–7.

49. Rodenas C, Lucas X, Tarantini T, et al. The effects of hoechst 33342 staining and the male sample donor on the sorting efficiency of canine spermatozoa. Reprod Domest Anim 2014;49(1):115–21.

50. Oi M, Yamada K, Hayakawa H, et al. Sexing of dog sperm by fluorescence in situ hybridization. J Reprod Dev 2013;59(1):92–6.

51. Wei YF, Chen FL, Tang SS, et al. Birth of puppies of predetermined sex after artificial insemination with a low number of sex-sorted, frozen-thawed spermatozoa in field conditions. Anim Sci J 2017;88(8):1232–8.

52. Daloglu MU, Lin F, Chong B, et al. 3D imaging of sex-sorted bovine spermatozoon locomotion, head spin and flagellum beating. Sci Rep 2018;8(1):15650.

53. Dai C, Zhang Z, Huang J, et al. Automated non-invasive measurement of single sperm's motility and morphology. IEEE Trans Med Imaging 2018;37(10):2257–65.

54. Tran QT, Jatsenko T, Poolamets O, et al. Chromosomal scan of single sperm cells by combining fluorescence-activated cell sorting and next-generation sequencing. J Assist Reprod Genet 2019;36(1):91–7.

Progesterone Analysis in Canine Breeding Management

Alan J. Conley, BVSc, MS, PhD, FRCVS, Dipl ACT (honorary)[a],*,
Kristine L. Gonzales, BS, DVM, Dipl ACT[b], Hollis N. Erb, DVM, MS, PhD[c],
Bruce W. Christensen, DVM, MS, Dipl ACT[d]

KEYWORDS

- Canine reproduction • Breeding management • Cesarian section
- Progesterone monitoring • Immunoassay • Point-of-care analysis

KEY POINTS

- Progesterone is a valuable addition to the clinical assessment of cycle stage for breeding, elective cesarian delivery, and reproductive management.
- Repeated monitoring of progesterone with consistent collection protocols, together with analytic precision, accuracy, and repeatability, are necessary.
- Quality control, calibration, validation, instrument maintenance, training, and reference concentration development in practices using point-of-care platforms are necessary for diagnostic reliability.

PROGESTERONE IN THE MANAGEMENT OF CANINE REPRODUCTION

Progesterone is required to establish pregnancy in mammals, and the decline in concentrations (or decreasing responsiveness of reproductive tissues) at the end of gestation precedes and initiates parturition in all species studied to date. However, progesterone concentrations have also become a widely used clinical biomarker in the reproductive management of the bitch. Use as biomarker includes estimating the likely time of ovulation and the fertile period for insemination based on increasing progesterone concentrations exceeding 2 ng/mL,[1–3] sometimes referred to as the "initial rise."[3] More recently, progesterone concentrations have been used in predicting gestation length and thereby the likely whelping date to ensure some measure of fetal maturation for elective cesarean deliveries.[4,5] Gestation length can be estimated simply from the initial rise in progesterone levels before the breeding, or by monitoring the actual

[a] Department of Population Health & Reproduction, School of Veterinary Medicine, University of California, Davis, CA 95616, USA; [b] Guide Dogs for the Blind, California Campus, PO Box 151200, San Rafael, CA 94915, USA; [c] Department of Population Medicine and Diagnostic Sciences, Cornell University College of Veterinary Medicine, Ithaca, NY 14853, USA; [d] Kokopelli Assisted Reproductive Services, Sacramento, CA, USA
* Corresponding author.
E-mail address: ajconley@ucdavis.edu

Vet Clin Small Anim 53 (2023) 931–949
https://doi.org/10.1016/j.cvsm.2023.05.007
0195-5616/23/© 2023 Elsevier Inc. All rights reserved.

preparturient decline in progesterone concentrations around the time whelping is anticipated. Regardless, the clinical decisions involved require rapid results from whatever analysis is readily available. This requirement has culminated in the development of point-of-care instruments to measure this steroid hormone within hours, but raises questions as to how reliable those results might be.[6] The technology that supports these platforms, the variability in the data generated, and the reliability of clinical interpretations and diagnostic utility may not be clear, even to practitioners with a high reproductive caseload (and experience interpreting them), for a variety of reasons. Practitioners may lack enough understanding of the inherent variability in progesterone concentrations underlying physiologic events (or how progesterone concentrations are determined analytically) to evaluate their value appropriately. The goal of this review is to provide an objective, mechanistic understanding and appreciation of the true value of serum or plasma progesterone determinations in clinical practice, specifically, why estimates vary among available methods and samples, to what degree the results can vary in the most clinically relevant concentration range, how this might influence decisions as to the optimum time to breed or schedule elective cesarean deliveries, and the likely practical impact on reproductive outcomes and efficiency. The article begins with a brief overview of the physiologic basis behind breeding practices and the inherent difficulty in defining a fertile period and then discusses the differences in assays and where it is that variability and a lack of reliability in the results arises.

Beginning more than a century ago,[7] studies into the canine estrous cycle[8] established the fundamental underlying reproductive physiology and endocrinology, which has been reviewed extensively many times.[9–24] No attempt will be made to try to replicate as thorough a literature review as is provided in those aforementioned articles. It is suffice to say that the stages of the cycle are prolonged and variable among and even within individuals,[25] as are the timing and duration of the luteinizing hormone (LH) surge,[9,26–28] the increase in progesterone levels,[28–30] and detected ovulation.[31,32] Oocytes are at the germinal vesicle stage when released at the time of ovulation[33,34] and mature to the secondary stage at a variable rate over 2 to 3 days in the oviducts[8] before fertilization is possible.[15] Because oocytes must mature to the secondary stage (complete first stage of meiosis with extrusion of the first polar body) before fertilization is possible, their viability after estimated ovulation is quite long[35] compared with other species.[36] In fact, pregnancies can still be established even after the cervix has closed if sperm are deposited directly into the uterine lumen.[37] Canine sperm also have prolonged longevity in the female reproductive tract, particularly after natural mating,[38] in part because of their retention in uterine crypts[39] and uterotubal junction,[24] especially so if fresh and unprocessed semen is used for insemination.[14] Practically speaking then, if the LH surge can exceed 2 days in a bitch, as can ovulation itself, added to which is an extended period of canine oocyte maturation before fertilization is even possible, and the unpredictable closure of the cervix as a barrier to vaginally deposited semen, the ability to predict the "fertile period"[14] becomes challenging. Sperm viability in the female reproductive tract being prolonged also suggests that the need to closely coordinate breeding with ovulation may be a less critical factor in reproductive efficiency in dogs than in other species. This fact is likely to be true unless the insemination dose is compromised because of the poor quality of fresh ejaculates or the result of processing for artificial insemination.[40,41]

Despite a multitude of experimental studies and advances in technologies, it is still not easy to determine the actual time of ovulation in the bitch with confidence. Therefore, breeding management strategies rely on indirect means of monitoring cycles such as vaginal cytology, vaginoscopy, or endocrine testing.[2] The canine ovary is encased in a bursa that prevents direct observation and confirmation of ovulation unless it is surgically exposed or[31,42] examined at laparotomy,[27] after ovariectomy,[43,44] or at necropsy.[32] Repeated ultrasound examination has also been used[45–48] with apparently increasing confidence in recent years.[34,49–52] Regardless, the practical difficulties of verifying ovulation visually have led to the use of hormones as proxies for estimating the time of ovulation, principally the initial rise in concentrations of not only progesterone[1,28,29,44,52,53] but also LH.[27,28,31,32,43,54] This method has been adopted widely by veterinarians over many years, even though the increase in progesterone levels may not always be clearly progressive. For instance, in 4 of 6 beagle bitches sampled multiple times a day, progesterone concentrations increased initially concomitant with a recognizable LH surge but then paused, not increasing for 3 days until an apparent luteal phase was finally initiated.[28] Therefore, although reasonable in most circumstances, it should still be acknowledged that the time of ovulation can only be approximated from progesterone or even LH determinations, which are typically monitored every other day at most. The duration from the first to last oocyte released is variable and can occur over days,[31,52] which may explain the sometimes-extended delays between the LH surge and the increase in progesterone associated with luteal formation as distinct from any initial increase from preovulatory luteinization.[28] Moreover, the broad clinical use of historically reported, specific hormone concentrations at any point in a cycle ignores the inherent biological and analytical variability in results from the differing assay protocols and platforms generating those data, as discussed later. Finally, although hormonal estimates are extensively used in breeding management, few data are available comparing, and explicitly evaluating, the reproductive outcomes of these various approaches in large patient cohorts of various breeds and body size.[3,41]

The most common proxy for assessing the likely time of the LH surge, ovulation, oocyte maturation, and (theoretical) the optimal time for insemination (fertile period) is the initial rise in progesterone concentrations associated with preovulatory luteinization. As an example of how this is used in practice, shown are the results obtained monitoring progesterone in carefully managed breeding colony of Labrador and golden retrievers at Guide Dogs for the Blind (**Fig. 1**). Samples were submitted to a

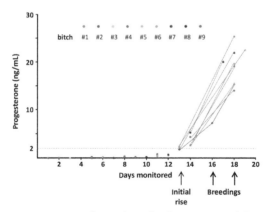

Fig. 1. Progesterone concentrations (ng/mL) in 6 bitches monitored during their cycles from appearance of a serosanguinous discharge to the initial rise above 2.0 ng/mL (*dotted line*; designated as d0) and the subsequent breedings (typically twice) 3 and 5 days later. Because cycle length varies considerably, the data have been aligned around the day of the initial rise for presentation purposes. All bitches became pregnant and delivered litters of normal size (7–9 pups). Progesterone concentrations greater than 10 ng/mL affirmed ovulation had taken place. All serum progesterone concentrations were analyzed on a chemiluminescence immunoassay platform at a commercial laboratory.

commercial laboratory for analysis of progesterone using a chemiluminescence platform, and results were returned the following day. The sequence of events from the appearance of a serosanguinous vaginal discharge to the time of insemination is depicted for several bitches, aligned around the initial rise in progesterone levels from less than 1.0 ng/mL to greater than 2 ng/mL.[3] These females were followed every 2 to 3 days by vaginal cytology and vaginoscopy until bred, twice, 2 days apart. Only progesterone concentrations are shown, although vaginal cytology was also conducted routinely. All breedings shown resulted in pregnancies, delivering litters of 7 to 9 pups. This facility manages ≈150 breedings per year with pregnancy rates approaching 97%, most from natural mating but some from transcervical insemination (TCI) with fresh or frozen semen also.

Progesterone is a steroid hormone in the chemical class known as pregnanes, which also includes the corticoids. As with cortisol, progesterone is not a species-specific molecule, even though normal reference ranges for progesterone differ markedly from species to species and vary widely according to the reproductive state or cycle stage within a species. Assays for progesterone do not need to be species specific (as they do for protein hormones), but they do need to be carefully validated for that species and the form of the sample (serum or plasma with whatever anticoagulant). It is a relatively stable hormone once serum or plasma have been removed from the red blood cells or clot and samples are frozen, but some assay platforms advise against the use of serum separator tubes just the same.[55–58] However, progesterone concentrations can be altered by exposure to blood cells after collection in both a time- and temperature-dependent fashion in some species.[59–61] Reimers and colleagues[59] reported no significant effect of storage overnight at 4°C or room temperature on progesterone concentrations in canine plasma, but others reported a slight decrease in the first 2 hours[62] or at 12 and 24 hours at room temperature.[63] Volkmann[61] also observed a decrease in serum progesterone levels but only if samples were refrigerated in the first 2 hours after collection not if kept at room temperature. Consequently, sample handling matters[62] but is likely to vary from practice to practice, whatever sample is taken and whatever assay protocol is followed. Therefore, rather than specific recommendations, consistency in whatever protocols are followed is likely of more importance in minimizing variability and thereby increasing the reliability of results in the monitoring of individual cycles. The pattern of the increase in concentration values over the course of days is more important than the actual numbers obtained on individual days.

WHY DO RESULTS OF PROGESTERONE DETERMINATIONS FROM DIFFERENT LABORATORIES (AND/OR INSTRUMENT PLATFORMS) DIFFER?

Progesterone can be measured relatively easily in all species, compared with protein hormones, most commonly by immunoassay of one sort or another. It may not be essential for clinicians to understand the details of methodologic differences across various assay platforms, protocols, and procedures. However, it is important to realize that the results can differ depending on the assay used (**Tables 1** and **2**), especially within the critically important 1 to 2 ng/mL concentration range,[3] enough to influence clinical decisions concerning days of insemination or gestation length potentially affecting outcomes (see **Fig. 1**). Knowing why estimates vary may help clinicians make more informed choices of where and how to measure progesterone for optimum management of the breeding bitch or how better to use and interpret those results. What is measured in systemic circulation is typically secreted by the corpora lutea in all mammals,[64] the placenta of some (although not canine) species,[65] and in dogs

Table 1
Commercially available assays for quantitative determination of progesterone concentrations in canine blood

Instrument	Accessibility	Assay Type	Antibody	Assay Signal Detection	Recommended Sample	Range (ng/mL)	References
IMMULITE (CLIA)	Reference laboratory	Immunoassay	Rabbit polyclonal	Chemiluminescence (CLIA)	Serum (not plasma)	0.2–40	5,88,89,97,100
Elecsys (E-CLIA)	Reference laboratory	Immunoassay	Biotinylated monoclonal	Electrochemiluminescence (E-CLIA)	Serum, plasma	0.05–60	72
Catalyst (CIA)	Point of care	Immunoassay	Unknown antibody	Chromogenic/colorimetric (CIA)	Serum (not serum separator), plasma	0.2–20	5,63,89,97,100
MINI VIDAS (ELFA)	Point of care	Immunoassay	Monoclonal	Enzyme-linked fluorescence (ELFA)	Serum, plasma	0.25–80	94,97
Tosoh (ELFA)	Point of care	Immunoassay	Unknown antibody	Enzyme-linked fluorescence (ELFA)	Serum, plasma (not EDTA or citrate)	0.5–45	98,99

Note that neither RIAs nor EIA/ELISA are included because they are constructed more variably among laboratories in general, tend to be validated and used more for research, and are not usually available commercially for canine samples. The assay platforms represented include CLIAs (IMMULITE platform), E-CLIA (Elecsys platform), CIA (Catalyst platform), and ELFA. Note, the most recent CLIA performed on IMMULITE 2000 yields lower progesterone concentrations than that performed on the original IMMULITE 1000 (see **Table 2**). References refer to studies comparing results between or among the listed instruments.

Abbreviations: ELFA, enzyme-linked fluorescent immunoassay; CIA, colorimetric immunoassay or chromogenic immunoassay; CLIA, chemiluminescence immunoassay; E-CLIA, electrochemiluminescence immunoassay; EDTA, ethylenediaminetetraacetic acid; EIA, enzyme-linked immunoassay; ELISA, enzyme-linked immunosorbent assay; RIA, radioimmunoassay.

Table 2
Peer-reviewed publications by the listed authors comparing results of progesterone determinations on canine samples assayed on different commercial and point-of-care instrument platforms

Reference #	Comparison	Results	Authors' Conclusions
Kutzler et al,[3] 2003	CLIA-1000 vs RIA	Variable within 0.5–2.0 ng/mL range by 7.2%–20.6%	"Did not find these differences to be clinically relevant to applications in canine reproduction"
Volkmann,[61] 2006	CLIA-1000 vs RIA	RIA = 1.5 × CLIA-1000	"Reduction in measured SPC [serum progesterone concentration] may cause the LH surge to be diagnosed (erroneously)"
Chapwanya et al,[70] 2008	CLIA-1000 vs RIA	Equivalent results by either method	CLIA "accurate and reliable method"
Brugger et al,[94] 2011	ELFA vs EIA	ELFA = 0.83 × RIA	ELFA "provides rapid and reliable results"
Nothling & De Cramer,[95] 2018	CLIA-1000 vs RIA	CLIA = 0.85 × RIA	"Large differences in progesterone value sometimes occur"; clinician should not see a progesterone value obtained in isolation
Gloria et al,[96] 2018	CLIA-2000 vs RIA vs EIA	CLIA-2000 (& EIA) = 1.5 × RIA	"RIA and ELISA not interchangeable"; CLIA/EIA could initiate 24–48h earlier insemination than RIA
Nothling & De Cramer,[71] 2019	CLIA-1000 vs RIA	CLIA-1000 < RIA	"Required a change in the target concentrations"
Schooley et al,[89] 2019	CLIA-1000 vs CLIA-2000 vs CIA vs LC-MS/MS	CIA = CLIA-1000 and LC-MS/MS; CLIA-2000 = 0.75 × LC-MS/MS	CLIA-2000 proportional bias, need for consistent analytical methodology
Bilbrough & Glavan,[88] 2019	CLIA-1000 vs CLIA-2000 vs LC-MS/MS	CLIA-1000 = 1.25 × CLIA-2000, CLIA-1000 = LC-MS/MS	Proportional bias in newer-generation assay
Tal et al,[72] 2020	CLIA-2000 vs E-CLIA vs RIA	CLIA-2000 = 0.45 x RIA; E-CLIA = 1.06 x RIA	Clinically relevant for CLIA but not for E-CLIA

Study	Methods compared	Results	Comments
Hisanaga,[97] 2021	CLIA-2000 vs CIA vs ELFA	ELFA > CIA > CLIA; CLIA = 0.44 × ELFA; CLIA = 0.58 × CIA; CIA = 0.73 × ELFA	Suggested "formulaic adjustments"
Zuercher et al,[100] 2021	CIA (2 sites) vs CLIA- 2000	CIA-1 = 1.42 × CLIA-2000; CIA-2 = 1.54 × CLIA-2000	Proportional bias, earlier increase, anticipated ovulation 1–2 days sooner than the actual ovulation, thus predicting insemination dates outside of the fertile window
Nothling et al,[5] 2022	CLIA-2000 vs CIA	CIA-1 < CLIA-2000	Bias became proportional >2 ng/mL
Østergård Jensen et al,[63] 2022	CLIA-? vs CIA vs LC- MS	CIA > LC-MS/MS > CLIA	Proportional error but advised against using "correction factor"

Note: IMMULITE platforms used the CLIA-1000 assay until superseded by the CLIA-2000 assay more recently. Differences between and among results are expressed as correction factors applied to concentrations determined by different methods where reported by the authors based on regression analysis.

Abbreviations: CIA, colorimetric/chromogenic immunoassay; CLIA, chemiluminescence immunoassay; ELFA, enzyme-linked immunofluorescence assay; LC-MS/MS, liquid chromatography-tandem mass spectrometry; RIA, radioimmunoassay.

by the stimulated adrenal gland.[66] In the bitch it is also secreted in significant amounts before ovulation by follicles[27,43] that are in the process of luteinization[67] induced by the preovulatory surge of LH. Progesterone concentrations reportedly exhibit a diurnal variation, being significantly higher in the evening than in the morning in bitches in proestrus and estrus before ovulation but higher in the morning samples after ovulation.[68] Higher progesterone concentrations were seen in the morning than in the evening samples in pregnant bitches.[69] Therefore, diurnal rhythms in progesterone appear to change with the reproductive state in the bitch for unknown reasons, and this poses yet another potential source of variability in progesterone concentrations and argues that consideration should be given to drawing blood at the same time of day in managing clinical cases, perhaps even fasted in the morning, for instance.

Historically, radioimmunoassay has been considered the gold standard in the numerous veterinary publications in which different progesterone analyses have been compared.[3,61,70–72] Most commercially available analyses and point-of-care instruments for progesterone still use immunoassays, but there are differences in the procedures and specific reagents they use and therefore in the results they generate.[73,74] Some of the earlier developed immunoassays used organic solvents to extract progesterone from samples (serum or plasma) before analysis.[75,76] Unless automated, other laboratories, and presumably all stand-alone clinical instruments, use straight serum or plasma because of the time, reagents, and additional technician time required for extraction. However, using unextracted serum or plasma means that assay reactions are conducted in an even more complex liquid matrix of proteins, ions, lipids, and even sulfated or glucuronidated (conjugated) steroids that can certainly interact or interfere with antibodies, thereby influencing results.[77] Differences in the sample matrix may explain in part why serum and plasma harvested from the same blood draw can give different results in the same assay. For instance, canine serum yielded significantly higher concentrations than plasma in an enzyme-linked immunoassay[68] and some assays may recommend using only serum or plasma accordingly.[61] And yet, commercially accessible assays marketed for human as well as veterinary diagnostics likely do not use canine serum (or plasma) in their standard curves to mitigate or minimize matrix effects. Research, reference, and specialized analytical laboratories employing mass spectrometry and/or immunoassays add serum or plasma appropriate to the species to their standards and calibrators before organically extracting samples for analysis of steroids such as progesterone[78,79] to control for these sample matrix effects that can differ among species.[80] Regardless, most laboratories would consider mass spectrometry to be a more robust gold standard than immunoassays[80,81]. Mass spectrometry analysis is automated and rapidly completed when compared with most immunoassays, resulting in short turnaround times, but it is expensive and generally not as readily available for veterinary practice.

Most assays for the clinical determination of progesterone are still immunoassays that vary primarily in the method of signal detection resulting from the competition between progesterone in the sample and the radiolabeled, enzyme-linked, or otherwise conjugated progesterone reagent added in the assay (**Fig. 2**). Some of the more commonly used assays available in reference laboratories, or as point-of-care platforms, are listed for comparison along with their major distinguishing technical characteristics (see **Table 1**). Other immunoassay platforms using alternative detection technologies also show promise.[82,83] Two of the key components of most immunoassays are the primary antibody (polyclonal antisera or monoclonal, whatever the case may be for that assay) and the assay standard curve. Steroids are small molecules that are not themselves immunogenic. To stimulate the generation of antibodies that are used in immunoassays, the target steroid must be conjugated to an

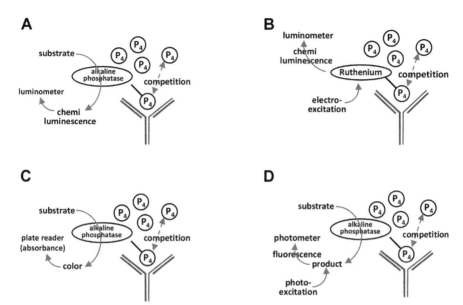

Fig. 2. Simplified schematic illustrating some of the basic methodologic differences among commercially available or accessible immunoassay platforms. (*A*) Chemiluminescence immunoassay, (*B*) electrochemiluminescence immunoassay, (*C*) colorimetric (chromogenic) immunoassay, and (*D*) enzyme-linked immunofluorescence assay.

immunogenic chemical group or even protein (bovine serum albumen for instance) to enhance immune stimulation.[80] The primary antibody (monoclonal) or antisera (polyclonal) of the assay recognizes the target analyte (eg, progesterone), but few laboratories or assay platforms use the same one. Antisera and monoclonal antibodies vary in their affinity for the steroid target and in their cross-reactivity with other steroids they may also recognize.[75,76,84–86] The antisera or antibodies used in each of these assays are as varied in their specificity as are any antisera stimulated by immunization, and it is why cross-reactivities are must be cited in peer-reviewed publications as part of the description of assay methodologies.[80,87] It also why information on cross-reactivity of antisera accompanies commercial assay kits and perhaps contributes to the differences in results (see **Table 2**) from newer generations of the same assay platform, like the IMMULITE chemiluminescence immunoassay (Siemens Medical Solutions Diagnostics, Los Angeles, CA).[88,89] Moreover, in some cases, antibody or antisera cross-reactivity can lead to wildly different, falsely elevated results from different assay platforms for the same analyte in the very same samples. This fact was vividly illustrated by progesterone determinations on serum from late pregnant mares where the same samples in different progesterone assays yielded results that were 10- to 100-fold different in some cases[90] due to the high concentrations of cross-reacting metabolites of progesterone present at this stage of equine gestation.[79] Cross-reactivity with common therapeutics, such as prednisolone, may also falsely indicate an elevated progesterone concentration in clinical samples, whereas others, such as altrenogest, may not (Conley, 2023, unpublished results). In any case, different assays generate results that are significantly different, enough to change a clinical interpretation in canine samples (Gonzales & Conley, 2023, unpublished observations), especially in the lower, historically adopted, 1 to 2 ng/mL range.[3] Notwithstanding these limitations, the clinical interpretation of progesterone results may be valid enough under certain circumstances if the assay is precise and repeatable in the clinically relevant range. Repeated sampling during a cycle and measurement on the same instrument, together with sufficient experience with that platform to be able to confidently identify trends (increases or decreases), may suffice regardless of the assay methodology.

Another major component of any quantitative assay is a standard curve that enables accurate quantification in a sample if the analyte of interest is present within a quantifiable range. Two characteristics are significant in this regard, the number of standard concentration points and the matrix in which they are constituted. The more points representing different concentrations, the better the quantitative estimate, although accuracy diminishes at both lower and higher concentrations as fitted curves become less linear. However, the more the number of points in the fitted curve, the greater is the time and cost added to the procedure and the fewer the samples that can be included in each analytical run, increasing the unit cost. Consequently, assays may include only a minimal number of points. Too few points in a standard curve and the results become only semiquantitative. In addition, standalone clinical instruments require regular attention to quality control or assessment[6,91,92] including frequent calibration, and, if not, results can suffer significant drift. Finally, standard curves are rarely constituted in simple serum or plasma of any species, let alone the serum or plasma (matrix) of the species being analyzed. As noted, commercial assays made for human diagnostics likely use a human serum or plasma matrix[93] that may not be optimum for determinations in samples from canine samples. Differences in the reaction mix between the standard curve and the sample introduces error into the analysis whether or not extraction is used. Again, this may be more consequential at lower concentrations within the clinically critical range of 1 to 2 ng/mL. For all these reasons and others, results for progesterone determinations can differ substantially, when using different instruments or assay platforms,[88–90] or even among commercial[74] or other laboratories using the same platform.[93] Comparisons among the more commonly used platforms (chemiluminescence immunoassay [CLIA], electrochemiluminescence immunoassay [E-CLIA], colorimetric [chromogenic] immunoassay) and enzyme-linked fluorescence immunoassay for canine progesterone determination[3,5,61,63,70–72,88,89,94–99] demonstrate that different platforms frequently yield significantly different results (summarized, see **Table 2**;[3,5,61,63,70–72,88,89,94–100]). Ultimately, it is more important that an analysis generates internally consistent, clinically interpretable, and clinically relevant results within the critical concentrations range than it is that absolute concentrations resulting from different assays or laboratories yield comparable values. However, in general, the standards of quality control, instrument maintenance, training, and reference concentration development that are needed in practices using point-of-care platforms[6,91,92] have been shown to fall short of compliance with professional guidelines.[101] Commercial laboratories conduct calibration checks using commercial calibrators every week or two at the most along with recommended daily, weekly, monthly, and quarterly maintenance procedures, which compensates for any possible drift.

Appropriate quality control and standard of care in laboratory practices can be achieved in a veterinary clinical setting, resulting in repeatable progesterone concentration values that can be interpreted in meaningful ways. As an example, 2 of the authors (B.W.C. and H.N.E.) compared progesterone concentrations generated from a point-of-care analyzer (TOS; Tosoh AIA-360, Tosoh Biosciences Inc, South San Francisco, CA, USA) and a reference laboratory (IMM; IDEXX Siemann's IMMULITE 2000, IDEXX Laboratories, Inc, Sacramento, CA, USA). Serum samples from 120 bitches ranging in age from 1.3 to 8.8 years and representing 40 breeds were collected. All bitches were fasted the morning of the blood collection. The blood was placed in a nonadditive tube ("red top tube"), allowed to sit and clot for 10 minutes, and then centrifuged at 1000 g for 10 minutes. The serum was divided into 2 aliquots. The first aliquot was placed in the freezer ($-20°$ C) until submission to a reference lab (IDEXX Laboratories, Inc) for analysis on the IMM. The second aliquot was immediately run on the in-house TOS and then placed in the freezer in case it was needed again. For statistical analysis purposes, results were grouped into the following ng/mL ranges, as determined by IMM (n): 0.2 to 0.49 (10), 0.5 to 0.9 (12), 0.91 to 1.5 (10), 1.51 to 2.5 (21), 2.51 to 3.5 (15), 3.51 to 4.5 (9), 4.51 to 5.5 (19), 5.51 to 6.5 (12), 6.51 to 7.5 (16), 7.51 to 8.5 (9), 8.51 to 9.5 (7), 9.51 to 10.5 (8), 10.51 to 11.5 (10), and 11.51 to 25.5 (55). The first 5 samples from each value range (n = 65) were run a second time through both TOS and submitted as a second, blinded sample (labeled with a unique name) to IMM to assess intra-assay repeatability.

The Shapiro-Wilk test indicated that all measurements of either first or second samples of the same assay were significant ($P \leq .0053$, indicating lack of adherence to a bell-shaped curve). Therefore, Spearman rank correlation was used with scatter diagrams to compare intra-assay progesterone measurements within split samples. (Rank-based tests calculate the rankings of each data value within the same variable, from lowest = rank 1 to highest = eg, rank 65 or rank 120). Split samples were available from 65 bitches, spread evenly throughout the IMM result ranges. The graphs and rank correlations were done separately for IMM and TOS.

The scatter diagrams for IMM and TOS are in **Fig. 3**A and B, respectively. The rank correlation for IMM is 0.988 ($P < .0001$), indicating that the split samples tend to take similar rankings between the first and second split samples. The values also visually fall along a rather tight straight line (at least below 20 ng/mL), so that the values within each pair tend also to be similar in ng/mL. The results for the TOS split samples suggest a similar level of repeatability visually, and the rank correlation = 0.995 ($P < .0001$). *Therefore, both IMM and TOS can be expected to provide repeatable measurements across the scales observed.* Using either IMM or TOS solely within one reproductive cycle would be expected to show measurements within "a couple of ng/mL" *unless* the progesterone levels within the bitch were truly changing.

However, the intermingling of the 2 assays within a cycle cannot be recommended. Values obtained on TOS were not numerically equivalent with those from the same samples run with IMM. Undetectable variation was noted at values less than 1 ng/mL, but as progesterone concentrations increased, the values reported with TOS increased at a faster rate than the same samples reported with IMM. The higher the value, the greater the difference and the greater the variation between the 2 assays.

Fig. 3C clearly demonstrates that the TOS values are typically higher than the IMM values (ie, "IMM minus TOS" was always and often dramatically negative). It is not easy to adjust one assay to the other, because of the spread of values along the imaginary line from upper left to lower right (compare these visually to the scattering in **Fig. 3**A and B). It is possible, however, to predict a relative range of values that might be obtained had a sample been submitted to a reference laboratory. For example, looking at **Fig. 3**C, one can see that a value of 10 ng/mL on TOS correlates with a range of 5 to 7 ng/mL on IMM; this gives a rough estimation of what might have been obtained had the sample actually been submitted for IMM evaluation. However, it should be noted that at any given value there are only a few data points, so the correlation is far from exact and the range of variation between assays is likely greater than detected with our sample size. It is much more important to note that because

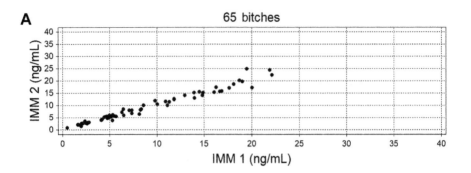

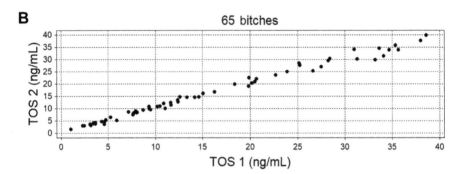

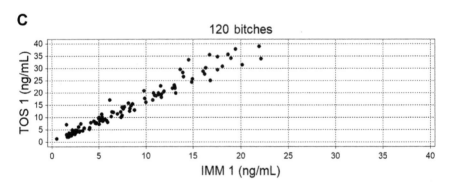

Fig. 3. (*A*) Scatter plot for 65 serum samples run twice each on IMM to compare intra-assay variation. The rank correlation is 0.988 (*P* < .0001), indicating that the split samples tend to take similar rankings between the first and second split samples. (*B*) Scatter plot for 65 serum samples run twice each on TOS to compare intra-assay variation. The rank correlation is 0.995 (*P* < .0001) indicating that the split samples tend to take similar rankings between the first and second split samples. (*C*) Scatter plot for 120 serum samples run on both TOS and IMM.

the intra-assay variation was low, tracking changes over time using the same assay will yield a much better idea of true change in progesterone concentrations than trying to point-match single values between assays. These estimations and the pattern of their increase over time, along with accompanying vaginoscopy, vaginal cytology evaluations, and (in some cases) LH testing, can then be used to make meaningful clinical assessments of the stage of estrous cycle and estimations of LH surge, ovulation, fertile period, best breeding dates, and dates for elective cesarean delivery.

A clinician with access to multiple assays could do essentially this same study without the formal statistical calculations. Only graph paper would be needed to plot values from the same assay on split samples.

In the clinical practice of one of the authors (B.W.C.), steps are taken to ensure high standards of laboratory practice, including daily commercial controls, new standard curves with every new batch of assay cups, and fresh reagents made according to manufacturer recommended schedules. Bitches are fasted before sample collection, and efforts are made to collect serum at the same time of day for each respective patient. Laboratory protocols for sample handling are followed consistently by having a dedicated laboratory technician assigned to sample handling. Following these practices, in the course of a year (2022), resulted in a TCI pregnancy rate of 91.5% using fresh semen (n = 71), 70.9% using chilled semen (n = 55), and 73.9% using frozen semen (n = 46). These values represent multiple breeds of dog at various ages and without factoring in semen quality, which ranged from very poor to excellent, or any fertility issues for the individual bitches. As such, these data should reflect a realistic level of performance at a well-run clinical practice.

Consistency in sample quality and type, collection timing, processing and analysis, and experience in interpreting changes among samples taken during proestrus and estrus should at least minimize some of the inherent sources of variability as long as the analysis is precise enough to produce internally consistent and reliable results over time; this is of concern with point-of-care analyzers[6] that require consistent quality control.[91] In the experience of the authors, the more parameters that can be assessed in a single sample by a single instrument, and the more rapidly results are generated on point-of-care instruments in particular, the less reliable the results are likely to be, at least for immunoassays. The benefits of immediate results must be weighed against the potential expense of poor reliability and outcomes. Decisions are best made by clinicians themselves in consultation with clients but with a comprehensive understanding of the variability possible in results of progesterone assays along with all available clinical information. On a more academic level, it is worrisome that publications comparing progesterone concentrations among various studies are discussed without consideration to differences in methodology (eg, see Ref.[102]). This concern applies equally to the general use of the 2 ng/mL (6.3 nM) of progesterone as a clinical landmark and proxy for the initial rise in breeding management. Other characteristics may prove as valuable. For example, a study of 1420 cycles in 1300 bitches using a commercial progesterone assay (E-CLIA) observed that bitches experiencing a slower rate of increase in progesterone whelped smaller litters.[53] More generally, however, the literature seems to lack studies comparing results among different assay platforms that have been evaluated by way of their impact on clinical outcomes in large-enough cohorts to draw valid conclusions. In other words, the potential benefits of progesterone determinations by whatever means (beyond those of other clinical parameters) on pregnancy rate, litter size, and neonatal viability have yet to be adequately quantified in canine practice.

SUMMARY

In conclusion, progesterone has proven itself to be a reasonable parameter to include when making breeding and other clinically relevant decisions in canine reproductive management, but different assays yield variable results. Commercially available assay instruments also require rigorous validation, maintenance, and quality control to ensure that results are reliable and reproducible. Established rules based on specific concentration targets are not equivalent when measured in different assays on specific instruments, and misinterpretation of single determinations, in particular, can pose significant problems. Progesterone determinations can be a valuable aid in making clinical determinations on the reproductive state of a bitch, perhaps becoming a standard of care, but frequent or repeated sampling is required so that significant trends can be recognized. Importantly, vaginal cytology, vaginoscopy, and even ultrasound imaging still provide extremely useful additional information. Even so, there remains a lack of evidence of the potential rewards in terms of their impact on reproductive outcomes of the various available assay platforms and what they add to other clinical assessments.

DISCLOSURES

The authors have no conflicts of interest to disclose. All funding and support related to the work presented was entirely intramural. Supplies were provided by Tosoh Bioscience, Inc, for generating some of the data in this article.

ACKNOWLEDGMENTS

The authors are especially grateful to Valerie Solerno, Rebecca Cotterman and Casey Caruso, and Drs Ned Place, Bill Vernau, Sophie Grundy, and Jim Kennedy for their technical input and advice on the article. The authors are grateful to Tosoh Biosciences, Inc, for supplying laboratory reagents for generating some of the data presented.

REFERENCES

1. Wright PJ. Application of vaginal cytology and plasma progesterone determinations to the management of reproduction in the bitch. J Small Anim Pract 1990; 31:335–40.
2. Johnston SD, Root Kustritz MV, Olson PNS. Breeding management and artificial insemination of the bitch. Canine and Feline Theriogenology. Philadelphia, PA: International Veterinary Information Service: W. B. Saunders; 2001. p. 41–65.
3. Kutzler MA, Mohammed HO, Lamb SV, et al. Accuracy of canine parturition date prediction from the initial rise in preovulatory progesterone concentration. Theriogenology 2003;60:1187–96.
4. England GC, Verstegen JP. Prediction of parturition in the bitch using semiquantitative ELISA measurement of plasma progesterone concentration. Vet Rec 1996;139:496–7.
5. Nothling JO, Joone CJ, Hegarty E, et al. Use of a point-of-care progesterone assay to predict onset of parturition in the bitch. Front Vet Sci 2022;9:914659.
6. Stern JK, Camus MS. Point-of-care instruments. Vet Clin North Am Small Anim Pract 2023;53:17–28.
7. Marshall FHA, Jolly WA. Contributions to the physiology of mammalian reproduction. Part I.-The estrous cycle in the dog. Part II.-The ovary as an organ of internal secretion. Proceedings of the Royal Society of London Series B-Biological Sciences 1905;cxcviii:395–8.
8. Evans HM, Cole HH. An introduction to the study of the oestrous cycle in the dog, vol. 9. Berkeley, CA: Memoirs of the University of California; 1931. p. 65–103.

9. Concannon PW. Endocrinologic control of normal canine ovarian function. Reprod Domest Anim 2009;44(Suppl 2):3–15.
10. Concannon PW, McCann JP, Temple M. Biology and endocrinology of ovulation, pregnancy and parturition in the dog. J Reprod Fertil Suppl 1989;39:3–25.
11. Jochle W, Andersen AC. The estrous cycle in the dog: a review. Theriogenology 1977;7:113–40.
12. Johnston SD, Root Kustritz MV, Olson PNS. The canine estrous cycle. Canine and Feline Theriogenology. Philadelphia: W. B. Saunders; 2001. p. 16–31.
13. Songsasen N, Wildt DE. Oocyte biology and challenges in developing in vitro maturation systems in the domestic dog. Anim Reprod Sci 2007;98:2–22.
14. England GC, Burgess CM, Freeman SL, et al. Relationship between the fertile period and sperm transport in the bitch. Theriogenology 2006;66:1410–8.
15. Tsutsui T. Gamete physiology and timing of ovulation and fertilization in dogs. J Reprod Fertil Suppl 1989;39:269–75.
16. Reynaud K, Fontbonne A, Marseloo N, et al. In vivo canine oocyte maturation, fertilization and early embryogenesis: a review. Theriogenology 2006;66: 1685–93.
17. Renton JP, Boyd JS, Eckersall PD, et al. Ovulation, fertilization and early embryonic development in the bitch (Canis familiaris). J Reprod Fertil 1991;93:221–31.
18. Verstegen-Onclin K, Verstegen J. Endocrinology of pregnancy in the dog: a review. Theriogenology 2008;70:291–9.
19. Hoffmann B, Riesenbeck A, Klein R. Reproductive endocrinology of bitches. Anim Reprod Sci 1996;42:275–88.
20. Hoffmann B, Busges F, Engel E, et al. Regulation of corpus luteum-function in the bitch. Reprod Domest Anim 2004;39:232–40.
21. Kowalewski MP. Endocrine and molecular control of luteal and placental function in dogs: a review. Reprod Domest Anim 2012;47(Suppl 6):19–24.
22. Olson PN, Husted PW, Allen TA, et al. Reproductive endocrinology and physiology of the bitch and queen. Vet Clin North Am Small Anim Pract 1984;14: 927–46.
23. Christie DW, Bell ET. Endocrinology of the oestrous cycle in the bitch. J Small Anim Pract 1971;12:383–9.
24. England GCW, Rijsselaere T, Campbell A, et al. Normal and abnormal response to sperm deposition in female dogs: a review and new hypotheses for endometritis. Theriogenology 2021;159:176–83.
25. Bouchard G, Youngquist RS, Vaillancourt D, et al. Seasonality and variability of the interestrous interval in the bitch. Theriogenology 1991;36:41–50.
26. Jones GE, Boyns AR, Cameron EH, et al. Plasma oestradiol, luteinizing hormone and progesterone during pregnancy in the Beagle bitch. J Reprod Fertil 1973; 35:187–9.
27. Smith MS, McDonald LE. Serum levels of luteinizing hormone and progesterone during the estrous cycle, pseudopregnancy and pregnancy in the dog. Endocrinology 1974;94:404–12.
28. de Gier J, Kooistra HS, Djajadiningrat-Laanen SC, et al. Temporal relations between plasma concentrations of luteinizing hormone, follicle-stimulating hormone, estradiol-17beta, progesterone, prolactin, and alpha-melanocyte-stimulating hormone during the follicular, ovulatory, and early luteal phase in the bitch. Theriogenology 2006;65:1346–59.
29. Christie DW, Bell ET, Horth CE, et al. Peripheral plasma progesterone levels during the canine oestrous cycle. Acta Endocrinol 1971;68:543–50.

30. Concannon PW, Hansel W, Visek WJ. The ovarian cycle of the bitch: plasma estrogen, LH and progesterone. Biol Reprod 1975;13:112–21.

31. Wildt DE, Chakraborty PK, Panko WB, et al. Relationship of reproductive behavior, serum luteinizing hormone and time of ovulation in the bitch. Biol Reprod 1978;18:561–70.

32. Phemister RD, Holst PA, Spano JS, et al. Time of ovulation in the beagle bitch. Biol Reprod 1973;8:74–82.

33. Holst PA, Phemister RD. The prenatal development of the dog: preimplantation events. Biol Reprod 1971;5:194–206.

34. Reynaud K, Fontbonne A, Marseloo N, et al. In vivo meiotic resumption, fertilization and early embryonic development in the bitch. Reproduction 2005;130: 193–201.

35. Tsutsui T, Takahashi F, Hori T, et al. Prolonged duration of fertility of dog ova. Reprod Domest Anim 2009;44(Suppl 2):230–3.

36. Dalbies-Tran R, Cadoret V, Desmarchais A, et al. A comparative analysis of oocyte development in mammals. Cells 2020;9:1–27.

37. Verstegen JP, Silva LD, Onclin K. Determination of the role of cervical closure in fertility regulation after mating or artificial insemination in beagle bitches. J Reprod Fertil Suppl 2001;57:31–4.

38. Doak RL, Hall A, Dale HE. Longevity of spermatozoa in the reproductive tract of the bitch. J Reprod Fertil 1967;13:51–8.

39. Karre I, Meyer-Lindenberg A, Urhausen C, et al. Distribution and viability of spermatozoa in the canine female genital tract during post-ovulatory oocyte maturation. Acta Vet Scand 2012;54:49.

40. Nishiyama T, Kinugasa T, Kimura T, et al. Determination of optimal time for mating by artificial insemination with chilled semen using luteinizing hormone surge as an indicator in beagles. J Am Anim Hosp Assoc 1999;35:348–52.

41. Hollinshead FK, Hanlon DW. Factors affecting the reproductive performance of bitches: a prospective cohort study involving 1203 inseminations with fresh and frozen semen. Theriogenology 2017;101:62–72.

42. Wildt DE, Levinson CJ, Seager SW. Laparoscopic exposure and sequential observation of the ovary of the cycling bitch. Anat Rec 1977;189:443–9.

43. Concannon P, Hansel W, McEntee K. Changes in LH, progesterone and sexual behavior associated with preovulatory luteinization in the bitch. Biol Reprod 1977;17:604–13.

44. Groppetti D, Aralla M, Bronzo V, et al. Periovulatory time in the bitch: what's new to know?: Comparison between ovarian histology and clinical features. Anim Reprod Sci 2015;152:108–16.

45. Renton JP, Boyd JS, Harvey MJ, et al. Comparison of endocrine changes and ultrasound as means of identifying ovulation in the bitch. Res Vet Sci 1992; 53:74–9.

46. Boyd JS, Renton JP, Harvey MJ, et al. Problems associated with ultrasonography of the canine ovary around the time of ovulation. J Reprod Fertil Suppl 1993;47:101–5.

47. Silva LDM, Onclin K, Verstegen JP. Assessment of ovarian changes around ovulation in bitches by ultrasonography, laparoscopy and hormonal assays. Vet Radiol Ultrasound 1996;37:313–20.

48. Hayer P, Gunzel-Apel AR, Luerssen D, et al. Ultrasonographic monitoring of follicular development, ovulation and the early luteal phase in the bitch. J Reprod Fertil Suppl 1993;47:93–100.

49. Hase M, Hori T, Kawakami E, et al. Plasma LH and progesterone levels before and after ovulation and observation of ovarian follicles by ultrasonographic diagnosis system in dogs. J Vet Med Sci 2000;62:243–8.
50. England GC, Russo M, Freeman SL. Follicular dynamics, ovulation and conception rates in bitches. Reprod Domest Anim 2009;44(Suppl 2):53–8.
51. Bergeron LH, Nykamp SG, Brisson BA, et al. An evaluation of B-mode and color Doppler ultrasonography for detecting periovulatory events in the bitch. Theriogenology 2013;79:274–83.
52. Tsuchida M, Komura N, Yoshihara T, et al. Ultrasonographic observation in combination with progesterone monitoring for detection of ovulation in Labrador Retrievers. Reprod Domest Anim 2022;57:149–56.
53. Hollinshead F, Hanlon D. Normal progesterone profiles during estrus in the bitch: A prospective analysis of 1420 estrous cycles. Theriogenology 2019; 125:37–42.
54. Onclin K, Murphy B, Verstegen JP. Comparisons of estradiol, LH and FSH patterns in pregnant and nonpregnant beagle bitches. Theriogenology 2002;57: 1957–72.
55. Reimers TJ, McCann JP, Cowan RG. Effects of storage times and temperatures on T3, T4, LH, prolactin, insulin, cortisol and progesterone concentrations in blood samples from cows. J Anim Sci 1983;57:683–91.
56. Smith RL. Effect of serum-separating gels on progesterone assays. Clin Chem 1985;31:1239.
57. Hilborn S, Krahn J. Effect of time of exposure of serum to gel-barrier tubes on results for progesterone and some other endocrine tests. Clin Chem 1987;33: 203–4.
58. Ferry JD, Collins S, Sykes E. Effect of serum volume and time of exposure to gel barrier tubes on results for progesterone by Roche Diagnostics Elecsys 2010. Clin Chem 1999;45:1574–5.
59. Reimers TJ, Lamb SV, Bartlett SA, et al. Effects of hemolysis and storage on quantification of hormones in blood samples from dogs, cattle, and horses. Am J Vet Res 1991;52:1075–80.
60. Hegstad-Davies RL. A review of sample handling considerations for reproductive and thyroid hormone measurement in serum or plasma. Theriogenology 2006;66:592–8.
61. Volkmann DH. The effects of storage time and temperature and anticoagulant on laboratory measurements of canine blood progesterone concentrations. Theriogenology 2006;66:1583–6.
62. Tahir MZ, Thoumire S, Raffaelli M, et al. Effect of blood handling conditions on progesterone assay results obtained by chemiluminescence in the bitch. Domest Anim Endocrinol 2013;45:141–4.
63. Østergård Jensen S, Öberg J, Alm H, et al. Validation of a dry-slide immunoassay for progesterone analysis in canine plasma in a clinical setting. Vet Clin Pathol 2022;51:524–32.
64. Rothchild I. The regulation of the mammalian corpus luteum. Recent Prog Horm Res 1981;37:183–298.
65. Geisert RD, Conley AJ. Secretion and metabolism of steroids in subprimate mammals during pregnancy. In: Bazer FW, editor. The endocrinology of pregnancy. New Jersey: Humana Press Inc.; 1998. p. 291–318.
66. Frank LA, Rohrbach BW, Bailey EM, et al. Steroid hormone concentration profiles in healthy intact and neutered dogs before and after cosyntropin administration. Domest Anim Endocrinol 2003;24:43–57.

67. Abel JH Jr, Verhage HG, McClellan MC, et al. Ultrastructural analysis of the granulosa–luteal cell transition in the ovary of the dog. Cell Tissue Res 1975; 160:155–76.

68. Thuroczy J, Wolfling A, Tibold A, et al. Effect of anticoagulants and sampling time on results of progesterone determination in canine blood samples. Reprod Domest Anim 2003;38:386–9.

69. Steinetz BG, Goldsmith LT, Hasan SH, et al. Diurnal variation of serum progesterone, but not relaxin, prolactin, or estradiol-17 beta in the pregnant bitch. Endocrinology 1990;127:1057–63.

70. Chapwanya A, Clegg T, Stanley P, et al. Comparison of the immulite and RIA assay methods for measuring peripheral blood progesterone levels in Greyhound bitches. Theriogenology 2008;70:795–9.

71. Nothling JO, De Cramer KGM. Comparison of progesterone assay by chemiluminescence or radioimmunoassay for clinical decision-making in canine reproduction. J S Afr Vet Assoc 2019;90:e1–6.

72. Tal S, Mazaki-Tovi M, Druker S, et al. Evaluation of two chemiluminescent assays compared with radioimmunoassay for serum progesterone measurement in bitches. Theriogenology 2020;147:116–23.

73. Munro CJ, Lasley BL. Non-radiometric methods for immunoassay of steroid hormones. Prog Clin Biol Res 1988;285:289–329.

74. Stanczyk FZ, Lee JS, Santen RJ. Standardization of steroid hormone assays: why, how, and when? Cancer Epidemiol Biomarkers Prev 2007;16:1713–9.

75. Shille VM, Stabenfeldt GH. Luteal function in the domestic cat during pseudopregnancy and after treatment with prostaglandin F2 alpha. Biol Reprod 1979; 21:1217–23.

76. Munro C, Stabenfeldt G. Development of a microtitre plate enzyme immunoassay for the determination of progesterone. J Endocrinol 1984;101:41–9.

77. Wood WG. "Matrix effects" in immunoassays. Scand J Clin Lab Invest Suppl 1991;205:105–12.

78. Scholtz EL, Krishnan S, Ball BA, et al. Pregnancy without progesterone in horses defines a second endogenous biopotent progesterone receptor agonist, 5alpha-dihydroprogesterone. Proc Natl Acad Sci U S A 2014;111:3365–70.

79. Legacki EL, Scholtz EL, Ball BA, et al. The dynamic steroid landscape of equine pregnancy mapped by mass spectrometry. Reproduction 2016;151:421–30.

80. Wudy SA, Schuler G, Sanchez-Guijo A, et al. The art of measuring steroids: Principles and practice of current hormonal steroid analysis. J Steroid Biochem Mol Biol 2018;179:88–103.

81. French D. Advances in bioanalytical techniques to measure steroid hormones in serum. Bioanalysis 2016;8:1203–19.

82. Fontbonne A, Maenhoudt C, Thoumire S, et al. Evaluation of surface plasmon field-enhanced fluorescence spectroscopy for rapid measurement of progesterone concentration in bitches. Am J Vet Res 2021;82:417–24.

83. Kunanusont N, Punyadarsaniya D, Ruenphet S. Accuracy and precision guidelines for optimal breeding time in bitches using in-house progesterone measurement compared with chemiluminescent microparticle immunoassay. Vet World 2021;14:585–8.

84. Niswender GD. Influence of the site of conjugation on the specificity of antibodies to progesterone. Steroids 1973;22:413–24.

85. Yoon DY, Choi MJ, Choe IS, et al. Influence of the conjugation site on the specificity of monoclonal antibodies to progesterone and on the performance of direct enzyme immunoassay. Biochem Mol Biol Int 1993;31:553–63.

86. Gani M, Coley J, Piron J, et al. Monoclonal antibodies against progesterone: effect of steroid-carrier coupling position on antibody specificity. J Steroid Biochem Mol Biol 1994;48:277–82.
87. Krasowski MD, Drees D, Morris CS, et al. Cross-reactivity of steroid hormone immunoassays: clinical significance and two-dimensional molecular similarity prediction. BMC Clin Pathol 2014;14:1–13.
88. Bilbrough G, Glavan T. Catalyst Progesterone for in-house measurement of progesterone in plasma from bitches. Westbrook, ME: IDEXX Corporation; 2019. p. 1–4.
89. Schooley E, Bilbrough G, Glavan T. Art of measuring progesterone: understanding immunoassays. Clinical Theriogenology 2019;11:627–31.
90. Wynn MAA, Esteller-Vico A, Legacki EL, et al. A comparison of progesterone assays for determination of peripheral pregnane concentrations in the late pregnant mare. Theriogenology 2018;106:127–33.
91. Hooijberg EH. Quality assurance for veterinary In-clinic laboratories. Vet Clin North Am Small Anim Pract 2023;53:1–16.
92. Flatland B, Freeman KP, Vap LM, et al. Asvcp. ASVCP guidelines: quality assurance for point-of-care testing in veterinary medicine. Vet Clin Pathol 2013;42:405–23.
93. Jones KL, Megahed AA, Diehl BN, et al. Analytical validation of the IMMULITE((R)) 2000 XPi progesterone assay for quantitative analysis in ovine serum. Animals (Basel) 2022;12:1–14.
94. Brugger N, Otzdorff C, Walter B, et al. Quantitative determination of progesterone (P4) in canine blood serum using an enzyme-linked fluorescence assay. Reprod Domest Anim 2011;46:870–3.
95. Nothling JO, De Cramer KGM. Comparing the values of progesterone in the blood of bitches as measured with a chemiluminescence immunoassay and a radioimmunoassay. Reprod Domest Anim 2018;53:1136–41.
96. Gloria A, Contri A, Carluccio A, et al. Blood periovulatory progesterone quantification using different techniques in the dog. Anim Reprod Sci 2018;192:179–84.
97. Hisanaga T. Comparison of three different analyzers to measure canine serum progesterone. Honors College. Corvallis: Oregon State University; 2021. p. 22.
98. Milani C, Boscato EL, Gabai G, et al. Analytical and clinical performance of a fluorescence enzyme immunoassay for progesterone and determination of ovulation day in bitches. J Vet Diagn Invest 2022;34:977–82.
99. Rota A, Vannozzi I, Marianelli S, et al. Laboratory and clinical evaluation of a FEIA method for canine serum progesterone assay. Reprod Domest Anim 2016;51:69–74.
100. Zuercher J, Boes KM, Balogh O, et al. Comparison of a point-of-care analyzer with a chemiluminescent immunoassay for serum progesterone measurement in breeding management of the bitch. Front Vet Sci 2021;8:660923.
101. Bell R, Harr K, Rishniw M, et al. Survey of point-of-care instrumentation, analysis, and quality assurance in veterinary practice. Vet Clin Pathol 2014;43:185–92.
102. Hinderer J, Ludeke J, Riege L, et al. Progesterone concentrations during canine pregnancy. Animals (Basel) 2021;11:1–25.

Incorporating Genetic Testing into a Breeding Program

Bart J.G. Broeckx, Msc Vet Med, Msc Stat Data Analysis, PhD

KEYWORDS

• Genetic diversity • DNA test • Penetrance • Genetic heterogeneity • Marker

KEY POINTS

- Every breeding program should start with defining their breeding goals.
- Improving a breeding population requires balancing genetic diversity and selection.
- Selection can be achieved with various methods, but DNA tests give a direct insight into the genetic constitution of an animal and the outcome of certain combinations.
- Even animals affected by a disease with an autosomal recessive inheritance pattern or studs affected by an X-linked recessive phenotype, do not always have to be excluded from breeding if a DNA-test is available: when properly combined with a suitable mating partner, not a single puppy in the next generation will express the phenotype.
- The best results can only be achieved when proper attention is given to environmental optimization and state-of-the-art diagnostic methods.

INTRODUCTION

Genetic testing is defined as the use of a laboratory test to examine an individual's DNA for variations.[1] In the dog, the rate at which variants associated with phenotypes are discovered has skyrocketed with well over 300 new variants identified the last decade (**Fig. 1**).[2] With currently close to 500 phenotype-associated variants in the database, genetic tests are increasingly available for various diseases. This has several consequences. Fast increasing numbers of DNA tests also imply that keeping track of which DNA tests are important is becoming more difficult. Furthermore, not all DNA tests are easy to interpret, even when it is a so-called simple Mendelian disease. One notorious example is testing for the coat color "Merle."[3–5] For Merle, not only the presence of the "Merle" allele but also the length of that allele determines the phenotype. The "Merle" phenotype can be broadly divided into several phenotypic clusters and there are indications that the length associated with a specific Merle phenotypic cluster might vary slightly between breeds. Furthermore, the expression depends on the background coat color; in dogs with a minimal amount of eumelanin in their coat,

Department of Veterinary and Biosciences, Laboratory of Animal Genetics, Faculty of Veterinary Medicine, Ghent University, Heidestraat 19, Merelbeke 9820, Belgium
E-mail address: Bart.Broeckx@ugent.be

Vet Clin Small Anim 53 (2023) 951–963
https://doi.org/10.1016/j.cvsm.2023.04.002
0195-5616/23/© 2023 Elsevier Inc. All rights reserved.

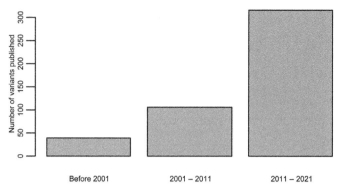

Fig. 1. The number of variants discovered per decade. The numbers per decade are based on the year of discovery, as reported in the Online Mendelian Inheritance in Animals database.[2]

expression of the "Merle" allele is hidden. Finally, the Merle allele is relatively instable, that is, its length can change from one generation to the next, but can also vary with the tissue sampled.

An increasing number of genetic tests also imply the probability that any individual dog will test positive for some genetic disease. When only 152 disease-associated variants were tested, 40% of the dogs carried already at least one copy of a disease variant.[6] It will thus not take long before phenotype- (and disease)-associated variants will be identified in every single dog. Combined, it is no surprise that 72% of the veterinarians believe that the importance of genetic testing will only increase the upcoming 5 to 10 years.[7]

Overall, it seems unlikely nowadays that a person responsible for managing a breeding program will not encounter any DNA test pertinent to their breed. In what follows, the focus will be on DNA tests used in breeding programs, supplemented with personal experiences of managing a breeding colony. Furthermore, practical examples illustrating some of the complexities are incorporated. This breeding program-oriented view of DNA tests represents of course only a subset of all the different applications of DNA tests. Some reference to the bigger picture is presented in the penultimate section.

THE PURPOSE OF THE BREEDING PROGRAM

Although this might seem an unnecessary step in the context of implementing genetic tests in breeding programs, a formal definition of the goal of the program is nonetheless essential. This is important for various reasons. First of all, if it is not defined, it is impossible to evaluate whether any progress is made. Second, especially when the breeding program is managed by a group and not by one individual, it is not necessarily true that everybody has the same goal or time interval to achieve it in mind. Third, it also allows a formal check whether the goal is actually ethically defendable. Defining what is ethically acceptable is of course a topic that on its own already can lead to quite some debate. In managing breeding programs, the following definition is what I currently adhere to: "*ethical breeding involves the use of healthy animals true to their breed in behavior and looks, and when applicable, showing a sustainable performance.*"[8,9]

THE ROLE OF GENETIC DIVERSITY

Although the focus is quite often oriented toward the diseases or phenotypes themselves, maintaining and/or improving genetic diversity is often neglected. The reasons are various. A reduced genetic diversity in itself is not visible, only the consequences (eg, increased disease prevalence) are. Furthermore, it is in itself also something which is not easy to explain. A rather vague understanding of the concept "genetic diversity" makes it of course difficult to convince others of the importance but also to implement it. Contributing factors are that genetic diversity can be based on various resources (eg, pedigrees or with genetic markers) and can be quantified and expressed variably.[10–12]

Practically, we use DNA test results to maximize genetic diversity and not to maximize the exclusion of animals. The reasons are that the genetic diversity is dangerously low in certain dog breeds, whereas the disease prevalence can be tremendously high at the same time.[10,13] Selecting against diseases for which there are no DNA tests implies excluding animals. To allow a maximal response for those phenotypes while maintaining sufficient genetic diversity, we try to avoid excluding animals for DNA test-based phenotypes whenever possible, as detailed further below.[13,14]

INTERPRETATION OF THE GENETIC TEST

Genetic test results can be interpreted at various levels. The first level is the dog itself. This level thus deals with the direct consequences of the genetic constitution of that individual and basically handles the question whether the dog will develop the disease or not. An easy example is the simple fully penetrant early-onset ataxia in Malinois caused by a mutation in the *SLC12A6* gene.[15] This is an autosomal recessive disease where all animals homozygous for the disease-causing allele demonstrate severe generalized hypermetric ataxia and a mild to moderate paraparesis, starting at the age of 3 to 6 months. Carriers and animals homozygous for the normal allele are entirely normal. Unfortunately, this dichotomized view (will the animal develop the disease? yes or no) is only valid for the simple fully penetrant disorders. Quite often, the situation is a lot more complex, as discussed further (section "Complications and considerations on genetic testing").

The second level handles the possible consequences of combining certain dogs. This level thus deals with the progeny, which is of course very important in breeding programs. Interpreting test results and implementing them in breeding programs are not always easy, as indicated by a recent questionnaire.[7] The number of correct answers varied strongly per respondent but did also depend on the inheritance pattern, with X-linked diseases scoring worst. As an aid, a short overview with all possible autosomal recessive, dominant, and X-linked dominant and recessive combinations and outcomes is provided in **Fig. 2**.

IMPROVING GENETIC DIVERSITY AND REDUCING DISEASE PREVALENCE

Closely linked to the second level in the previous paragraph, yet still distinct, is the question whether a specific dog should be used or excluded in a breeding program. In this specific case, the focus will lie entirely on the results of genetic tests. As mentioned further, it is however important to take "the whole picture" into account.

Genetic tests offer unique possibilities; they allow the immediate elimination of disease-associated variants in one generation because they not only ensure the identification of affected individuals but also of carriers. Taking into account however that every single individual at least carries disease-associated variants and that the number of variants known to be associated with diseases will only increase, applying this approach will result in the immediate elimination of all dogs at some point. As such, it is clearly not how DNA tests should be used. What is important is that the knowledge of the genotype of an individual animal makes it possible to combine dogs in such a way that there is a zero percent chance of affected progeny based on that specific

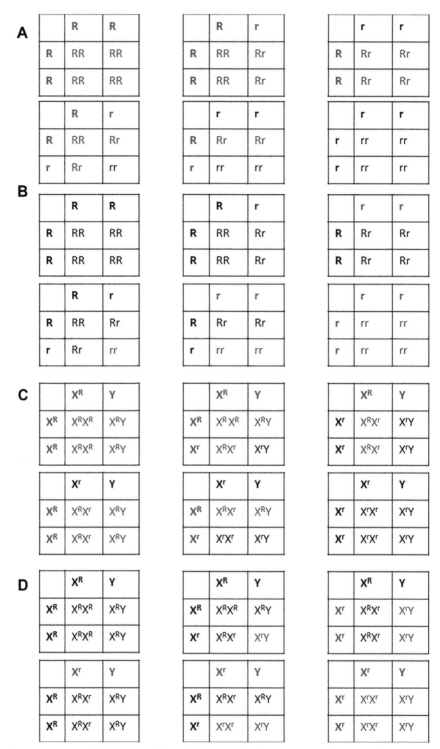

Fig. 2. Overview of all the possible combinations for (*A*) autosomal dominant, (*B*) autosomal recessive, (*C*) X-linked dominant, and (*D*) X-linked recessive diseases for one specific locus

mutation, even when the dog itself is affected. Various examples are depicted in **Fig. 2**; a combination of a dog genetically "affected" with an autosomal recessive disease with a dog homozygous for the wild-type allele will result in litters without any puppy developing the disease. Similarly, a stud affected with an X-linked recessive disease can actually father litters where no phenotypically affected puppies will be born from but only when combined with the correct bitch. Although this might seem a strange strategy at first, this is actually not strange when the issues related to genetic diversity (see before) are taken into account. As the genetic diversity in several breeds is tremendously low, excluding animals will actually be in the long run far more dangerous than mating them wisely, that is, using combinations that will never result in affected progeny. The reason for this strategy becomes clear when various tests are combined, as demonstrated in section "A practical example."

There are two remarks that have to be made when the "avoid exclusion maximally" strategy is used. First, unfortunately, the observation that using genetically affected dogs is an option is not valid for every single disease; it is only valid for autosomal recessive (both sexes) and for X-linked recessive diseases (studs). As depicted in **Fig. 2**, every other situation where an affected individual is used can actually lead to affected progeny. A second remark is that the possibility to use an animal that actually has a disease genetically is only truly an option if this does not result in welfare issues (1) for the dog itself and (2) for the puppies. An example is degenerative myelopathy. This autosomal recessive disease has a late onset, with the earliest symptoms sometimes being seen at an age of 5 years, but usually dogs are a lot older.[16] Furthermore, there are no indications that pregnancy affects disease progression. As a phenotypically healthy young (<5 years) bitch is not affected in its possibilities to care for the puppies and neither the puppies themselves are harmed, there thus seems to be no contraindications to use such a bitch. An example where this would not be acceptable is the aforementioned example of the *SLC12A6*-associated ataxia. An affected Malinois bitch would simply not be able to properly take care of the puppies and might not even live long enough to get through a normal gestation.

A PRACTICAL EXAMPLE

To demonstrate the use of genetic tests in a breeding program, a practical example will be given. This example deals with a breeding program that aims to breed assistance dogs for various assistance dog organizations. It breeds Labrador Retrievers and started from zero and had to grow to a demand of at least 100 puppies annually.

In line with the aforementioned framework, the goal of the breeding program was first defined. This so-called mission statement is *"to optimize the physical and behavioral characteristics of future assistance dogs based on scientific knowledge and with respect for animal welfare."*[17] Practically, this involved first checking the reasons for rejection of assistance dogs. This turned out to be mainly related to orthopedic

←——————————————————————————————

with two alleles "R" and "r." For phenotypes inherited dominantly, "R" is considered the allele responsible for the dominant phenotype; for phenotypes inherited recessively, "r" is considered the allele responsible for the recessive phenotype. For X-linked diseases, a distinction per sex is made. The genotypes in bold are the parents, the ones without are the progeny. Animals in red are genetically affected (ie, predisposed to develop the disease), whereas animals in black are not. Being genetically affected does not necessarily imply that the disease is phenotypically visible, for example, when the penetrance is less than 100%.

diseases (hip and elbow dysplasia) and being not suitable due to behavior issues.[18] There were no rejections reported due to diseases where there were genetic tests available for. As such, the general mission statement was translated to reducing the number of rejections for the aforementioned orthopedic and behavior phenotypes. For diseases where there are genetic tests available, this implies (1) to continue to avoid that affected puppies (= puppies genetically "at risk" to develop the disease) are born, while (2) trying to not reduce genetic diversity based on genetic test results as this is important for the long-term health of the breeding program and as selection for the important phenotypes will either way result in a reduction of the number of animals suitable for breeding.

The next step after the goal has been defined is to identify those diseases that (potentially) segregate in the population and where the focus will be on here, for which there are genetic tests. Based on a combination of sources (1) the "Online Mendelian Inheritance in Animals" database,[2] (2) PubMed, (3) other breeding programs with a similar goal, a list of DNA tests was identified (**Table 1**). A couple years after the initiation of the program, the variant responsible for Stargardt was identified.[19] This variant was immediately included in the program. The project started with four bitches and has grown to nine in the meantime.

At the start of the program, two of four bitches were heterozygous for a disease (one for exercise-induced collapse [EIC] and one for Stargardt). In agreement with the aim to avoid reducing genetic diversity, these bitches were not excluded but mated with studs that were homozygous wild type for the test for which the bitch was a carrier. As the start of the program, 22 litters or 138 puppies were born. None of these puppies were genetically affected by any of the diseases tested for (ie, they did not have a variant in a zygosity that would imply an at risk state to develop the disease). Of the current bitches, there are two of nine that carry a disease (both Stargardt). None of the candidate bitches had to be excluded from breeding along the process.

This is a short example that indicates how genetic diseases can be avoided, without having to exclude potential brood bitches. Not excluding dogs based on their genetic test results did not lead to an increase of the allelic frequencies of disease-associated variants (EIC: started at an allelic frequency of 12.5% and now is 0%; Stargardt started at an allelic frequency of 12.5%, and now is 11.1%), neither to puppies that are genetically at risk to develop the disease (= 0/138). This allowed at the same time the successful selection against various other diseases. In more detail, the prevalence of the orthopedic disorders hip and elbow dysplasia is now 19% lower than in the population of dogs bred outside the program.

Two remarks have to be made. First, these results indicate indeed that not excluding animals can lead to a success without any concession in terms of quality or welfare. It

Table 1
Overview of the diseases for which a genetic test is implemented in a breeding program for assistance dogs based on a population of Labrador Retrievers

Phenotype	Mode of Inheritance	Reference
Centronuclear myopathy	AR	Pelé et al,[39] 2005
Exercise-induced collapse	AR	Patterson et al,[40] 2008
Hereditary nasal parakeratosis	AR	Jagannathan et al,[41] 2013
Progressive rod-cone degeneration	AR	Zangerl et al,[42] 2006
Stargardt disease	AR	Mäkeläinen et al,[19] 2019

Abbreviation: AR, autosomal recessive.

is, however, important that the option to not exclude any animal was a consequence of that all diseases inherited autosomal recessive. If this would not have been the case, if one disease would have been autosomal dominant, for example, animals would have been excluded. Second, one might wonder what would have happened if the two dogs that initially carried a disease would have been excluded from breeding and whether this would have led to better results. This would have reduced the number of puppies tremendously (57 less, bred directly from them or from their descendants), the number of bitches currently available (six instead of nine) and there would still be one bitch carrying a disease due to the introduction of a Stargardt allele through a collaboration for semen exchange (ie, the allelic frequency of Stargardt would only be marginally smaller with an allelic frequency of 8.3%, whereas the result for EIC would remain the same). In short, the demands would not have been met for several additional years, whereas there would have been no direct improvement in terms of health.

COMPLICATIONS AND CONSIDERATIONS ON GENETIC TESTING

So far, little attention has been given to factors that might complicate the choice for the correct DNA test and the interpretation of DNA test results. In reality, factors such as reduced penetrance and genetic heterogeneity make both the choice of test and the consequent interpretation less than straightforward. Furthermore, some commercially available tests have a low sensitivity and/or specificity (eg, some marker-based tests) or might just be plain wrong (eg, tests based on variants where the association with the phenotype turns out to be invalid). Technological advancements allow simultaneous mass testing of variants, but this can give a false sense of security. Overall, it can thus be quite challenging, especially when these factors occur jointly.

Penetrance

From time to time, genetic test results do not match the observed phenotype. One of the possible explanations is reduced penetrance. Penetrance, defined as the probability of observing a specific phenotype, given a certain genotype, can range between 0 and 1.[20] A penetrance of 1, that is, 100% of the dogs with that genotype show the phenotype, is generally no problem. The affected dogs can be distinguished from the non-affected dogs. It becomes more cumbersome when penetrance is reduced. Unfortunately, this is not rare. Examples are EIC, Stargardt disease, and degenerative myelopathy.[16,19,21] The fact that genetically affected dogs do not necessarily show the phenotype might lead to owners' disbelief in genetic test results and noncompliance with breeding guidelines. Although reasons for not expressing the phenotype can be various (eg, the animal is too young, is not physically tested enough to cross the threshold), the consequences are that sometimes surprisingly high numbers of genetically but not phenotypically affected dogs are found. Especially in those cases, it is important to use the aforementioned approach where only those dogs for which there is no choice but to exclude them are actually excluded and all the other ones are retained for breeding (but of course wisely combined).

Genetic Heterogeneity

Genetic heterogeneity implies that different variants at the same locus (= allelic heterogeneity) or at different loci (= locus heterogeneity) can result in the same or similar phenotypes. Practically, this makes it more difficult to select the correct genetic test. Although, for example, with degenerative myelopathy, there are only two different variants known, there are diseases for which the number of disease-associated loci is far higher.[22] One illustration is the glomerular basement membrane disorders. Grouped under the name "hereditary nephropathy,' there are four different collagen IV mutations, each one unique for one breed (or a very specific mixed breed).[23–26] Although choosing the wrong test is a waste of money, much worse is that it can lead to a false sense of security, which in turn, can also affect client or clinician confidence in the accuracy of genetic tests. The key message is to carefully check what exactly is tested and to which detail. Unfortunately, it is not always clear which variant is actually tested, neither before the test is conducted nor thereafter, that is, based on the test result. A recent study substantiated this as 44% of the veterinarians found it "rather difficult" to "very difficult" to select the appropriate test.[7] When in doubt, the most obvious solution is contacting the laboratory that performed the test, and this is especially true when there are multiple tests available.

Unvalidated and Invalid Genetic Tests

The translation of research results to a genetic test suitable for a breeding program can be difficult. Researchers often focus on the association but not necessarily immediately on the clinical use. This can also be very complex, especially when the diseases themselves are multifactorial, that is, the phenotype is the result of a combination of genes and environmental influences. Laboratories that offer genetic tests are at the same time in a race to implement variants as soon as possible. The responsibility to offer validated tests is of course a shared responsibility. It is at the same time also not easy. For the moment, there are no guidelines specifically developed for dogs on variant classification. Although the American College of Medical Genetics Guidelines used to classify variants in human genetics seem to have their merit, they are not entirely ideal.[27] One example is that they do not take the canine breeding history into account. This implies that they cannot deal with the high allelic frequencies that disease-causing variants can have in dogs. Currently, variant guidelines for cats and dogs are being developed, but no consensus has been published so far.

The statement that not necessarily every commercially or patented test actually should be implemented is substantiated by the example of a patented test on canine hip dysplasia; the (independent) validation study demonstrated an opposite association than the one found in the original article.[28] Discrepancies between the first publication and subsequent validation studies are not uniquely linked to the dog, as exemplified by a variant that was first suggested to be associated with hypertrophic cardiomyopathy in the cat, which subsequently turned out to be common and not linked.[29,30] The key message is thus to evaluate the scientific evidence of every single DNA test before the implementation in the breeding program.

Marker-Assisted Tests

Identifying the so-called disease-causing variant is not always easy. Often, it involves performing genome-wide association studies (GWASs). In a GWAS, large numbers of single-nucleotide variants (SNVs) are tested for a statistical association with a phenotype. Although these SNVs can be directly causing the phenotype theoretically, this is seldom the case.[31] Usually, the SNVs genotyped in a GWAS are in linkage disequilibrium with the actual phenotype-causing variant.[31] Although they thus do not directly cause the phenotype, they are statistically associated with it, which makes them a marker. This is also why a GWAS is usually followed downstream by sequencing in an attempt to identify the disease-causing variant. This is not always successful, and sometimes, these markers are thus already implemented in DNA tests and commercially available. This has various consequences. First, as the disease-associated variant is not genotyped, but an associated marker, the strength of the association with the phenotype can vary. Second, the association can be population-specific and will also reduce in time due to recombination.[32] Third, the interpretation can be extremely difficult not only at the level of the individual animal (what is the probability that the animal will actually develop the disease?) but also for the breeding program (should we exclude every "at risk" animal?). These considerations, together with the observation that some markers, are extremely prevalent (eg, a marker found to be associated with adult-onset deafness segregated at frequencies >20% in the control population[33]), indeed suggest being careful. Although markers are thus very interesting from a research point of view, they do raise an important (ethical) question, that is, whether and when should they be made commercially available[13]? The answer can of course not be generalized to yes or no but requires thorough balancing of the pros and cons for each marker individually. The aforementioned development of criteria for variant classification might aid to make it more clear-cut on which variants to commercialize and/or implement in a breeding program.

Mass Testing

Similar to human medicine, larger panels and even whole exome and whole genome sequencing are commercially available nowadays, next to the more traditional individual gene tests. These technological advancements allow genetic testing at an unprecedented scale but also raise some important points of consideration that warrant additional attention. First, impressive reports with a long list of variants that were tested for might give the idea that every variant that is actually important for the breeding population must have been reported. This is not necessarily the case. There are of course various reasons why an important variant might not have been tested. It might have to do with patents but also with the technique used to genotype. Array-based DNA tests are for example fixed once designed. Practically, this implies that every variant discovered after the design of the array will not be genotyped. This can be solved by running additional single-gene tests, but usually, this also means that testing facilities using this technique do not have the latest variants. Whole exome and whole genome sequencing have the advantage that they are "unbiased" in their approach, so the sequencing data can be searched for the presence of newly discovered disease-causing variants after the initial design and sequencing and in general, the vast majority of variants should have been genotyped. Practically, mass testing implies the need to thoroughly check the test results not only for what has been reported but also on what might be missing. This is a shared responsibility; ideally, the laboratory offering the test should follow the publication of new variants closely and also report what is not tested.

With trends indicating a shift toward large panel testing, an additional point of consideration is how to deal with incidental or secondary findings (ie, findings that are not related to the indication for ordering the sequencing but that may nonetheless be of medical value or utility to the ordering physician and the patient).[1] Although this is mainly important in clinical genetics (ie, related to diagnostics), in a screening content it might also occur. Usually, the variants that segregate or are potentially important in the breeding population are known. However, when testing large numbers of dogs and variants, occasionally unexpected variants can be found in breeds where the genotype-phenotype association has not been reported. To the investigators' knowledge, contradicting (and thus breed-specific) associations have not yet been reported in the dog; however, in mice even entirely opposite associations have been demonstrated.[34] This again implies the necessity to thoroughly check everything on implementation of tests, but also the laboratory ideally should mention whether genotype–phenotype associations have been established in a specific breed.

DISCUSSION
General Considerations

The increased discovery and thus implementation of genetic tests raises various questions. Is the target audience (owners, breeders, and veterinarians) sufficiently trained to interpret the results? If not, what are the knowledge gaps and how can they be resolved? Although there are a lot of uncertainties in terms of the knowledge of breeders and owners, a study has been performed on veterinarians.[7] This study indicated a wide variability on the knowledge of genetic diseases and correct interpretation of DNA test results. This is of course not uniquely linked to veterinary medicine. Observations in human medicine have identified issues with inaccurate information/interpretation of test results, inappropriate or wrong ordering of genetic tests, medical mismanagement, and so on.[35] This is where genetic counsellors in human medicine jump in and which has also recently been advocated in veterinary medicine.[36] In breeding programs, a similar recommendation has been made; ideally, the person in charge of the program should be somebody who is trained in animal breeding/genetics or there should be direct access to a consultant when this knowledge is not available within the breeding program.[37]

The Bigger Picture

Although the focus of this article is obviously "genetic tests"-oriented, there is much more to consider in breeding programs. Aside from the aforementioned caveats involving genetic tests, in general, genetic tests are not the most complicated part of breeding programs. It is far more complex when genetic tests are not available. When that is the case, genotypes have to be derived from the phenotype, which is at best an informed guess. This can be improved tremendously by using statistical techniques, such as estimated breeding values, and so on.

Aside from the genetic technique used to identify the most optimal breeders, there also has to be attention on applying the most optimal techniques for phenotyping. Just one example is the incorporation of laxity-based techniques to diagnose canine hip dysplasia or computed tomography for elbow dysplasia.[18,38] Finally, it is not seldomly the case that multifactorial diseases or phenotypes are part of the goal of breeding programs. For these phenotypes, it is important to not neglect the environmental part as the best results will only be achieved when that part is also optimized.[37]

SUMMARY

Genetic tests are widespread nowadays and are extremely helpful in avoiding genetic diseases. Implementation in a breeding program is however not always easy due to various complicating factors and requires someone with the necessary skills as a wrong use can lead to at best an unnecessary decrease of the number of dogs in the breeding program, but at worst to a program that cannot function anymore. Within a breeding program, genetic tests complement other selection methods against or in favor of other phenotypes perfectly.

CLINICS CARE POINTS

- Prior to implementation in a breeding program, always check the validity of any genetic test.
- A long list of tests does not necessarily implies that everything that is important was actually tested, neither that everything which has been tested, is actually important.

- It is important to differentiate test results from clinical symptoms: while they can be closely linked, this is not necessarily the case and especially when they are not closely linked, decision-making has to be done extra precautious.

DISCLOSURE

The author declares there is no conflict of interest.

REFERENCES

1. National Human Genome Research Institute. Talking Glossary of Genomic and Genetic Terms. Published December 16, 2022. Available at: https://www.genome.gov/genetics-glossary#G. Accessed December 19, 2022.
2. Nicholas FW. Online Mendelian Inheritance in Animals (OMIA): a comparative knowledgebase of genetic disorders and other familial traits in non-laboratory animals. Nucleic Acids Res 2003;31(1):275–7.
3. Ballif BC, Emerson LJ, Ramirez CJ, et al. The PMEL gene and merle (dapple) in the dachshund: cryptic, hidden, and mosaic variants demonstrate the need for genetic testing prior to breeding. Hum Genet 2021;140(11):1581–91.
4. Murphy SC, Evans JM, Tsai KL, et al. Length variations within the Merle retrotransposon of canine PMEL: Correlating genotype with phenotype. Mobile DNA 2018; 9(1). https://doi.org/10.1186/s13100-018-0131-6.
5. Ballif BC, Ramirez CJ, Carl CR, et al. The PMEL gene and merle in the domestic dog: a continuum of insertion lengths leads to a spectrum of coat color variations in Australian shepherds and related breeds. Cytogenet Genome Res 2018. https://doi.org/10.1159/000491408.
6. Donner J, Anderson H, Davison S, et al. Frequency and distribution of 152 genetic disease variants in over 100,000 mixed breed and purebred dogs. PLoS Genet 2018;14(4):e1007361.
7. Bogaerts E, den Boer E, Peelman L, et al. Veterinarians' competence in applying basic genetic principles and daily implementation of clinical genetics: a study in a university environment. J Vet Med Educ 2022;49(6):799–806.
8. Olsson IAS, Gamborg C, Sandøe P. Taking ethics into account in farm animal breeding: What can the breeding companies achieve? J Agric Environ Ethics 2006;19(1):37–46.
9. Farstad W. Ethics in animal breeding. Reprod Domest Anim 2018;53:4–13.
10. Wijnrocx K, Franc L, Stinckens A, et al. Half of 23 Belgian dog breeds has a compromised genetic diversity , as revealed by genealogical and molecular data analysis. J Anim Breed Genet 2016;133:375–83.
11. Leroy G. Genetic diversity, inbreeding and breeding practices in dogs: Results from pedigree analyses. Vet J 2011;189(2):177–82.
12. Leroy G, Verrier E, Meriaux JC, et al. Genetic diversity of dog breeds: Within-breed diversity comparing genealogical and molecular data. Anim Genet 2009; 40(3):323–32.
13. Mellersh C. DNA testing and domestic dogs. Mamm Genome 2012;23(1–2): 109–23.
14. Hedhammar ÅA, Indrebø A. Rules, regulations, strategies and activities within the Fédération Cynologique Internationale (FCI) to promote canine genetic health. Vet J 2011;189(2):141–6.

15. van Poucke M, Stee K, Sonck L, et al. Truncating SLC12A6 variants cause different clinical phenotypes in humans and dogs. Eur J Hum Genet 2019; 27(10). https://doi.org/10.1038/s41431-019-0432-3.

16. Coates JR, Wininger FA. Canine degenerative myelopathy. Vet Clin North Am Small Anim Pract 2010;40(5):929–50.

17. Purpose Dogs VZW Mission statement. Available at: https://purpose-dogs.be/en/home-2/. Accessed May 12, 2023.

18. Bogaerts E, Moons CPH, van Nieuwerburgh F, et al. Rejections in an non-purpose bred assistance dog population: Reasons, consequences and methods for screening. PLoS One 2019;14(6):e0218339.

19. Mäkeläinen S, Gòdia M, Hellsand M, et al. An ABCA4 loss-of-function mutation causes a canine form of stargardt disease. PLoS Genet 2019;15(3). https://doi.org/10.1371/journal.pgen.1007873.

20. Broeckx BJG, Coopman F, Verhoeven GEC, et al. Toward the most ideal case-control design with related and unrelated dogs in whole-exome sequencing studies. Anim Genet 2016;47(2). https://doi.org/10.1111/age.12400.

21. Minor KM, Patterson EE, Keating MK, et al. Presence and impact of the exercise-induced collapse associated DNM1 mutation in Labrador retrievers and other breeds. Vet J 2011;189(2):214–9.

22. Wininger Fa, Zeng R, Johnson GS, et al. Degenerative myelopathy in a bernese mountain dog with a novel SOD1 missense mutation. J Vet Intern Med 2011; 25(5):1166–70.

23. Zheng R, Thorner PS, Marrano P, et al. Canine X chromosome-linked hereditary nephritis: a genetic model for human X-linked hereditary nephritis resulting from a single base mutation in the gene encoding the α5 chain of collagen type IV. Proc Natl Acad Sci U S A 1994;91(9):3989–93.

24. Cox ML, Lees GE, Kashtan CE, et al. Genetic cause of X-linked Alport syndrome in a family of domestic dogs. Mamm Genome 2003;14(6):396–403.

25. Nowend KL, Starr-Moss a N, Lees GE, et al. Characterization of the genetic basis for autosomal recessive hereditary nephropathy in the english springer spaniel. J Vet Intern Med 2012;26(2):294–301.

26. Davidson AG, Bell RJ, Lees GE, et al. Genetic cause of autosomal recessive hereditary nephropathy in the english cocker spaniel. J Vet Intern Med 2007;21(3): 394–401.

27. Richards S, Aziz N, Bale S, et al. Standards and guidelines for the interpretation of sequence variants: a joint consensus recommendation of the American College of Medical Genetics and Genomics and the Association for Molecular Pathology. Genet Med 2015;17(5). https://doi.org/10.1038/gim.2015.30.

28. Manz E, Tellhelm B, Krawczak M. Prospective evaluation of a patented DNA test for canine hip dysplasia (CHD). PLoS One 2017;12(8):e0182093.

29. Schipper T, Å O, Longeri M, et al. The TNNT2:c.95-108G>A variant is common in Maine Coons and shows no association with hypertrophic cardiomyopathy. Anim Genet 2022;53(4):526–9.

30. McNamara JW, Schuckman M, Becker RC, et al. A Novel Homozygous Intronic Variant in TNNT2 Associates With Feline Cardiomyopathy. Front Physiol 2020; 11. https://doi.org/10.3389/fphys.2020.608473.

31. Bush WS, Moore JH. Chapter 11: Genome-Wide Association Studies. PLoS Comput Biol 2012;8(12):e1002822.

32. Nicholas F.W., Nicholas F.W., Chapter 15: Selection within populations, *Introduction to veterinary genetics*, 3rd edition, 2010, John Wiley & Sons Ltd, West Sussex, UK, 235–248.

33. Yokoyama JS, Lam ET, Ruhe AL, et al. Variation in genes related to cochlear biology is strongly associated with adult-onset deafness in border collies. PLoS Genet 2012;8(9). https://doi.org/10.1371/journal.pgen.1002898.

34. Bourdi M, Davies JS, Pohl LR. Mispairing C57BL/6 substrains of genetically engineered mice and wild-type controls can lead to confounding results as it did in studies of JNK2 in acetaminophen and concanavalin a liver injury. Chem Res Toxicol 2011;24(6):794–6.

35. Bensend TA, Veach PMC, Niendorf KB. What's the harm? Genetic counselor perceptions of adverse effects of genetics service provision by non-genetics professionals. J Genet Couns 2014;23(1):48–63.

36. Moses L, Niemi S, Karlsson E. Pet genomics medicine runs wild. Nature 2018; 559:470–2.

37. Leighton EA. Secrets for producing high-quality working dogs. J Vet Behav Clin Appl Res 2009;4(6):212–5.

38. Broeckx BJG, Vezzoni A, Bogaerts E, et al. Comparison of three methods to quantify laxity in the canine hip joint. Vet Comp Orthop Traumatol 2018;31:23–9.

39. Pelé M, Tiret L, Kessler JL, et al. SINE exonic insertion in the PTPLA gene leads to multiple splicing defects and segregates with the autosomal recessive centronuclear myopathy in dogs. Hum Mol Genet 2005;14(11):1417–27.

40. Patterson EE, Minor KM, Tchernatynskaia A v, et al. A canine DNM1 mutation is highly associated with the syndrome of exercise-induced collapse. Nat Genet 2008;40(10):1235–9.

41. Jagannathan V, Bannoehr J, Plattet P, et al. A Mutation in the SUV39H2 gene in labrador retrievers with hereditary nasal parakeratosis (HNPK) provides insights into the epigenetics of keratinocyte differentiation. PLoS Genet 2013;9(10). https://doi.org/10.1371/journal.pgen.1003848.

42. Zangerl B, Goldstein O, Philp AR, et al. Identical mutation in a novel retinal gene causes progressive rod-cone degeneration (PRCD) in dogs and retinitis pigmentosa in man. Genomics 2006;88(5):551–63.

Ophthalmic Disease and Screening in Breeding Dogs

Kathryn A. Diehl, MS, DVM, DACVO[a],*, Sonia Kuhn Asif, DVM, DACVO[b],
Freya Mowat, BVSc, PhD, DECVO, DACVO, MRCVS[c,d]

KEYWORDS

- Breed-screening • Orthopedic foundation for animals
- Companion animal eye registry • Inherited • Ophthalmic • Canine • Incidence

KEY POINTS

- The Orthopedic Foundation for Animals Companion Animal Eye Registry is operated to reduce the incidence of comfort- and vision-threatening inherited ophthalmic conditions.
- A document written by the American College of Veterinary Ophthalmologists (ACVO) genetics committee called *Ocular Disorders Presumed to be Inherited in Purebred Dogs* guides certification and breeding recommendations of screening ophthalmic examination findings.
- Serial screening ophthalmic examinations by Diplomates of the ACVO, with breeding recommendations, have decreased the incidence of some inherited ophthalmic disorders in dogs.

CANINE BREED SCREENING OPHTHALMIC EXAMINATION

The American College of Veterinary Ophthalmologists (ACVO) and the Orthopedic Foundation for Animals (OFA) work jointly to operate the Companion Animal Eye Registry (CAER). Through screening ophthalmic examinations and certifications with associated breeding recommendations, the goal is to reduce the incidence of comfort- and vision-threatening inherited ophthalmic conditions in animals, mainly purebred dogs.

HISTORY AND CURRENT ORGANIZATION

In 1970, Dolly Trauner established the Society for the Investigation of Hereditary Defects in Dogs. This group performed pedigree analyses and determined coefficients of

---

[a] Department of Small Animal Medicine and Surgery, University of Georgia College of Veterinary Medicine, 2200 College Station Road, Athens, GA 30602, USA; [b] Blue Pearl Veterinary Eye Care, 3783 Pine Lane, Bessemer, AL 35022, USA; [c] Department of Surgical Sciences, School of Veterinary Medicine, University of Wisconsin-Madison, 1300 University Avenue, Madison, WI 53704, USA; [d] Department of Ophthalmology and Visual Sciences, School of Medicine and Public Health, 1300 University Avenue, Madison, WI 53704, USA
* Corresponding author.
E-mail address: kadiehl@uga.edu

Vet Clin Small Anim 53 (2023) 965–983
https://doi.org/10.1016/j.cvsm.2023.04.003   **vetsmall.theclinics.com**
0195-5616/23/© 2023 Elsevier Inc. All rights reserved.

inbreeding to reduce the likelihood that dogs affected with inherited diseases would be bred. However, progress was limited by resistance of owners of affected dogs to make pedigrees available. In 1974, Mrs Trauner established the Canine Eye Registry Foundation (CERF) in an attempt to mediate the lack of pedigree information. The goals for CERF were to promote recognition of inherited ophthalmic conditions in dogs and implement methods for control of these via breeding practices (G Aguirre, personal communication, January 2023). This involved in ophthalmic examinations of breeding dogs, which eventually became exclusively performed by Diplomates of the ACVO (DACVO) and the Veterinary Medical Database through 2013 and OFA beginning 2012 to present, as registry and certifying organizations for these CERF and CAER examinations, respectively.

The American Board of Veterinary Ophthalmologists standardizes and oversees the residency training programs and certification of DACVO. Performing and interpreting ophthalmic examinations are foundational to the practice of veterinary ophthalmology and are thus a focus of the training and credentialing process, though residents may or may not be exposed to CAER examinations specifically. Once diplomate status is conferred to candidates, they receive an orientation to the nuances of breed screening CAER ophthalmic examinations. This is provided by the OFA CAER program manager and either the ACVO-OFA liaison or a member of the ACVO genetics committee. The ACVO-OFA liaison and ACVO genetics committee members are all ACVO board-certified veterinary ophthalmologists (DACVO). The OFA CAER program manager, ACVO-OFA liaison, and members of the ACVO genetics committee are also available to answer examiner, owner, and breed club questions regarding these examinations.

Ocular Disorders Presumed to be Inherited in Purebred Dogs

The ACVO genetics committee, with the help of OFA personnel and registry information, compiles and evaluates information regarding known and presumed inherited ophthalmic conditions in dogs to generate the document *Ocular Disorders Presumed to be Inherited in Purebred Dogs*, often referred to solely as *The Blue Book*.[1] It is available online via the ACVO (acvo.org) and OFA (ofa.org/diseases/eye-disease/blue-book/) Web sites and serves as a resource for veterinarians and owners, and as the guide for diagnostic coding of CAER examination findings and ultimately certification and breeding recommendations. *The Blue Book* is updated annually based on registry data and relevant published literature reviewed by the ACVO genetics committee. Evidence-based breed club requests, available genetic tests, and ACVO genetics committee discretionary recommendations may also generate updates to *The Blue Book*.[1,2]

American Kennel Club-recognized breeds are each given a specific "page" within *The Blue Book* if warranted by breed CAER data and scientific information. There, specific ophthalmic disorders are listed for each breed if examined dogs are reported in sufficient numbers to detect presumed inherited ophthalmic conditions via registry data or if scientific studies or a genetic test has identified inherited ophthalmic conditions. Sufficient numbers are defined as an incidence $\geq 1\%$ of the examined population with a minimum of five affected animals per 5-year period or 50 or more affected animals in a 5-year period regardless of the population of dogs examined.[1] Descriptive information about the listed disorder is provided, including the mode of inheritance or genetic mutation if known and cited with appropriate references.[1]

In addition, breeding advice is given for each listed disorder of each breed. "Breeder option" conditions are either unlikely inherited, though the possibility cannot yet be definitively ruled out (eg, suspect not inherited/significance unknown cataracts) or suspected or known to be inherited but not of significant potential threat to ocular comfort or vision in either the individual dog or potential offspring.[1] Awareness of such conditions and status enables and empowers breeders to responsibly breed away from the condition as indicated, hence the designation "breeder option." A "no" or do not breed recommendation is listed on the breed page for disorders with very strong evidence of heritability and significant potential threat to ocular comfort or vision in either the individual or the offspring.[1] "No" breeding advice for a given disorder in a given breed may also be stated per breed club request at the discretion of the ACVO genetics committee. Finally, certain CAER examination diagnoses generate "no" breeding advice irrespective of whether or not the disorder is listed on the dog's Blue Book breed page because they have both strong evidence of heritability and frequently result in ocular pain and/or blindness in the offspring and sometimes the individual (**Table 1**).

Each breed "page" concludes with its associated complete ocular disorders report, which lists prevalence of all diagnoses for reported examined dogs of the breed.

OPHTHALMIC EXAMINATION PROCESS AND CERTIFICATION

To enhance sensitivity of detection of inherited conditions, which are frequently not congenital, the ACVO recommends serial *annual* ophthalmic examinations of dogs in active breeding lines of all breeds,[1] though some breed clubs have their own recommendations based on specific concerns for their breeds. Serial examination with associated breeding advice by the German panel of veterinary ophthalmologist has been shown to reduce the incidence of certain inherited ophthalmic disorders (cataract, progressive retinal atrophy [PRA]) in German dachshunds.[3]

A breed screening CAER ophthalmic examination thoroughly assesses features of the orbits, eyelids, and globes (from corneas to retinas and optic nerves) and is performed by a DACVO using slit lamp biomicroscopy and binocular indirect ophthalmoscopy. It is performed after pharmacologic mydriasis (pupil dilation) to best allow thorough evaluation of the peripheral/entire lenses and ocular fundi. Dogs of certain breeds with known inherited disorders of the iris should be examined before dilation to best allow thorough evaluation of the anterior segment for the following disorders: dalmatian—iris hypoplasia/sphincter dysplasia; Australian shepherd, miniature American shepherd/miniature Australian shepherd, and toy Australian shepherd—iris coloboma.[1] They should subsequently be dilated and otherwise examined fully as above. *All* findings of the breed screening CAER ophthalmic examination, though with a focus on those potentially significant to breeding (ie, known, suspected, or possibly inherited), are noted by the diplomate examiner on a specific CAER examination form (**Fig. 1**). This allows most appropriate documentation and communication and ultimately appropriate and consistent diagnosis/coding and certification with breeding

---

Table 1
Unequivocal "no" breeding recommendation conditions[1]

- Keratoconjunctivitis sicca (KCS or dry eye)
- Certain forms of persistent pupillary membranes (PPM) and associated findings (iris to iris and iris to cornea PPM, iris sheets, and endothelial opacity/no strands)
- Lens subluxation or luxation
- Retinal detachment
- Geographic or detached retinal dysplasia
- Optic nerve coloboma or hypoplasia

- Glaucoma
- Cataracts without an obvious, reasonable, non-inherited explanation
- Persistent hyperplastic primary vitreous (PHPV)/persistent hyperplastic tunica vasculosa lentis (PHTVL)
- Generalized or diffuse retinal atrophy/retinal degeneration (eg, the inherited progressive retinal atrophies [PRA])

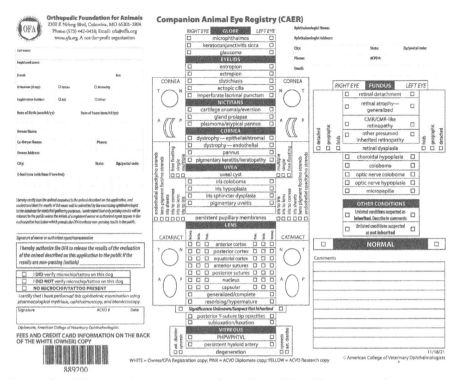

Fig. 1. The CAER ophthalmic examination form. (*From* OFA; with permission.)

recommendations dictated by the ACVO genetics committee via *The Blue Book* through OFA.

It should be noted that a Schirmer tear test (STT), fluorescein staining, tonometry, gonioscopy, high-resolution ultrasonographic imaging for evaluation of the iridocorneal angle, electroretinography, and streak retinoscopy to determine refractive error are not components of the routine CAER examination. Certainly, these ophthalmic diagnostic tests may provide additional information relevant to the breed screening CAER ophthalmic examination (ie, diseases they test for may be inherited) or the individual canine patient being examined (ie, they may warrant intervention to reduce risk of ocular discomfort and or visual impairment). They may thus be performed at the discretion of the examiner or request of the owner and documented as "comments" on the examination form. In addition, in some cases (eg, where KCS is suspected but cannot be confirmed solely via examination findings), such tests (in this case, an STT) may be requested or required to be performed before an official diagnosis can be given and thus a certificate or other result generated at OFA. However, because these additional ophthalmic examination components are not included in the vast majority of CAER examinations, early cases where physical ophthalmic examination signs are not yet present could be missed.[1]

With input from the ACVO Vision for Animals Foundation Canine Glaucoma Consortium, the ACVO genetics committee and OFA have created a separate gonioscopy examination form. Although currently only in the data collection phase, the goal of this form is to establish a standardized database for additional information related to the iridocorneal angle/aqueous humor outflow and potential risk factors for glaucoma in purebred and breeding dogs. Like the general breed screening CAER ophthalmic examination, the ultimate goals of this additional arm of the program are to promote recognition and allow understanding of predispositions to inherited primary glaucoma in dogs (ie, are there predictable iridocorneal angle factors and examination findings?) and make evidence-based breeding recommendations to reduce such. At present, if performed, gonioscopy and any other iridocorneal angle assessment findings may be written in as comments on the CAER form as above or a gonioscopy form may be completed.

Although examiners provide and document gonioscopic findings to owners and may interpret and make breeding recommendations regarding these results, no certification or recommendation is provided by OFA/ACVO as both performing that examination itself and interpreting what it means for the individual dog and its breed lines is complicated and lacks consensus. Dogs having had gonioscopy performed and documented on a CAER or gonioscopy form submitted to OFA receive a denotation on their CAER certificates that it was done, but again, no official interpretation or recommendations occur.

It is important to note that like most physical examination subsets, breed screening CAER ophthalmic examinations are phenotypic. Dogs may be carriers of inherited conditions or even genetically affected but not (yet) displaying the phenotype as many non-congenital inherited diseases manifest later in life, often after dogs have been bred. In these cases, CAER examinations could be normal despite the possibility of dogs passing on problematic genes and ultimately disorders. Many genetic defects with ophthalmic ramifications are not yet known or do not have an available genetic test. In addition, available genetic testing is very specific (eg, may rule in or out one form of inherited retinal degeneration but not others), whereas the phenotypic screening CAER examination, which looks at the entire ophthalmic system, is broad. Therefore, it is recommended that dogs in active breeding lines receive phenotypic CAER examinations that are complemented with genetic testing for specific disorders in dogs of known affected breeds.

Given the screening nature of CAER examinations, they attract a biased population and generate biased, likely underestimated, data regarding the true incidence of disorders in affected dog breeds. Dogs with ophthalmic disorders that cause noticeable pain and or vision loss, or even just obviously visible lesions may not be presented for and diagnosed via CAER examinations as their severity may have already necessitated veterinary attention. Asymptomatic but phenotypically present conditions are more likely to be detected on this type of examination.

Owner copies of completed CAER examination forms may be submitted to OFA for registry and certification. A database is created from this registry along with CAER examination form research copies which capture instances of examined dogs where owners do not submit results. A review by the ACVO-OFA liaison will clarify unclear diagnoses and cross-reference findings with any previous examinations on file. Ultimately, diagnoses are finalized and certificate codes and breeding recommendations are generated per *The Blue Book* guidelines and breed pages. Although forms may be submitted any time, certification and breeding recommendations expire a year after the date of the examination to encourage serial screening and enhance the sensitivity of detecting inherited conditions.

SELECTED SPECIFIC CONDITIONS SCREENED FOR ON A COMPANION ANIMAL EYE REGISTRY EXAMINATION

Common or otherwise particularly problematic conditions from each section of the CAER form are described and discussed below.

Multiple canine eyelid conditions are likely inherited, though the causative mutations are unknown. These adnexal disorders usually generate a "breeder option" breeding recommendation when diagnosed on a CAER examination because they are complexly inherited and cause less severe pathology than disorders where breeding is not recommended.

- A distichia is abnormal eyelashes that emerge through the eyelid margin, most commonly through the meibomian gland orifices (**Fig. 2**). They are usually asymptomatic but can cause squinting, tearing, and corneal ulceration in some instances.
- Entropion is an inward rolling of the eyelid margin that causes irritation and corneal ulceration when periocular hair rubs on the ocular surface. In contrast, ectropion is an outward rolling of the eyelids that can cause ocular surface irritation via exposure. Both entropion and ectropion are likely influenced by multiple factors related to facial conformation and therefore may be inadvertently selected for as breeders seek a desired appearance in their dogs. At the request of their breed clubs, entropion in the Rhodesian ridgeback and rottweiler has been designated as a "no" breeding recommendation.[1]

Corneal disorders with a presumed or known genetic basis in dogs vary in their clinical significance and therefore also in CAER breeding recommendations.

- Chronic superficial keratitis, also known as pannus, is an immune-mediated corneal disease characterized by vascularization, fibrosis, pigmentation, and infiltrate often to the extent of pink proliferative tissue formation (**Fig. 3**). Pannus of the nictitans can occur in isolation (plasmoma or atypical pannus) or concurrent with corneal disease and is manifested by a pink nodular appearance to the normally smooth pigmented third eyelid conjunctiva. Blindness can occur when corneal disease is severe. A genetic basis is suspected in German shepherds (GSD), greyhounds, Belgian tervurens, Belgian sheepdogs, and Maremma sheepdogs due to breed predilections and sufficient incidence in CAER data.[1,4–6] A CAER examination diagnosis of pannus receives a "no" breeding recommendation. This has seemingly improved breeding practices and decreased incidence of the condition in GSD presented for CAER examinations: in 2013, 150 GSD were examined and 2% were affected with plasmoma, 1.3% with corneal pannus; in 2022, 209 were examined and 0% and 0.5% were affected with plasmoma and corneal pannus, respectively. (J Pautz, personal communication of breed data report, January 2023).

Epithelial-stromal corneal dystrophy is characterized by the accumulation of white to gray opacities, most often lipid, within one or more corneal layers (**Fig. 4**). It rarely

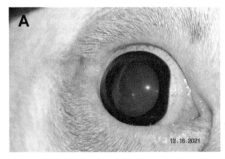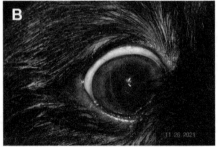

Fig. 2. Distichia in the right eye of a 2-year-old spayed-female boxer (*A*) and the right eye of a 1.5-year-old spayed-female shih tzu (*B*). These were bilateral in both cases.

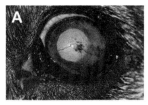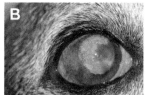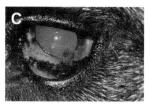

Fig. 3. Pannus in the left eye of a 6-year-old spayed-female German shepherd (*A*), the right eye of a 4-year-old neutered-male greyhound (*B*). Pannus and atypical pannus in the left eye of 5-year-old neutered-male German shepherd (*C*). These were all bilateral.

causes pain or blindness and usually does not require treatment; therefore, for most breeds, this diagnosis receives a breeding recommendation of "breeder option." This still allows breeding practices to select away from the disorder, and the cavalier King Charles spaniel (CKCS) provides an example of a commonly affected breed with decreasing incidence in dogs presented for CAER examinations: in 2013, with 2520 CKCS examined, 10% were affected with corneal dystrophy; in 2022, with 3192 CKCS examined, 7.6% were affected (J Pautz, personal communication of breed data report, January 2023). Exceptions to the breeder option recommendation for corneal dystrophy include "Sheltie corneal dystrophy" in the Shetland sheepdog, which carries a "no" breeding recommendation because the disease results in an unstable overlying tear film and often painful corneal erosions warranting treatment,[1,7] and the Siberian husky where the inheritance is presumed to be autosomal recessive and the opacities are often more severe, potentially resulting in vision impairment.[1,8–11]

- Endothelial corneal dystrophy results in progressive corneal edema. When severe, this disease causes pain via chronic corneal ulcerations and vision impairment from corneal opacification. Predispositions have been identified in the basenji, Boston terrier, chihuahua, and dachshund; therefore, a "no" breeding recommendation is made for these breeds due to the presumption of hereditary disease.[1,8] Based on sufficient incidence in CAER data, endothelial corneal dystrophy is also listed as a disorder for the petit basset griffon vendeen with a "breeder option" breeding recommendation.[1] Corneal endothelial *degeneration*, which is usually age-related and may present similarly clinically, does not generate any specific breeding recommendations.
- Macular corneal dystrophy is a unique form of corneal dystrophy in Labrador retrievers with autosomal recessive inheritance from a mutation in the CHST6

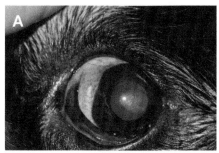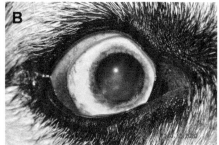

Fig. 4. Epithelial-stromal corneal dystrophy in the left eye of a 6-year-old neutered-male cavalier King Charles spaniel (*A*) and the right eye of a 4-year-old male Siberian husky (*B*). These were bilateral in both cases.

gene.[12] This disease usually affects dogs aged 4 to 6 years and is characterized by bilateral stromal grey–tan circular corneal opacities of varying size with potential associated vascularization.[13] A commercial genetic test is available, and a "no" breeding recommendation is made if this disorder is diagnosed on a CAER examination.

- Pigmentary keratitis, also known as pigmentary keratopathy, is defined as the deposition of superficial corneal pigment which is usually accompanied by fibrosis and vascularization (**Fig. 5**). It is most often a problem in brachycephalic dogs, especially pugs, where ocular surface irritation and exposure from facial conformation such as medial lower eyelid entropion and macropalpebral fissure (wide eyelid openings) may play a role.[14] As with the previously discussed adnexal disorders, selection for a certain facial appearance may result in an increased prevalence of pigmentary keratitis. However, one study in pugs did not find an association between facial conformation and corneal pigmentation and therefore surmised that the disorder may have its own genetic basis separate from corneal pigmentation secondary to irritation and exposure considerations.[15] This disorder is categorized as "breeder option" as it is not fully understood, does not threaten ocular comfort, and though may be vision impairing when severe, often is milder. Again, this still allows breeding practices to select away from the disorder, and the incidence in pugs presented for CAER examinations went from 73.3% (of 101 dogs examined) in 2013 to 46.2% affected (of 173 dogs examined) in 2022 (J Pautz, personal communication of breed data report, January 2023).

Uveal disorders vary in severity and breeding recommendations.

- Uveal cysts are fluid-filled semitransparent circular structures arising from the epithelium of the posterior iris or ciliary body (**Fig. 6**). They can be variably pigmented, vary in size, and remain attached or break free to float in the anterior chamber. Cysts may rupture and deposit pigment on intraocular tissues. Uveal cysts rarely cause clinical problems and in all breeds are receive a breeding recommendation of "breeder option." However, in the golden retriever, uveal cysts may be associated with pigmentary uveitis and secondary glaucoma, and they may be associated with glaucoma in the great dane and American bulldog.[16–19]
- Pigmentary uveitis is a poorly understood and potentially devastating condition that occurs in middle-aged to older golden retrievers[16] and carries an OFA

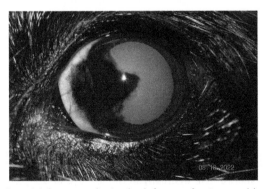

Fig. 5. Pigmentary keratitis/keratopathy in the left eye of a 4-year-old neutered-male shih tzu. Note the typical "wedge" of nasal corneal pigment, in this case without vascularization.

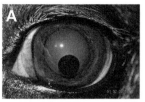
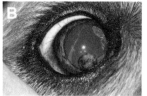
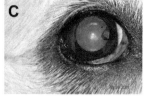

Fig. 6. Solitary, heavily pigmented, free-floating (in the anterior chamber) uveal cyst in the left eye of a 6-year-old neutered-male Boston terrier (*A*). Solitary, mildly-pigmented, free-floating uveal cyst, along with multiple, lightly pigmented uveal cysts "peeking" around the nasal pupillary margin from behind, in the right eye of a 5-year-old neutered-male golden retriever (*B*). Multiple, mildly pigmented uveal cysts at the nasal pupillary margin in the right eye of an 8-year-old spayed-female golden retriever with pigmentary uveitis and secondary glaucoma in the contralateral eye (*C*). Note the relatively heavily pigmented iris, and focal dense pigment on the superior-nasal anterior lens capsule, which is a remnant from a ruptured and deflated previous additional uveal cyst.

"no" breeding recommendation (**Fig. 7**). It begins with the presence of radial pigment deposition on the anterior lens capsule and can progress to cause posterior synechiae, secondary cataract, and in its most advanced form, secondary glaucoma.[20,21] This disease has been associated with the presence of uveal cysts, though not all golden retrievers with uveal cysts will progress to develop pigmentary uveitis.[17,21,22] As dogs in the initial stage of this disease are often asymptomatic, screening ophthalmic examinations may allow earlier detection and altered breeding practices. At later stages, affected dogs are usually recognized when clinical signs prompt veterinary attention. However, elimination of this disease has been challenging because it does not yet have a genetic test and affected dogs are usually not diagnosed until after they may have been bred. This said, with recognition and earlier diagnosis of the disorder, the incidence in golden retrievers presented for CAER examinations has decreased: 2% (of 6458 dogs examined) in 2013 to 1.1% affected (of 9619 dogs examined) in 2022 (J Pautz, personal communication of breed data report, January 2023).

- An iris coloboma is a congenital full-thickness defect of the iris that occurs as a developmental anomaly. It can occur anywhere in the iris though most commonly occurs at the most ventral aspect (typical coloboma) from failure of closure of the

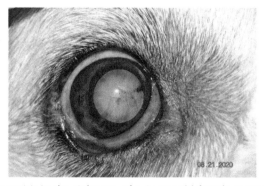

Fig. 7. Pigmentary uveitis in the right eye of a 9-year-old female-spayed golden retriever. Note the diffuse radial pigment deposition on the anterior lens capsule and early secondary cataract.

optic fissure. Iris colobomas are coded as "breeder option" except for in the Australian shepherd, miniature American shepherd/miniature Australian shepherd, and toy Australian shepherd where a "no" breeding recommendation is made due to their potential association with more serious abnormalities in other parts of the eye.[1] This has seemingly affected breeding practices and slightly decreased incidence of the condition in Australian shepherds presented for CAER examinations: in 2013, 3742 were examined and 1.5% were affected; in 2022, 3582 were examined and 0.9% were affected (J Pautz, personal communication of breed data report, January 2023).

- Congenital partial thickness iridal defects are marked as iris hypoplasia on the CAER form and are considered "breeder option" for all breeds.
- Persistent pupillary membranes (PPMs) are remnants of the fetal anterior segment vascular system that have failed to regress by 3 months postnatally. They can occur unilaterally or bilaterally in a variety of forms: strands that originate from the surface of the iris and connect to the iris (iris–iris PPM), lens (iris–lens PPM), or cornea (iris–cornea PPM), as endothelial corneal opacities without strands (**Fig. 8**), or most severely as iridal sheets within the anterior chamber. PPMs that contact the lens frequently cause cataract and those that contact the cornea cause corneal opacity. The mildest form, iris–iris PPMs, is coded "breeder option," but for all other forms, a "no" breeding recommendation is made as they can cause vision impairment and or because of potential heritability and more severe forms in offspring. PPMs are found in multiple breeds but have been especially significant in the basenji, where they may also be associated with optic nerve colobomas[23,24] and the (English) mastiff and Pembroke Welsh corgi breeds.[1] The incidence of iris-to-iris PPMs in Pembroke Welsh corgis presented for CAER examinations decreased from 17.2% (of 529 dogs examined) in 2013 to 14% affected (of 810 dogs examined) in 2022. The incidence of iris-to-lens PPMs in basenjis presented for CAER examinations decreased from 7.7% (of 221 dogs examined) in 2013 to 1.1% affected (of 272 dogs examined) in 2022. The incidence of endothelial corneal opacities without strands from previous PPMs in

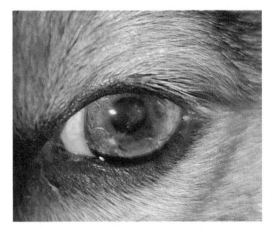

Fig. 8. Iris-to-iris persistent pupillary membranes (PPM) and endothelial opacities no strands (remnants of iris-to-cornea PPM) in the left eye of a 4-month-old male corgi. The contralateral eye was equivocally microphthalmic and had iris-to-cornea PPM with associated corneal endothelial leukoma and overlying corneal edema from focal endothelial dysfunction in the region of PPM adherence.

mastiffs presented for CAER examinations decreased from 3% (of 201 dogs examined) in 2013 to 1.9% affected (of 160 dogs examined) in 2022 (J Pautz, personal communication of breed data report, January 2023).

Disorders of the lens can result in ocular discomfort and vision impairment via opacification, intraocular inflammation, and secondary glaucoma. Many severe lens conditions result in a "no" breeding recommendation.

- Lens luxation is a potentially blinding disorder in dogs but fortunately one of the few anterior segment disorders that has a well-defined genetic etiology. An autosomal recessively inherited mutation in *ADAMTS17* causes the development of abnormal lens zonules which break prematurely.[25] As a result, the lens becomes loose and can move anteriorly or posteriorly out of position to increase susceptibility to glaucoma, corneal edema, uveitis, and retinal detachment. This mutation is widespread across breeds but is especially prevalent in terriers and other dogs bred for short stature.[26,27] This gene has also been associated with primary open angle glaucoma in a growing number of breeds, including the shar-pei, basset hound, petit basset griffon vendeen, and basset fauve de Bretagne.[27–30] Subtle signs of lens instability, such as a deep anterior chamber, vitreous in the anterior chamber and abnormal movement of the iris or lens with rapid eye movements (iridodonesis and phacodonesis, respectively) may be found on a CAER examination before more devastating disease occurs when the lens has become completely luxated. A "no" breeding recommendation is made for this condition. Commercial genetic testing is available.
- A cataract is an opacity of the lens, and the most common presumed etiology of clinically significant cataracts in dogs is heredity. Hereditary cataracts can occur in any part of the lens and vary in size/extent. In general, a cataract that is suspected to be hereditary (without other reasonable, likely explanation such as developmental vascular contact, trauma, age, or previous inflammation, and so forth, typical in location, shape, and so forth) on a CAER examination receives a "no" breeding recommendation. There are some exceptions to this such as posterior Y-suture tip opacities, which are not considered a true cataract, and nuclear fibrillar/pulverulent cataracts, which may be inherited and/or senile. These lesions do not progress to cause vision impairment and are not associated with risk of more severe forms in offspring. Therefore, these cataract types are coded as "breeder option," with posterior Y-suture tip opacities receiving their own specific code (E2). In GSD presented for CAER examinations, the incidence of nuclear cataracts decreased from 6% in 2013 with 150 dogs examined to 4.3% in 2022 with 209 dogs examined (J Pautz, personal communication of breed data report, January 2023).

Mutations in the *HSF4* gene have been associated with cataract development as an autosomal codominant trait in the Australian shepherd, miniature American shepherd/miniature Australian shepherd, and toy Australian shepherd (*HSF4-2*), and an autosomal recessive trait in the Boston terrier, Staffordshire bull terrier, French bulldog, and miniature pinscher (*HSF4-1*).[1,31–34] However, in most breeds, the specific gene or genes involved in cataract formation remain unknown. In addition, other genes may be involved within known *HSF4* affected breeds.

Posterior polar cataracts, which are presumed hereditary in multiple breeds, are small, often triangular, and usually do not significantly impact vision in the animal in which they occur (**Fig. 9**). However, they may be associated with more severe forms of cataract in offspring, and hence, a "no" breeding recommendation is made for this

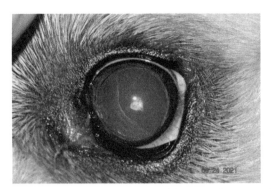

Fig. 9. Posterior polar cataract in the left eye of a 3-year-old female golden retriever presented for CAER examination. This was bilateral.

diagnosis on a CAER examination.[35] This has seemingly affected breeding practices and decreased incidence of the condition in dogs presented for CAER examinations of several breeds: golden retrievers [4.1% (of 6458 dogs examined) in 2013 to 3.2% (of 9619 dogs examined) in 2022]; cocker spaniels [4.3% (of 1129 dogs examined) in 2013 to 3.1% (of 1085 dogs examined) in 2022]; Siberian huskies [4.9% (of 984 dogs examined) in 2013 to 3.8% (of 993 dogs examined] in 2022; and greater Swiss mountain dogs [5.2% (of 115 dogs examined) in 2013 to 1.9% (of 105 dogs examined) in 2022] (J Pautz, personal communication of breed data report, January 2023).

Another form of cataract, in the equatorial cortex, may be inherited or not. Its incidence has decreased in greater Swiss mountain dogs (6.1% of 115 dogs examined to 2.9% of 105 dogs examined) and Boston terriers (2.8% of 533 dogs examined to 1.7% of 773 dogs examined) presented for CAER examinations in 2013 and 2022, respectively (J Pautz, personal communication of breed data report, January 2023).

Cataracts can occur secondary to nonhereditary causes, such as trauma, aging, uveitis, nutritional deficiencies, and specific metabolic diseases such as diabetes mellitus and hypocalcemia. For those cataracts that the examiner suspects not to be genetic in origin, "significance unknown/suspect not inherited" can be marked on the CAER form and those dogs may receive a breeder option code (E1).

The vitreous, retina, pigmented epithelium, choroid, sclera, and optic nerve comprise the posterior aspect/segment of the globe. These tissues mediate initiation of the visual pathway, transmission of visual information to the brain, recycling of visual pigments, and provision of nutrients/metabolite removal for the metabolically active photoreceptors. Inherited or presumed inherited disorders of these structures are common and can be congenital (retinal dysplasias, collie eye anomaly, optic nerve hypoplasia, or coloboma) or adult-onset (PRA, multifocal retinopathy). Although genetic tests for some conditions are available, there are many potentially inherited conditions for which no genetic diagnosis (and therefore test) exists. Hence, genetic testing cannot replace yearly hereditary eye disease screening, particularly for posterior segment conditions. For breeding dogs, a clinical diagnosis of a potentially inherited retinal disorder could be confirmed with genetic testing, but a "clear" genetic test does not exclude an inherited component. Most inherited conditions of the canine posterior segment have an autosomal recessive mode of inheritance, although dominant conditions and recessive conditions with additional modifier genes have been described. The CAER examination system does not currently administer breeding recommendations based solely on genetic testing, and owners should seek expert advice from ophthalmologists and theriogenologists when making breeding decisions based on these outcomes. Genetic test results may help further inform or modify a phenotypic CAER examination diagnosis and breeding recommendations.

Vitreous Conditions

- Liquefaction of the vitreous is common in aging, but earlier onset vitreous degeneration occurs in specific breeds. The genetics of this condition are not defined but it is presumed inherited in the Italian greyhound, Brussels griffon, shih tzu, whippet, and bichon frise, as well as other breeds based on sufficient incidence in CAER data and references.[1,36] Although this theoretically predisposes dogs to retinal detachment, glaucoma, and lens luxation, in a study of these dogs diagnosed with vitreous degeneration on CAER examinations, no such association with these ocular comorbidities nor cataract was found.[36] In Italian greyhounds, Brussels griffons, and whippets, from 2013 to 2022, incidence of one form of vitreous degeneration (syneresis) in dogs presented for CAER examinations decreased from 26% to 4.3% (in 192 and 94 Italian greyhounds examined), 20% to 14.3% (in 60 and 63 Brussels griffons examined), and 4.5% to 2.4% (in 355 and 594 whippets examined) (J Pautz, personal communication of breed data report, January 2023).
- A group of congenital conditions relate to persistence of the fetal lens vasculature in the vitreous (persistent hyaloid artery [PHA], persistent hyperplastic primary vitreous or persistent hyperplastic tunica vasculosa lentis [PHPV/PHTVL]). These vessels can contribute to cataract formation and/or vitreal hemorrhage if patent. PHPV/PHTVL is best documented as a presumed inherited disorder in Doberman pinschers and Staffordshire bull terriers, though the genetics of the disorder are not defined.[1,37–44] CAER examinations seem to have decreased the incidence of these conditions in these breeds in that the incidence of PHA in Staffordshire bull terriers presented for CAER examinations decreased from 3.4% in 2013 (88 dogs examined) to 2% in 2022 (99 dogs examined), and the incidence of PHPV/PHTVL in Doberman pinschers presented for CAER examinations decreased from 1.2% in 2013 (172 dogs examined) to 0.7% in 2022 (287 dogs examined) (J Pautz, personal communication of breed data report, January 2023).

Congenital Retina/Choroid/Optic Nerve Conditions

- Retinal dysplasias vary from mild (retinal folds manifesting as small multifocal areas of retinal thickening and/or thinning) (Fig. 10), moderate (larger, geographic areas of retinal thickening and/or thinning) to severe (complete detachment of the retina with visual impairment). Although commonly diagnosed clinically in many breeds, mutations have been described in only two genes, COL9A2 (Labrador retriever) and COL9A3 (Samoyed and northern Inuit), which also cause an oculo-skeletal dysplasia.[45] Limb deformities include shortened forelimbs with valgus deformity, and ocular abnormalities include cataract, multifocal retinal dysplasia, vitreous degeneration, and retinal detachment. Diagnosis of the more severe forms of retinal dysplasia (geographic/complete) on a CAER examination will result in a "no" breeding recommendation. Retinal folds vary in their recommendation from "breeder option" to "no" based on the breed affected and can be downgraded from a "no" to a "breeder option" for the three already mentioned breeds affected by COL9A2 and COL9A3 mutations if a negative genetic test can be provided.[1] The Labrador retriever provides an example of decreased incidence of retinal dysplasia–folds: 1.5% of 6741 dogs examined for CAER examinations in 2013 were affected versus 0.8% of 6374 dogs in

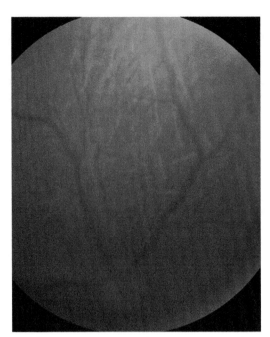

Fig. 10. Extensive retinal folds in the right eye of an 8-week-old English springer spaniel presented for CAER litter screening examination. Multiple puppies in the litter were affected with retinal folds or geographic retinal dysplasia in one or both eyes.

2022. The English springer spaniel was similar with a decreased incidence from 3.2% (of 1618 dogs examined for CAER examinations) in 2013 to 2.2% (of 1077 dogs) in 2022 (J Pautz, personal communication of breed data report, January 2023).

- Collie eye anomaly is most prevalent in collies and related breeds. Phenotypes range from inadequate development of the choroid (choroidal hypoplasia) to defects of the choroid, sclera, and/or optic nerve (coloboma/staphyloma) to complete retinal detachment (with or without hemorrhage) that may be blinding. Mildly affected animals will have no detectable vision impairment. It is important to screen for this condition in puppies, as the development of pigmentation and the tapetum can sometimes mask milder versions of the condition (the "go normal" phenomenon), limiting clinical detection in adulthood. A mutation in the gene *NHEJ1* is known to be associated with choroidal hypoplasia; however, the genes responsible for colobomas are unknown.[46] A clinical or genetic diagnosis of collie eye anomaly results in a "no" breeding recommendation.
- Optic nerve hypoplasia is a maldevelopment of the optic nerve that results in visual impairment. It is characterized by a very small optic nerve head and blindness or severely impaired vision and can occur unilaterally or bilaterally. Although inheritance is likely autosomal recessive, there may be incomplete penetrance, and the genetics of this condition have not been defined. Commonly affected breeds include the miniature poodle, Belgian tervuren, and shih tzu.[1] Micropapilla is a related condition where a small optic nerve head is observed clinically but without vision impairment. A diagnosis of optic nerve hypoplasia results in a "no" breeding recommendation, whereas a diagnosis of micropapilla results in a breeder option recommendation.

Adult-Onset Retina/Choroid/Optic Nerve Conditions

- Multifocal retinopathy is characterized by numerous distinct (ie, multifocal), roughly circular patches of elevated retina with accumulation of material that produces gray-tan-pink colored lesions (multifocal bullous retinal detachments). These lesions, looking somewhat like blisters, vary in location and size, although typically they are present in both eyes of the affected dog. Infrequently or chronically, this disorder can impair vision. There are several forms of canine multifocal retinopathy from known mutations in the *BEST1* gene with commercially available genetic tests. Breeding recommendations vary from "breeder option" to "no" based on breed, and commonly affected breeds include the bullmastiff (English) mastiff, American bulldog, great Pyrenees, coton de Tulear, Finnish Lapphund, Lapponian herder, and Australian shepherd.[1,47–53] The miniature American shepherd/miniature Australian shepherd, toy Australian shepherd, boerboel, Brazilian terrier, bulldog, cane corso, dogue de Bordeaux, perro de presa canario, and other breeds may also be affected.[48,52,53]
- PRA is a group of hereditary diseases that cause bilaterally symmetric, progressive degeneration of the retinal photoreceptors. More commonly, rod photoreceptors are affected by gene mutations, although cone disorders are described. Cone dysfunction and/or degeneration can also be a consequence of rod dysfunction and or degeneration. Dogs will typically present with night vision changes before onset of vision changes in daylight or bright light. Age of onset and rate of progression are highly variable, underpinning the necessity to perform CAER examinations yearly. On the CAER form, PRA is denoted as "retinal atrophy–generalized." The most well-known genetic mutation associated with PRA is the autosomal recessively inherited *prcd* mutation, though over 20 different mutations have been discovered to cause this disease in a variety of breeds and many more are yet to be discovered.[34,53,54] A clinical diagnosis of PRA results in a "no" breeding recommendation. Because not all PRA causative genes are known, genetic testing may be used to complement but not circumvent a clinical diagnosis. The English cocker spaniel provides an example of decreased incidence of PRA in dogs presented for CAER examinations: 2.6% of 116 dogs examined in 2013 versus 0.7% of 268 dogs in 2022 (J Pautz, personal communication of breed data report, January 2023).

SUMMARY

The incidence of comfort- and vision-threatening inherited canine ophthalmic conditions can be reduced with the use of screening examinations and certifications with associated breeding recommendations provided by collaboration between the ACVO and OFA in the form of CAER examinations. The document *Ocular Disorders Presumed to be Inherited in Purebred Dogs* (known as "*The Blue Book*") is the primary reference for these recommendations and can be viewed online.

DISCLOSURE

The authors have no commercial or financial conflicts of interest to disclose. Drs KA Diehl and S Kuhn have no funding sources to disclose. Dr F Mowat acknowledges salary funding from an NIH, United States K08 award: K08EY028628.

ACKNOWLEDGMENTS

The authors would like to acknowledge and thank Dr Gustavo Aguirre for assistance recounting historical information. They would also like to acknowledge and thank Ms Erika Werne—OFA CAER Program Manager, and Mr Jeff Pautz—OFA Chief Information Officer for assistance with CAER breed data acquisition and analysis.

REFERENCES

1. Genetics committee of the American College of Veterinary Ophthalmologists. Ocular disorders presumed to be inherited in purebred dogs. 13th ed. Columbia, MO: American College of Veterinary Ophthalmologists; 2021.
2. American College of Veterinary Ophthalmologists. American College of Veterinary Ophthalmologists: Operational and committee policies and procedures, 2021, p.35-38.
3. Koll S, Reese S, Medugorac I, et al. The effect of repeated eye examinations and breeding advice on the prevalence and incidence of cataracts and progressive retinal atrophy in German dachshunds over a 13-year period. Vet Ophthalmol 2017;20:114–22.
4. Peiffer RL Jr, Gelatt KN, Gwin RM. Chronic superficial keratitis. Vet Med Small Anim Clin 1977;72(1):35–7.
5. Jokinen P, Rusanen EM, Kennedy LJ, et al. MHC class II risk haplotype associated with canine chronic superficial keratitis in German Shepherd dogs. Vet Immunol Immunopathol 2011;140(1–2):37–41.
6. Chavkin MJ, Roberts SM, Salman MD, et al. Risk factors for development of chronic superficial keratitis in dogs. J Am Vet Med Assoc 1994;204(10):1630–4.
7. Crispin SM, Barnett KC. Dystrophy, degeneration and infiltration of the canine cornea. J Small Anim Pract 1983;24(2):63–83.
8. Cooley PL, Dice PF 2nd. Corneal dystrophy in the dog and cat. Vet Clin North Am Small Anim Pract 1990;20(3):681–92.
9. Waring GO 3rd. Inheritance of crystalline corneal dystrophy in Siberian Huskies. J Am Anim Hosp Assoc 1986;22:655.
10. MacMillan AD, Waring GO 3rd, Spangler WL, et al. Crystalline corneal opacities in the Siberian Husky. J Am Vet Med Assoc 1979;175:829–32.
11. Waring GO, Elkins MB, Spangler W. Oval lipid corneal opacities in beagles and crystalline lipid corneal opacities in Siberian Huskies. Metab Pediatr Ophthalmol 1979;3:203–13.
12. Tetas Pont R, Downs L, Pettitt L, et al. A Carbohydrate Sulfotransferase-6 (CHST6) gene mutation is associated with Macular Corneal Dystrophy in Labrador Retrievers. Vet Ophthalmol 2016;19(6):488–92.
13. Busse C, Kafarnik C, Linn-Pearl R, et al. Phenotype of macular corneal dystrophy in labrador retrievers: a multicenter study. Vet Ophthalmol 2019;22(3):294–304, published correction appears in Vet Ophthalmol. 2020 May;23(3):592.
14. Maini S, Everson R, Dawson C, et al. Pigmentary keratitis in pugs in the United Kingdom: prevalence and associated features. BMC Vet Res 2019;15(1):384.
15. Labelle AL, Dresser CB, Hamor RE, et al. Characteristics of, prevalence of, and risk factors for corneal pigmentation (pigmentary keratopathy) in Pugs. J Am Vet Med Assoc 2013;243(5):667–74.
16. Townsend WM, Gornik KR. Prevalence of uveal cysts and pigmentary uveitis in Golden Retrievers in three Midwestern states. J Am Vet Med Assoc 2013;243(9):1298–301.

17. Holly VL, Sandmeyer LS, Bauer BS, et al. Golden retriever cystic uveal disease: a longitudinal study of iridociliary cysts, pigmentary uveitis, and pigmentary/cystic glaucoma over a decade in western Canada. Vet Ophthalmol 2016; 19(3):237–44.

18. Spiess BM, Bolliger JO, Guscetti F, et al. Multiple ciliary body cysts and secondary glaucoma in the Great Dane: a report of nine cases. Vet Ophthalmol 1998; 1(1):41–5.

19. Pumphrey SA, Pizzirani S, Pirie CG, et al. Glaucoma associated with uveal cysts and goniodysgenesis in American Bulldogs: a case series. Vet Ophthalmol 2013; 16(5):377–85.

20. Townsend WM, Huey JA, McCool E, et al. Golden retriever pigmentary uveitis: challenges of diagnosis and treatment. Vet Ophthalmol 2020;23(5):774–84.

21. Sapienza JS, Simó FJ, Prades-Sapienza A. Golden Retriever uveitis: 75 cases (1994-1999). Vet Ophthalmol 2000;3(4):241–6.

22. Esson D, Armour M, Mundy P, et al. The histopathological and immunohistochemical characteristics of pigmentary and cystic glaucoma in the Golden Retriever. Vet Ophthalmol 2009;12(6):361–8.

23. Barnett KC, Knight GC. Persistent pupillary membrane and associated defects in the Basenji. Vet Rec 1969;85(9):242–8.

24. Roberts SR, Bistner SI. Persistent pupillary membrane in Basenji dogs. J Am Vet Med Assoc 1968;153(5):533–42.

25. Farias FH, Johnson GS, Taylor JF, et al. An ADAMTS17 splice donor site mutation in dogs with primary lens luxation. Invest Ophthalmol Vis Sci 2010;51(9):4716–21.

26. Gould D, Pettitt L, McLaughlin B, et al. ADAMTS17 mutation associated with primary lens luxation is widespread among breeds. Vet Ophthalmol 2011;14(6): 378–84.

27. Jeanes EC, Oliver JAC, Ricketts SL, et al. Glaucoma-causing*ADAMTS17* mutations are also reproducibly associated with height in two domestic dog breeds: selection for short stature may have contributed to increased prevalence of glaucoma. Canine Genet Epidemiol 2019;6:5.

28. Oliver JAC, Rustidge S, Pettitt L, et al. Evaluation of ADAMTS17 in Chinese Shar-Pei with primary open-angle glaucoma, primary lens luxation, or both. Am J Vet Res 2018;79(1):98–106.

29. Oliver JA, Forman OP, Pettitt L, et al. Two independent mutations in ADAMTS17 are associated with primary open angle glaucoma in the basset hound and basset fauve de bretagne breeds of dog. PLoS One 2015;10(10):e0140436, published correction appears in PLoS One. 2016;11(5):e0156192.

30. Forman OP, Pettitt L, Komáromy AM, et al. a novel genome-wide association study approach using genotyping by exome sequencing leads to the identification of a primary open angle glaucoma associated inversion disrupting ADAMTS17. PLoS One 2015;10(12):e0143546.

31. Mellersh CS, McLaughlin B, Ahonen S, et al. Mutation in HSF4 is associated with hereditary cataract in the Australian Shepherd. Vet Ophthalmol 2009;12(6): 372–8.

32. Mellersh CS, Graves KT, McLaughlin B, et al. Mutation in HSF4 associated with early but not late-onset hereditary cataract in the Boston Terrier. J Hered 2007; 98(5):531–3.

33. Mellersh CS, Pettitt L, Forman OP, et al. Identification of mutations in HSF4 in dogs of three different breeds with hereditary cataracts. Vet Ophthalmol 2006; 9(5):369–78.

34. Donner J, Anderson H, Davison S, et al. Frequency and distribution of 152 genetic disease variants in over 100,000 mixed breed and purebred dogs. PLoS Genet 2018;14(4):e1007361, published correction appears in PLoS Genet. 2019 Jan 18;15(1):e1007938.

35. Kraijer-Huver IM, Gubbels EJ, Scholten J, et al. Characterization and prevalence of cataracts in labrador retrievers in The Netherlands. Am J Vet Res 2008;69(10): 1336–40.

36. Krishnan H, Diehl K, Stefanovski D, et al. Vitreous degeneration and associated ocular abnormalities in the dog. Vet Ophthalmol 2020;23(2):219–24.

37. van der Linde-Sipman JS, Stades FC, Wolff-Rouen-daal D. Persistent hyperplastic tunica vasculosa lentis and persistent hyperplastic primary vitreous in the Doberman Pinscher: Pathologic aspects. J Am Anim Hosp Assoc 1983; 19:791.

38. Stades FC. Persistent hyperplastic tunica vasculosa lentis and persistent hyperplastic primary vitreous (PHTVL/PHPV) in ninety closely related Pinchers. J Am Anim Hosp Assoc 1980;16:739.

39. Stades FC. Persistent hyperplastic tunica vasculosa lentis and persistent hyperplastic primary vitreous in Doberman Pinschers: genetic aspects. J Am Anim Hosp Assoc 1983;19:957.

40. Stades FC, Boeve MH, van den Brom WE, et al. The incidence of PHTVL/PHPV in Dobermans and the results of breeding rules. Vet Q 1991;13:24.

41. Anderson DE. The incidence of PHTVL/PHPV in Dobermans and the results of breeding. J Hered 1991;82:21.

42. Boeve MH, Stades FC. Persistent hyperplastic tunica vasculosa lentis and primary vitreous (PHTVL/PHPV) in the dog: A comparative review. Prog Vet Comp Ophthalmol 1992;2:163.

43. Curtis R, Barnett KC, Leon A. Persistent hyperplastic primary vitreous in the Staffordshire Bull Terrier. Vet Rec 1984;115:385.

44. Leon A, Curtis R, Barnett K. Hereditary persistent hyperplastic primary vitreous in the Staffordshire Bull Terrier. J Am Anim Hosp Assoc 1986;22:765–74.

45. Goldstein O, Guyon R, Kukekova A, et al. COL9A2 and COL9A3 mutations in canine autosomal recessive oculoskeletal dysplasia. Mamm Genome 2010; 21(7–8):398–408.

46. Parker HG, Kukekova AV, Akey DT, et al. Breed relationships facilitate fine-mapping studies: a 7.8-kb deletion cosegregates with Collie eye anomaly across multiple dog breeds. Genome Res 2007;17(11):1562–71.

47. Guziewicz KE, Zangerl B, Lindauer SJ, et al. Bestrophin gene mutations cause canine multifocal retinopathy: a novel animal model for best disease. Invest Ophthalmol Vis Sci 2007;48(5):1959–67.

48. Zangerl B, Wickström K, Slavik J, et al. Assessment of canine BEST1 variations identifies new mutations and establishes an independent bestrophinopathy model (cmr3). Mol Vis 2010;16:2791–804.

49. Grahn BH, Philibert H, Cullen CL, et al. Multifocal retinopathy of Great Pyrenees dogs. Vet Ophthalmol 1998;1(4):211–21.

50. Grahn BH, Cullen CL. Retinopathy of Great Pyrenees dogs: fluorescein angiography, light microscopy and transmitting and scanning electron microscopy. Vet Ophthalmol 2001;4(3):191–9.

51. Grahn BH, Sandmeyer LL, Breaux C. Retinopathy of Coton de Tulear dogs: clinical manifestations, electroretinographic, ultrasonographic, fluorescein and indocyanine green angiographic, and optical coherence tomographic findings. Vet Ophthalmol 2008;11(4):242–9.

52. Hoffmann I, Guziewicz KE, Zangerl B, et al. Canine multifocal retinopathy in the Australian Shepherd: a case report. Vet Ophthalmol 2012;15(Suppl 2): 134–8, 0 2.
53. Donner J, Kaukonen M, Anderson H, et al. Genetic panel screening of nearly 100 mutations reveals new insights into the breed distribution of risk variants for canine hereditary disorders. PLoS One 2016;11(8):e0161005.
54. Online Mendelian Inheritance in Animals, OMIA. Sydney School of Veterinary Science. Available at: https://omia.org/. Accessed January 27, 2023.

Cardiac Disease and Screening in Breeding Dogs

Michael Aherne, MVB (Hons 1), GradDipVetStud, MS, MANZCVS (Small Animal Surgery), DACVIM (Cardiology)

KEYWORDS

- Dog • Breed screening • Cardiac disease • Congenital heart disease
- Acquired heart disease • Echocardiography • Heart murmur

KEY POINTS

- The overall prevalence of cardiac disease in dogs is relatively high and is estimated to be approximately 11% of the total canine population; the lifetime incidence of certain age-associated cardiac diseases approaches 100%.
- Many of the common cardiac diseases exhibit complex modes of inheritance, which may also differ between breeds for the same condition. Many cardiac diseases also display variable penetrance and so disease severity in offspring may not be reliably predicted by the disease severity in parents for certain conditions.
- Breed screening programs that aim to reduce the prevalence of specific cardiac diseases in certain breeds are largely based on early identification of disease phenotypes in order to prevent dogs from entering, or to remove dogs from, the breeding pool.
- Data on outcomes of breeding screening programs are limited but overall, they seem to have a positive effect on either reducing the prevalence, or increasing the age of onset, for several cardiac diseases in certain breeds of dogs.

INTRODUCTION/HISTORY/DEFINITIONS/BACKGROUND

In the late 1800s, as breeding and showing dogs became popular, Kennel Clubs were founded in the United Kingdom (UK) and in the United States of America (USA) to govern dog showing and breeding, register dogs, and establish the first stud books.[1] Selective breeding of dogs has resulted in wide phenotypic variation within the species. However, a consequence of selective breeding is loss of genetic variation as well as entrapment of certain disease alleles within specific breeds and lineages.[1,2] Canine health and well-being are considered very important for the image of dog breeding, and pet owners consider health-related matters to be essential in selection of a puppy's breeder and litter.[3] At least 396 health conditions with known or suspected genetic causes have been identified in pedigree dogs.[1]

Department of Small Animal Clinical Sciences, University of Florida College of Veterinary Medicine, 2015 Southwest 16th Avenue, Gainesville, FL 32610, USA
E-mail address: maherne@ufl.edu

Vet Clin Small Anim 53 (2023) 985–1012
https://doi.org/10.1016/j.cvsm.2023.05.001
vetsmall.theclinics.com
0195-5616/23/© 2023 Elsevier Inc. All rights reserved.

The overall estimated prevalence of heart disease in dogs is approximately 11% and may perhaps be even higher depending on various factors such as geographic location and endemic disease burden (eg, heartworm disease).[4,5] Most of this is attributable to acquired cardiac disease, whereas canine congenital cardiac disease has an estimated overall prevalence of 0.13% to 1.62%.[6–11]

Many cardiac diseases demonstrate significant breed associations with modes of inheritance and, in some cases specific genetic causes, established for certain conditions. Breed screening programs have been used in some canine breeds in an effort to remove undesirable traits associated with disease development from the breeding pool and reduce disease prevalence within specific breeds. This review provides a discussion of most common congenital and acquired cardiac diseases in dogs and the breed screening programs that have been used to reduce the prevalence of some of these conditions in certain breeds.

Congenital Cardiac Diseases

Among the most commonly reported congenital cardiac conditions in dogs are pulmonic stenosis (PS), subvalvular aortic stenosis (SAS), patent ductus arteriosus (PDA), ventricular septal defect (VSD), atrial septal defect (ASD), mitral valve dysplasia (MVD), and tricuspid valve dysplasia (TVD),[5,9,11–15] although various other congenital cardiac malformations can also be encountered. Geographical differences may also influence the relative proportions and prevalence of any of these conditions. For example, PDA is reported with a higher frequency in referral centers in North America and Australia when compared with those in Europe.[9]

Pulmonic stenosis

Pulmonic stenosis is a congenital malformation characterized by obstruction to right ventricular outflow as a result of pulmonic valve leaflet thickening or fusion or the presence of a discrete narrowing along the pulmonic outflow tract. It can manifest as subvalvular, valvular, and supravalvular forms depending on the exact location of the lesion. Valvular PS, however, is the most commonly encountered form in dogs.[16,17] Commonly affected breeds include Boxers, English Bulldogs, French Bulldogs, German Shepherd Dogs, Beagles, West Highland White Terriers, American Staffordshire Terriers, Pitbull Terriers, Cocker Spaniels, Miniature Schnauzers, Whippets, and mixed-breed dogs.[9,11,14–16,18] The estimated prevalence of PS in a referral hospital setting is reported to be approximately 0.37% to 0.41% of all hospital admissions[11,18] and 6.1% of all cardiology service admissions.[18] Pulmonic stenosis accounts for approximately 20.4% to 34.1% of congenital heart disease cases diagnosed in dogs.[9–12,14,15]

Two morphologies of valvular PS have been described. Type A morphology is characterized by fusion and systolic doming of the pulmonic valve leaflets. Type B morphology is characterized by hypomotile and thickened valve leaflets with pulmonary annular hypoplasia. Intermediate PS is used to describe morphologies between type A and type B.[17,19] Evaluation for the presence of PS includes 2-dimensional echocardiographic assessment of the pulmonic valve and right ventricular outflow tract for the presence of structural lesions on 2-dimensional imaging in conjunction with Doppler echocardiographic assessment of right ventricular/pulmonic outflow tract velocities.[19]

Conclusive evidence regarding the inheritance of PS in commonly affected breeds is limited; however, a pedigree analysis in a family of English Bulldogs suggests an autosomal recessive mode of inheritance in this breed. No genetic variants associated with the development of PS have been reported in dogs to date.[18]

Dogs with PS typically have a crescendo-decrescendo (ejection) murmur with point of maximal intensity at the left cardiac base, which may also radiate to the right cardiac base.[16] The severity of PS is determined from Doppler echocardiographic measurement of pulmonic outflow tract velocities and is classified based on the calculated peak pressure gradient across the obstruction as either mild ($\leq$49 mm Hg), moderate (50–80 mm Hg), or severe (>80 mm Hg).[19] Depending on the severity of PS, a variable degree of right ventricular concentric hypertrophy may also be appreciated on echocardiography. Systolic flattening, and occasionally paradoxical motion of the interventricular septum, may also be noted in dogs with more severe forms of PS; however, these findings are not specific to this condition and may also be observed with other causes of right ventricular pressure overload such as pulmonary hypertension. Poststenotic dilation of the main pulmonary artery is also frequently observed and results from turbulence associated with the increased blood velocities required to cross the stenotic valve.[16] Clinical signs associated with PS include weakness, lethargy, exercise intolerance, collapse, syncope, abdominal distension, abnormal jugular venous distension/pulsation, and other signs associated with right-sided congestive heart failure.

Mild-to-moderate forms of PS are generally associated with favorable long-term prognoses. Dogs with severe PS have an increased risk for death from the condition[17,20] unless treated, with an up to 25-fold increase in risk reported for dogs in this category.[20] The presence of clinical signs, younger age at diagnosis,[17] and concurrent tricuspid regurgitation[20] have also been shown to be associated with poorer outcomes in dogs with PS. Transcatheter balloon valvuloplasty is widely considered the treatment of choice for this condition and has been shown to alleviate clinical signs and prolong survival in dogs with severe PS.[17,21,22]

Subvalvular and valvular aortic stenosis

Subvalvular aortic stenosis is a congenital cardiac disease characterized by left ventricular outflow tract obstruction as a consequence of the presence of nodules, a ridge, or a ring of fibrous tissue below the aortic valve.[23–25] Supravalvular, valvular, and dynamic subvalvular forms of aortic stenosis have also been documented in dogs; however, discrete fibromuscular SAS is the most common form in this species.[24] Breeds predisposed to SAS include Boxers, Newfoundlands, Golden Retrievers, German Shepherd Dogs, Rottweilers, Dogues de Bordeaux, Bull Terriers, and Bullmastiffs.[9,14,15,23–25] Although a congenital condition, the progressive nature of the disease means that phenotypic manifestations of the condition may not become evident until the dog has reached skeletal maturity; the full severity of the condition cannot be truly appreciated until an individual has reached this point.[23,25] Because of changes in severity over time as the dog matures, it is recommended that dogs are at least 12 months of age before being evaluated for the presence of SAS and perhaps even older in some giant breeds to ensure full skeletal maturity has been reached.

Echocardiographic evaluation of SAS includes assessment of the left ventricular outflow tract for the presence of structural subvalvular lesions on 2-dimensional imaging and, especially in the absence of discrete structural lesions, assessment of left ventricular/aortic outflow tract velocities.[19,26] In order to reduce false-negative results, it is recommended to perform aortic outflow tract velocity measurements by continuous-wave Doppler from a subcostal position because variation in placement and alignment of the Doppler echocardiographic transducer can affect this measurement.[19,27] However, there is no firm consensus on a single agreed-upon cut-off value of aortic outflow tract velocities for the diagnosis of SAS, and this results in an equivocal range.[25] In the author's clinical practice, and in the absence of structural lesions on 2-dimensional echocardiography, dogs with aortic outflow tract velocities less than or equal to 1.9 m/s are considered normal, whereas dogs with aortic outflow tract velocities greater than 2.4 m/s are considered affected with SAS; dogs with aortic outflow tract velocities between these 2 values are met with diagnostic uncertainty. The effect of emotional stress on peak aortic velocities has been demonstrated[28] and may contribute to aortic velocity measurements in the equivocal range although this is considered unlikely to cause a truly unaffected dog to reach the threshold to be considered truly affected.[25]

Subvalvular aortic stenosis is most commonly seen in large and medium breed dogs and is only rarely identified in small or toy breeds.[15,25] The estimated prevalence of this condition in referral hospital settings is reported to be approximately 0.3% to 0.4% of all hospital admissions[11,18] and 4.7% of all cardiology service admissions.[18] Among dogs diagnosed with congenital cardiac disease, SAS is reported to account for 14.6% to 35.2% of congenital cases.[9,10,12,14,15]

The mode of inheritance for canine SAS is complex and variable. Several studies on the mode of SAS inheritance have been performed. In Newfoundlands, the findings of such studies suggest either an autosomal-dominant or a polygenic inheritance.[18,23,29] An autosomal-recessive inheritance has been reported for Golden Retrievers, Rottweilers, and Bullmastiffs,[18] as well as being suspected in Dogues de Bordeaux.[30] Based on the modes of inheritance reported, and in the absence of a genetic test, reducing the prevalence of SAS in affected dog breeds may be challenging especially in dog breeds with recessive modes of inheritance.[25] A single codon insertion in the *PICALM* gene was identified in a family of North American Newfoundlands with SAS.[31] This gene has been the only genetic variant associated with SAS in dogs reported to date, and it has not been determined if this is causative or simply an association.[25] A replication study in a cohort of European Newfoundlands affected with SAS failed to find an association between the *PICALM* gene variant and SAS in that cohort; however, phenotypic criteria differed between both studies, which may account for differences in results.[25,31,32] Based on genome-wide association studies in Golden Retrievers, Newfoundlands, and Rottweilers, a locus in chromosome 13 has been implicated as a candidate region for distinct or shared genetic variants that may be associated with SAS in dogs; however, further investigation with targeted or whole-genome sequencing methods is required.[25]

Dogs with aortic stenosis typically have a crescendo-decrescendo (ejection) murmur with point of maximal intensity at the left cardiac base, which, in severe cases, may radiate distally up the carotid arteries. Using Doppler echocardiographic measurements of aortic outflow tract velocities, SAS severity is classified based on the calculated peak pressure gradient across the obstruction as either mild ($\leq$49 mm Hg), moderate (50–80 mm Hg), or severe (>80 mm Hg).[19] Dogs with severe SAS typically have reduced life expectancy and are 16 times more likely to die suddenly than dogs with mild or moderate SAS.[24] Sudden death typically occurs within the first 2 to 3 years from diagnosis. Sudden death is believed to be associated with arrhythmias arising from myocardial ischemia as a consequence of ventricular outflow tract obstruction and subsequent concentric hypertrophy. Dogs with mild or moderate SAS typically have a normal life expectancy although dogs in the moderate category may experience variable clinical signs.[24] Clinical signs associated with SAS include weakness, lethargy, exercise intolerance, collapse, syncope, dyspnea/tachypnea, and other signs associated with left-sided congestive heart failure. Dogs with SAS of any severity are also at risk for the development of infective endocarditis.[24]

Patent ductus arteriosus

The ductus arteriosus is a normal fetal vascular communication between the main pulmonary artery and the aorta, allowing blood to bypass the nonfunctioning lungs during fetal development. It normally closes within hours following birth as a response to increased oxygen tension.[33] Failed closure of this vascular canal results in patent ductus arteriosus. In most of the patients with PDA, this results in left-to-right shunting of blood from the aorta into the pulmonary artery due to the normal pressure gradient that exists between these vessels after birth. The degree of shunting is determined by the size of the ductal orifice, and most often this will result in a volume overload being imposed on the lungs and the left heart, which results in increased pulmonary vascularity, and enlargement of the left atrium and left ventricle.[33] If the degree of shunting is sufficient, then left-sided, or occasionally generalized, congestive heart failure (CHF) may develop as early as 1 week of age up to several years old depending on ductal size.[33]

In a smaller proportion of dogs with PDA, pulmonary vascular disease may develop within the initial month of life and is akin to persistent fetal circulation.[33] This disease results in pulmonary hypertension of a sufficient degree to cause bidirectional or right-to-left flow through the PDA, which is then termed a reverse PDA. A reverse PDA results in shunting of deoxygenated blood from the pulmonary artery into the aorta, causing tissue hypoxia of the caudal portion of the body and may also result in right-sided CHF due to the effects of pulmonary hypertension on the right side of the heart.

The prevalence of PDA in dogs with congenital heart disease is reported to be between 8.5% and 31.9%.[9,11,12,14,15] Predisposed breeds for this condition include Poodles, Dachshunds, Maltese Terriers, German Shepherd Dogs, Doberman Pinschers, and mixed-breed dogs.[9,11,14,15] A female sex predilection has also been identified for this congenital malformation.[8,14,34] Patent ductus arteriosus is a highly heritable condition[35]; however, a precise genetic cause has not yet been identified.

Dogs with left-to-right shunting PDAs typically have a very characteristic continuous heart murmur that is most prominent in the left axillary region cranial to the heart base and may often be accompanied by a palpable continuous thrill. In dogs with equalizing diastolic pressures (eg, pulmonary hypertension) the murmur may be abbreviated to transsystolic, or even systolic, versus continuous.[33] Dogs with reverse PDAs typically do not have a murmur, which can make them more diagnostically challenging to identify, although occasionally a soft diastolic murmur caused by pulmonic insufficiency or a split second heart sound may be noted in these dogs. Clinical signs associated with PDA typically reflect the onset of left-sided congestive heart failure and include dyspnea, tachypnea, cough, weakness, lethargy, exercise intolerance, and collapse. In dogs with right-to-left shunting due to significant pulmonary vascular changes, clinical signs attributable to systemic tissue hypoxia or right-sided congestive heart failure may be noted.

Ventricular septal defect

Failure of partitioning between the left and right ventricles during embryologic development results in a congenital malformation known as a VSD. In the absence of other concurrent conditions, VSDs typically result in left-to-right shunting of blood across the defect. The size of the VSD and the pulmonary vascular resistance determine the magnitude of shunting and thus the hemodynamic consequences that result.[8,36] Various methods for describing and categorizing VSD lesions exist and may be based on either the location of the defect within the septum, the structures bordering the defect, or a combination of both.[37] Supracristal VSDs (also known as conoseptal, subarterial, or infundibular VSDs) are found below the right and noncoronary aortic valve cusps in the outlet region of the interventricular septum. Membranous VSDs are located within the membranous portion of the interventricular septum just below the aortic valve cusps; however, if the defect extends to the dorsal part of the muscular portion of the septum, these defects are described as paramembranous, perimembranous, or conoventricular. Muscular VSDs are located entirely within the muscular interventricular septum and may involve the inlet, outlet, or trabecular parts of the septum. Finally, atrioventricular canal type VSDs include the inlet of the right interventricular septum immediately beneath the atrioventricular valve apparatus.[36] Paramembraneous VSDs are the most common VSD type encountered in dogs.[8,36]

Ventricular septal defects account for approximately 4.8% to 14% of congenital heart defects in dogs.[9–12,14,15] These defects are frequently seen concurrently with other congenital defects, with almost half of dogs diagnosed with VSD having at least one other congenital malformation, with the most common concomitant abnormality being PS, either alone or as part of a complex congenital heart disease known as tetralogy of Fallot.[14,36] Among the most commonly reported breeds diagnosed with VSDs are French Bulldogs, Maltese Terriers, Pinschers, Fox Terriers, Jack Russell Terriers, English Bulldogs, German Shepherd Dogs, Labrador Retrievers, Keeshonds, as well as mixed-breed dogs.[9,11,14,36,38] Precise genetic causes for VSDs have not, as of yet, been identified; however, various modes of inheritance have been suggested in several different breeds. An autosomal recessive mode of inheritance has been suggested for VSDs resulting from conotruncal malformations in a family of beagles.[39] Meanwhile, the mode of inheritance has been suggested to be autosomal dominant with incomplete penetrance or polygenic in a family of English springer spaniels.[40] Studies of VSDs in Keeshonds with conotruncal defects initially suggested polygenic inheritance,[41] which was later believed to a single-gene autosomal recessive trait,[42] but most recently the trait seems to be oligogenic.[43]

Dogs with small VSDs are generally asymptomatic; however, those with large defects or concomitant pathology may have variable clinical signs. Left-to-right shunting paramembranous defects classically have a right-sided systolic murmur. Occasionally, a systolic ejection murmur associated with relative PS may also be appreciated at the left heart base, and less frequently a split second heart sound may also be noted.[8] Prognosis for patients with isolated VSDs is generally good with approximately 75% of animals remaining subclinical for the condition at 9.6 years of age[36]; however, individual survival times very much depend on the size of defect and the resulting degree of shunting. Rarely, spontaneous closure of small VSDs may occur in dogs.[44,45] Various open surgical and transcatheter methods of VSD closure have been successfully performed in this species.[36,46–49]

Atrial septal defect

An ASD is a communication between both atria as a result of failed partitioning of the interatrial septum during embryologic development. Atrial septal defects are classified based on their location within the interatrial septum with 3 types of ASD described.[50] Ostium primum ASDs are typically large defects that are located in the lower apical portion of the atrial septum and result from incomplete closure between the septum primum and the endocardial cushions.[50,51] Ostium secundum type defects are located within the fossa ovalis and are the most common ASD type encountered in dogs.[51,52] Ostium secundum ASDs can also be further subclassified as types Ia through Id and type II, depending on their exact morphologic characteristics.[53] Sinus venosus type ASDs are located high in the dorsal atrial septum near the junction with the cranial vena cava[51,54] and are rare in dogs.[8] Two additional abnormal congenital interatrial communications may occur but are not true ASDs, although they may be improperly classified as such, because the structures of the interatrial septum have formed normally in these situations. An unroofed coronary sinus results when there is failed formation of the wall between the left atrium and the coronary sinus.[51,55] In the case of patent foramen ovale, the interatrial septal structures form normally, but do not seal, which can allow the foramen ovale to be pushed or stretched open.[8]

The prevalence of atrial septal defects is reported to be between 0.7% and 3.7% of dogs with congenital cardiac defects.[8–10,12,14,15] Similar to VSDs, ASDs may also frequently occur in conjunction with other congenital defects. Between 33% and 60% of dogs with ASD are reported to have at least one additional concomitant abnormality.[9,14,15] The most commonly reported breeds affected with ASD include Boxers, Cavalier King Charles Spaniels (CKCS), German Shepherd Dogs, Labrador Retrievers, Doberman Pinschers, and Samoyeds.[8,50] A precise genetic cause for canine ASDs has not been identified.[8]

The direction and degree of shunting through an ASD depends on the size of the defect and the relative resistances in the systemic and pulmonary circulations.[8] Blood typically shunts left-to-right; however, in the setting of conditions that increase right atrial or right ventricular pressures such as PS, TVD, or pulmonary hypertension, right-to-left shunting through the defect may occur.[8] Right-to-left shunting is reported to occur in approximately 8% of cases.[50] A soft systolic left basilar heart murmur associated with relative PS is the most common clinical sign noted in dogs with isolated ASDs.[8,50] Rarely, a soft diastolic murmur associated with relative tricuspid stenosis may be noted.[8] Small defects are generally asymptomatic. Associated clinical signs may include dyspnea, tachypnea, exercise intolerance, weakness, cyanosis, and syncope, and these signs are typically only identified in adult animals.[50] The prognosis for secundum type ASDs is generally good, and the condition is usually well compensated.[8,50] Prognosis for primum ASDs is usually more guarded, and these have a higher likelihood to result in congestive heart failure (right-sided or biventricular) or pulmonary hypertension.[8] Similar to VSDs, various open surgical and transcatheter methods of ASD closure have been described in dogs.[53,54,56,57]

Mitral valve dysplasia

Congenital malformation of the mitral valve apparatus and its associated structures is known as MVD; this can result in a variable degree of mitral regurgitation and less commonly stenosis of the mitral valve. Valve abnormalities noted with MVD may include thickened valve leaflets, particularly at the leaflet tips; diastolic doming of the leaflet tips resulting in a "hockey stick" appearance; abnormally long or short valve leaflets, occasionally with a cleft; abnormally thick, short, or long chordae tendineae; tethered valve leaflets; direct insertion of papillary muscles into valve leaflets; and papillary muscle malformations.[8,58,59] Stenosis of the mitral valve may also been seen in dogs with MVD.[60] Rarely, MVD may also result in obstruction of the left ventricular outflow tract.[61]

Among dogs with congenital cardiac malformations, the prevalence of canine MVD is reported to be between 1.6% and 8.5%.[9,11,12,14,15] Breed predispositions for MVD exist for English Bull Terriers, Great Danes, German Shepherd Dogs, and Dalmatians.[8,58–60,62,63] Of dogs with mitral stenosis as part of their mitral valve complex, English Bull Terriers and Newfoundland are also overrepresented.[59,60] A genetic basis for MVD in dogs has not been identified.

The degree of mitral regurgitation or stenosis present determines the degree of left-sided volume loading and the presence and severity of clinical signs. Left-sided congestive heart failure can result in dogs with severe MVD. Typically, dogs with

MVD have a systolic left apical murmur of variable intensity and consistent with mitral regurgitation.[8,59] Rarely, a soft diastolic murmur may be noted in cases with mitral stenosis. Other clinical signs that may be noted in dogs with MVD may also include dyspnea, tachypnea, weakness, lethargy, exercise intolerance, and syncope. Arrhythmias including atrial fibrillation and, less frequently, ventricular premature complexes may also be noted and are typically a consequence of left-sided cardiomegaly.[8,59]

Tricuspid valve dysplasia

Tricuspid valve dysplasia is used to collectively describe several various congenital abnormalities of the tricuspid valve that can result in tricuspid regurgitation or rarely stenosis.[64,65] Associated malformations of the tricuspid valve that may be noted in cases of TVD include focal or diffuse valve leaflet thickening, underdevelopment or undifferentiation of chordae tendineae and papillary muscles, incomplete separation of valve components from the ventricular wall, focal agenesis of valvular tissue, and "Ebstein's anomaly", which is an apical displacement of the basal attachment of the tricuspid leaflets with resultant atrialization of the right ventricle.[8,64–68]

The prevalence of TVD in canine populations is reported to be between 2% and 7.9% of dogs with congenital heart disease.[9–12,14,15] Labrador Retrievers seem to be particularly predisposed to this condition with high heritability in this breed.[69] Other overrepresented breeds include Golden Retrievers, Dogues de Bordeaux, Boxers, German Shepherd Dogs, English Bulldogs, and Border Collies.[9,14,15,65,66,68,70] In Labrador Retrievers, the condition is autosomal dominant with incomplete penetrance and maps to chromosome 9.[71] An autosomal recessive mode of inheritance is proposed for Dogues de Bordeaux.[30]

Patients with TVD usually have a right-sided systolic murmur associated with tricuspid regurgitation. Rarely, in cases with tricuspid stenosis, a soft diastolic murmur may be appreciated. Murmur intensity is not correlated with the severity of TVD.[8,65,66] The presence and severity of clinical signs largely depend on the degree of tricuspid regurgitation or stenosis present. In severely affected dogs, right-sided congestive heart failure can occur. In addition to right apical murmurs, clinical signs associated with the presence of TVD may also include jugular venous distension and pulsation, weakness, lethargy, exercise intolerance, weight loss, syncope, peripheral edema, and ascites.[8,65–68] Splintering of the QRS complex on electrocardiography is reported in up to 60% of dogs with TVD.[72] Cardiac arrhythmias are reported in 16% to 22% of dogs with TVD and may include atrial fibrillation, supraventricular tachycardia, and ventricular premature complexes.[8,65,68,73] Interestingly, there is a high prevalence of accessory pathway–mediated supraventricular tachycardias in Labrador Retrievers and Boxers, both breeds predisposed to TVD, and a similar prevalence is also described in humans with Ebstein's anomaly.[73–76]

Acquired Cardiac Diseases

Myxomatous mitral valve disease

Myxomatous mitral valve disease (MMVD) is the most common cardiac disease affecting dogs. It has an estimated prevalence of about 10% in the overall canine population presenting to primary care veterinary practices.[77] Globally, it is the most common heart disease in dogs and is responsible for approximately 75% of heart disease in this species.[77,78] Synonyms for MMVD include chronic valvular disease, degenerative mitral valve disease, and endocardiosis.[79] Although the mitral valve is predominately affected, the tricuspid valve is also affected in at least 30% of dogs with the condition.[79] The disease is believed to result from dysregulation of valvular extracellular matrix remodeling via changes in transforming growth factor-beta and serotonin

signaling pathways.[77,80,81] Progressive degeneration of the atrioventricular valve apparatus eventually results in thickening of the valve leaflets, impaired leaflet coaptation,
and valvular regurgitation of varying magnitudes; this in turn imposes a volume overload
on the ipsilateral atrium and ventricle, which can result in enlargement of these chambers, increase cardiac work, and eventually lead to ventricular dysfunction.[77]

Disease prevalence for MMVD is variable depending on age. The prevalence of the
condition approaches 100% in older, small breed dogs, and the incidence of this disease over the course of a lifetime in most breeds is nearly 100%.[79] Small breed dogs
have a higher disease prevalence although larger breeds can also be affected with
MMVD. However, disease progression in larger breeds is usually faster with more
overt myocardial dysfunction than in smaller breeds.[77,82] Breeds predisposed to
developing MMVD include CKCS, King Charles Spaniels, Dachshunds, Poodles,
Cocker Spaniels, Miniature Schnauzers, Pomeranians, Chihuahuas, and Whippets.[79,83,84] Early onset of the disease is common in certain breeds including CKCS
and Dachshunds.[81] In a study of apparently healthy North American Whippets, echo-
cardiographically confirmed mitral regurgitation was identified in 21% of breeding age
(2–5 years) dogs.[85] Males also have a higher prevalence of the disease than
females.[79,83–85]

Myxomatous mitral valve disease exhibits a very high level of heritability.[81,86]
Despite this, the genetic etiopathogenesis of this disease is incompletely understood.
The evidence to date suggests a polygenic dominant mode of inheritance.[81,87] Two
loci have been identified as being associated with MMVD in CKCS[88]; however, the
precise genetic causes underlying the condition remain to be determined.[81]

The clinical effects of canine MMVD are variable depending on the degree of
valvular regurgitation and consequential volume overload imposed on the heart chambers ipsilateral to the affected valves. Because the mitral valve is most commonly
affected by this condition, left-sided cardiac changes are most common. Myxomatous
mitral valve disease is most often characterized by a left apical systolic murmur that is
constant in intensity.[83] The loudness of the murmur is variable depending on a variety
of factors including the degree of valvular insufficiency, the direction of the regurgitant
jet, and thoracic conformation. Right apical systolic murmurs may be appreciated in
dogs with significant tricuspid regurgitation as a result of valvular degeneration. The
American College of Veterinary Internal Medicine has developed a staging system
to classify the severity of morphologic changes and clinical signs caused by MMVD
in dogs.[77] In dogs with severe MMVD, congestive heart failure may develop. Clinical
signs in severely affected dogs include dyspnea, tachypnea, coughing, weakness,
lethargy, exercise intolerance, and syncope.[77–79,83] Echocardiography is recommended for definitive diagnosis of MMVD.[77,78] Thoracic radiography is recommended to
ascertain the hemodynamic effects of the valve disease, especially if left-sided
congestive heart failure is suspected.[77]

Dilated cardiomyopathy
Hereditary or primary idiopathic dilated cardiomyopathy (DCM) is an acquired cardiac
disease of dogs characterized by progressive systolic myocardial dysfunction leading
to dilation of the ventricles, particularly the left ventricle. Left-sided congestive heart
failure, and sudden cardiac death are the primary outcomes of this condition in
dogs.[89] It is the second most common heart disease in dogs.[89–91] Various infectious
and systemic diseases, toxicities, nutritional causes, and tachycardia-induced
myocardial injury can result in similar morphologic cardiac changes (ie, nonhereditary
or secondary DCM) and must be excluded before a diagnosis of primary idiopathic
DCM is made.[92]

Of these causes of secondary DCM, diet-associated DCM in particular has garnered some attention in recent years. The US Food and Drug Administration (FDA) issued an alert in 2018 about a potential link between nontraditional, boutique, exotic ingredient, and/or grain-free diets and DCM development in dogs not typically genetically prone to the disease.[93] To date, the FDA has received more than 1100 reports of apparently diet-associated DCM,[94] and approximately 90% of diets fed to DCM cases reported to the FDA were labeled "grain-free."[95] It is important to note that only an association has been identified, and no definitive causative factor has been proved as of yet. The grain-free nature of a diet might not be an issue per se but rather the foodstuffs used to replace grains in such diets might play a role in the development of diet-associated DCM. A large proportion of diets fed to dogs with diet-associated DCM contain one or more pulses (peas, lentils, chickpeas, beans) and to a lesser extent potatoes or sweet potatoes in higher proportions (ie, listed in the top 10 ingredients) than traditional diets.[95–99] Differences in biochemical compounds between DCM-associated and DCM-unassociated diets have been identified, with peas contributing to the largest difference between diet groups.[100] It has been hypothesized that, in many cases, diet-associated DCM is more likely the result of excessive levels of a nutrient or biochemical compound rather than deficiency, and several excessive compounds have been identified that could contribute to DCM development through various mechanisms.[99,100] Furthermore, certain genetic factors might also have a role in the development of diet-associated DCM in certain breeds. For example, associations between certain diets and taurine deficiency, a known nutritional cause of secondary dilated cardiomyopathy, has previously been identified in several dog breeds, including the Golden Retriever, Newfoundland, American Cocker Spaniel, English Setter, and Labrador Retriever,[96,101–104] and it is suggested that genetic differences might play a role in the susceptibility of certain breeds to developing taurine deficiency–associated DCM.[96] It is certainly possible that genetic factors might also influence the development of secondary DCM due to other causes. Further investigation to identify definitive causative factors in diet-associated DCM is ongoing. In the author's practice, it is recommended to feed diets selected based on the guidelines of the World Small Animal Veterinary Association's Global Nutrition Committee.[105]

Dogs with DCM are sometimes categorized by the clinical stage of the disease as either being in the "occult" or preclinical stage of the disease or the "overt" or clinical stage of the disease. Occult DCM describes dogs without current clinical signs attributable to heart disease that have morphologic or electrical cardiac changes evident on echocardiography and/or electrocardiography. Dogs with overt DCM are those dogs that have manifested clinical signs as a result of their heart disease. In some breeds, the presence of ventricular arrhythmias is associated with an increased risk for developing overt DCM.[106] A staging system for classification of DCM in dogs based on morphologic and clinical findings similar to the system developed for classification of MMVD has also been proposed.[92]

The overall prevalence of DCM in the general canine population is estimated to be between 0.5% and 1.1%.[107] Breed-specific disease (primary idiopathic DCM) is primarily responsible for the high incidence of this condition in dogs.[89] Breeds with an increased prevalence of this condition include Doberman Pinschers, Great Danes, Irish Wolfhounds, Boxers, Portuguese Water Dogs, Newfoundlands, Welsh Springer Spaniels, and Cocker Spaniels.[89,91,92,107–109] In Doberman Pinschers, DCM has an autosomal dominant mode of inheritance with both age-related and incomplete penetrance.[89] To date, 2 genetic mutations have been associated with DCM in Doberman Pinschers, named DCM1 and DCM2.[89,91]

The DCM1 mutation is a splice site mutation of the pyruvate dehydrogenase kinase 4 (PDK4) gene, which has been shown to interfere with cellular energetics.[110] Doberman Pinschers with the DCM mutation (homozygous and heterozygous) have been shown to be 10 times more likely to develop DCM compared with wild-type dogs.[89] The DCM2 mutation is a missense mutation in the titin (TTN) gene, which is associated with decreased active tension and Z disc streaming in the sarcomere; however, the precise mechanisms by which this mutation plays a role in the pathophysiology of DCM is incompletely understood.[111] Doberman Pinschers with only the DCM2 mutation (homozygous or heterozygous) have been shown to be 21 times more likely to develop DCM than wild-type individuals, and this increases to 30 times more likely if the DCM2 mutation is combined with a copy of the DCM1 mutation.[89] In a North American cohort of Doberman Pinschers, the DCM2 variant seems to be more common than the DCM1 variant.[112] Meanwhile, in European cohorts of Doberman Pinschers another genetic locus on chromosome 5 has been associated with the development of DCM although the precise genetic cause has yet to be identified.[113] Furthermore, an association between the DCM1 mutation and development of DCM was not identified in these European cohorts.[114] In addition, Doberman Pinschers without the DCM1 or DCM2 mutations may also be encountered, exhibiting a classic DCM phenotype. These findings speak to the likelihood of additional genetic heterogeneity having a role in the development of this condition.[89]

In Standard Schnauzers, a familial, early onset form of DCM with an autosomal recessive mode of inheritance has been identified.[115] Subsequent genetic analysis identified a variant in the gene encoding RNA-binding motif protein 20 (RBM20) that is highly associated with DCM and premature death in both Standard Schnauzers and Giant Schnauzers. Homozygosity of this genetic variant in Standard Schnauzers is associated with an approximately 80% reduction in lifespan and seems to have a worldwide distribution in this breed.[116]

A mutation in the phospholamban gene has recently been identified to be associated with an autosomal dominant familial DCM and sudden cardiac death in Welsh Springer Spaniels. The mutation is named R9H and seems to have a high penetrance in the cohort of dogs studied, with all mutation-positive dogs developing DCM.[117]

Boxer dogs with a deletion mutation in the striatin gene, particularly individuals homozygous for the genetic variant, have a high association with the development of DCM.[118] Striatin is a protein that contributes to the integrity of the desmosome in cardiac myocytes, and this mutation has also been associated with the development of arrhythmogenic right ventricular cardiomyopathy (ARVC) in this breed.[119] These findings suggest that DCM and ARVC in Boxers may have a common etiopathogenesis and may be different manifestations of the same disease.[118]

Additional loci have also been identified in association with the development of DCM in other breeds including Irish Wolfhounds[120,121] and Portuguese Water Dogs[122]; however, precise genetic causes have not been determined in these or other breeds. Data in Irish Wolfhounds suggest that the risk for DCM is influenced by multiple rather than individual genetic factors.[121]

Screening for canine DCM is typically recommended to start at 3 to 4 years of age.[92,109] Annual screening is recommended over the lifetime of an individual dog because the disease has a slow onset that may be age-related, and so one-time screening is not sufficient to rule out future development of DCM.[92,109] Genetic testing for DCM1 and DCM2 mutations in Doberman Pinschers is available through North Carolina State University. Because no mutations identified in association with DCM have been shown to have complete penetrance, and individuals without genetic mutations can also develop the disease, the results of genetic testing should not be used in place of standard screening with echocardiography and, in breeds with known associations between the presence of arrhythmias and DCM development, Holter monitor analysis. The results of genetic testing may help inform breeders on selection of dogs for breeding purposes.[92]

Holter monitor analysis is recommended to screen for ventricular arrhythmias in certain breeds, such as Boxers, Doberman Pinschers, and Great Danes.[92,109] In Doberman Pinschers, less than 50 single ventricular premature complexes (VPCs) in 24 hours are considered to be normal; however, detection of any number of VPCs may be a cause for concern.[106,109] Holter recordings demonstrating more than 300 VPCs in 24 hours, or 2 subsequent recordings within 12 months showing 50 to 300 VPCs in 24 hours, are considered diagnostic of occult DCM in Doberman Pinschers regardless of the concurrent echocardiographic findings.[109] In other breeds, a cut-off value of greater than 100 VPCs in 24 hours is suggested for diagnosis of DCM.[92]

Screening for the presence of DCM should also include thorough echocardiographic examination to evaluate systolic myocardial function and to determine the presence and severity of any secondary structural changes, that is, chamber dilation as a result of volume overload. Echocardiographic measurements should be compared with breed-specific reference intervals, where available. Left ventricular volumetric assessments are recommended to be performed using Simpson's method of discs.[92,109,123] Increased values for end-systolic left ventricular volume, end-systolic left ventricular diameter, and increased E-point septal separation indicate systolic myocardial dysfunction. Volume overload is indicated by increased values for end-diastolic left ventricular volume and end-diastolic left ventricular diameter. Reduced values for fractional shortening, ejection fraction, and sphericity index are also considered supportive for the diagnosis of DCM.[92,123]

Ancillary cardiac biomarkers testing such as N-terminal pro-B-type natriuretic peptide (NT-proBNP) or cardiac troponin I (cTnI) may have utility for DCM screening in settings where echocardiography or Holter monitor analysis is unavailable or not feasible; however these have not been shown to replace standard screening.[92,109,124] For NT-proBNP, cut-off values of greater than 550 to 626 pmol/L[124,125] are considered indicative for the presence of DCM in Doberman Pinschers, whereas a cut-off value of greater than 900 pmol/L is considered to indicate cardiac enlargement in other breeds.[126] With regard to cTnI, cut-off values vary depending on the specific assay used. A cut-off value to predict presence of DCM in Doberman Pinschers of greater than 0.22 ng/mL was identified using a first-generation cTnI assay,[127] whereas cut-off values of greater than 0.056 to 0.113 mg/mL have been identified using high-sensitivity cTnI assays.[124,128] Elevations in cTnI are not specific to DCM and may also result from myocarditis and various other systemic diseases. The results of cTnI analysis should therefore be interpreted in the context of the patient's clinical presentation.

When present, clinical signs associated with DCM typically are reflective of either left-sided myocardial failure or arrhythmogenesis. Common clinical signs include dyspnea, tachypnea, coughing, weakness, lethargy, exercise intolerance, and syncope. Sudden death may be encountered in dogs with ventricular arrhythmias.[129] Atrial arrhythmias including atrial fibrillation may also be identified and are usually a consequence of atrial dilation.[130–132]

Arrhythmogenic right ventricular cardiomyopathy

ARVC is an acquired myocardial disease characterized by replacement of myocardial tissue (typically that of the right ventricle) with fibrofatty infiltrates, which provides a substrate for ventricular arrhythmias, which are the dominant clinical manifestation of the disease.[89,133] Occasionally supraventricular arrhythmias may also be noted.[134] Less commonly, right ventricular systolic dysfunction and dilation of the right heart chambers may manifest in some dogs with ARVC.[134,135] There may also be geographic variation in the manifestations of ARVC, with the myocardial dysfunction form of the disease being more prevalent in Boxers in the UK,[136] whereas the arrhythmogenic form is more prevalent in Boxers in the USA.[135]

Boxer dogs are significantly overrepresented in studies of ARVC in dogs, so much so that the term "Boxer cardiomyopathy" was once used to describe the condition.[136] The estimated prevalence of ARVC in Boxers is approximately 9%.[135] Isolated cases of ARVC have also been observed in other breeds, most notably in English Bulldogs.[134] A deletion mutation in the striatin gene is associated with the development of ARVC in Boxers and is an autosomal dominant trait.[119] Penetrance of this genetic mutation is variable and is approximately 40% to 60% for heterozygous dogs and 80% to 100% for homozygous dogs.[89,119] Striatin is a protein located in the intercalated disc region that colocalizes to plakophilin-2 and other desmosomal proteins that have also been associated with the development of ARVC in humans.[89,119] Furthermore, ARVC may also develop in dogs without the striatin mutation, indicating there is a degree of genetic heterogeneity and suggesting other causative mutations may also be associated with development of the condition.[89,137]

Most dogs with ARVC do not develop phenotypic manifestations until they reach middle age, and it is suggested to begin annual screening for the condition at approximately 4 years of age.[92,135] Both Holter monitor analysis and echocardiographic examination are recommended for screening of ARVC. In Boxers, more than 300 VPCs in 24 hours is considered confirmatory for the diagnosis of ARVC, whereas 100 to 300 VPCs in 24 hours is considered suspicious for the presence of the condition, and it is considered more likely if increased complexity (couplets, triplets, rapid coupling rates) is also noted.[92,135] Thorough echocardiographic examination should be performed with particular attention paid to the systolic myocardial function, of not only the right ventricle, but also of the left ventricle, as the latter may also be affected in some forms of the condition.[136]

Clinical signs of ARVC are variable and reflective of the predominant form of the cardiomyopathy present in an individual, and a proportion of the dogs with the condition will be asymptomatic. Typical clinical signs resulting from ARVC include frequent cardiogenic syncope and occasionally sudden death in some dogs.[89,134,135] If systolic myocardial dysfunction is present then signs of right-sided or biventricular congestive heart failure may be noted.[89,118,135]

BREED SCREENING PROGRAMS
Orthopedic Foundation for Animals–the Canine Health Information Center Cardiac Database

In North America, breed screening databases for a variety of genetic and hereditary conditions are administered and maintained by the Orthopedic Foundation for Animals–The Canine Health Information Center (OFA-CHIC). The OFA-CHIC is a private nonprofit foundation that formed a voluntary dysplasia control database in 1966. Today the OFA-CHIC operates under the following objectives.

- To collate and disseminate information concerning orthopedic and genetic diseases of animals.
- To advise, encourage, and establish control programs to lower the incidence of orthopedic and genetic diseases.
- To encourage and finance research in orthopedic and genetic disease in animals.

- To receive funds and make grants to carry out these objectives.[138]

The OFA-CHIC also provides a certification program whereby a dog achieves OFA-CHIC certification if it has been screened for every disease recommended by the parent club for that breed, and those results are publicly available in the database.[139]

In conjunction with the American College of Veterinary Internal Medicine Cardiac Health Committee, the OFA-CHIC maintains 2 separate and distinct cardiac databases: the Basic Cardiac Database (BCD) and the Advanced Cardiac Database (ACD).

Basic cardiac database

The BCD is an auscultation-only examination that can be performed by any veterinarian, including general practitioners. The resulting OFA clearance number designates the expertise of the examiner by assigning appropriate suffixes (P = General Practitioner, S = Specialist, C = Cardiologist). The minimum age for clearance is 12 months. Because acquired heart disease may develop later, these evaluations are valid for 1 year from the time of examination, and annual examinations are recommended. Inclusion of the examination results in the database is solely at the discretion of the dog owners.[140]

Advanced cardiac database

The ACD provides 2 levels of clearance: congenital cardiac disease and adult-onset cardiac disease. Echocardiographic examination by a board-certified veterinary cardiologist is a mandatory requirement of the advanced cardiac application (ACA). As with the BCD, the minimum age for clearance is 12 months, with clearance from congenital cardiac disease being lifelong and clearance from adult-onset cardiac disease being valid for 1 year. Because of well-documented arrhythmogenic disorders and scientific data to support the predictive value of Holter testing in Boxers and Doberman pinschers, there is also a mandatory requirement for Holter testing in these 2 breeds. Holter testing must be performed within 90 days of echocardiographic examination, and interpretation of the Holter results must be performed by a board-certified veterinary cardiologist. The ACA form is a hardcopy triplicate form that must be obtained from the OFA by a board-certified cardiologist that is registered with the OFA. Anonymized results of the examination are provided directly to OFA by the examining cardiologist for improved statistical tracking. In addition, the dog owner may voluntarily submit their copy of the form for obtaining clearances.[140]

At the time of writing, data evaluating the outcomes of the OFA-CHIC cardiac databases for breed screening over time in various breeds have not been assessed.

Italian Boxer Club Breed Screening Program

The Italian Boxer Club established a mandatory national breed screening program for congenital heart disease in Boxer dogs in 1999.[141] This screening program requires Boxer dogs to undergo both cardiac auscultation and echocardiographic examination by a board-certified veterinary cardiologist[141,142] in accordance with established guidelines for echocardiographic studies of suspected SAS and PS.[19] Major and minor criteria were established for definitive diagnosis of each of these conditions. For SAS, the major criterion is overt echocardiographic evidence of overt structural abnormalities in the left ventricular outflow tract, whereas the minor criterion is turbulent aortic flow, determined by pulsed wave Doppler, with peak velocity on continuous wave Doppler obtained from the subcostal view of greater than 2 m/s, when averaged over 3 cardiac cycles during sinus rhythm. For PS, the major criterion is overt echocardiographic evidence of overt structural abnormalities in the right ventricular outflow tract, whereas the minor criterion is turbulent pulmonic flow, determined by pulsed-wave Doppler, with peak velocity on continuous-wave Doppler of greater than 1.6 m/s, when averaged over 3 cardiac cycles during sinus rhythm. For any individual dog, a definitive diagnosis of either SAS or PS is made if both the major and minor criteria for the respective disease are fulfilled. Dogs that fulfill only minor criteria without echocardiographic evidence of structural outflow tract obstruction are considered free of SAS or PS if peak aortic or pulmonic flow velocities are less than 2.3 or 1.8 m/s, respectively.[141] The severity of SAS or PS lesions is classified based on the calculated peak pressure gradient across the obstruction as either mild ($\leq$49 mm Hg), moderate (50–80 mm Hg), or severe (>80 mm Hg).[19]

Over the initial 6 years of this breeding program (January 1999 to December 2004), a total of 1283 Boxers were examined, with congenital heart disease identified in 165 (12.86%) dogs. Of these Boxers with congenital heart disease, SAS was diagnosed in 109 (66.1%) dogs, PS was diagnosed in 40 (24.2%) dogs, and 13 (7.9%) dogs had both conditions currently.[141] When the results of these first 6 years of the breed screening program were compared with a study of 500 randomly chosen Boxers among training dogs at regional Boxer Club centers before the breeding program's implementation,[143] the prevalence of both isolated and concurrent forms of SAS and PS within the total study populations was reduced from 17.8% to 12.68%. When the subpopulations of dogs diagnosed with heart disease in both studies were compared, the frequency of isolated SAS was similar (66.1% vs 64.1%), the frequency of isolated PS was increased (24.2% vs 10.1%), and the frequency of concurrent SAS and PS was significantly reduced (7.9% vs 24.7%).[141] When considering all forms of SAS and PS within the study populations, the findings suggest an effect of breed screening on the prevalence of these conditions, although the effect seems more pronounced for SAS versus PS.[141] However, it is important to note that comparisons between both studies are limited due to distinct differences between the study populations, and so direct comparison may not be appropriate.

A subsequent analysis of the cardiovascular and echocardiographic examinations from the 1283 Boxers screened in the initial 6 years of the Italian breed screening program was undertaken to investigate the role of auscultatory and echocardiographic traits as risk factors for the development of SAS and PS and to estimate heritability (h^2) of echocardiographic findings, murmur severity, and diagnosis of SAS and PS.[142] This study found that murmur, peak outflow tract velocity, and valve annulus area were risk factors for SAS and PS occurrence and displayed moderate h^2 estimates, suggesting these are candidate indicator traits that may have utility in breed screening to reduce the severity of these cardiac diseases.[142] Another study evaluating the prevalence of congenital heart disease in dogs presenting to a referral center in Italy between 1997 and 2017 showed that the probability of a Boxer being diagnosed with PS decreased from 35% in 1997 to 23.8% in 2017 and further supports the effects of the screening program.[15]

Swedish Kennel Club/Special Club for Cavalier King Charles Spaniels Breed Screening Program

In 2001, the Swedish Kennel Club and the Special Club for Cavalier King Charles Spaniels established a breed screening program aiming to reduce MMVD in the Swedish CKCS population. All CKCS, and not just those with good breeding characteristics, are recommended to undergo annual cardiac examination. A cardiac health certificate is provided if no evidence of cardiac disease is identified on auscultation by a veterinary specialist. Registration of dogs is not permitted unless both parents have obtained a certificate of cardiac health within 12 months before mating and have no other restrictions to breeding.[144] Before 2017, dogs were not allowed to breed until

4 years of age provided they were free of any cardiac murmurs on auscultation within 8 months before mating. However, dogs were allowed to breed at 2 years old, if the dog and both its parents are examined and no murmurs were detected. Male dogs with normal cardiac auscultation at 7 years of age were allowed to breed without further heart evaluation. Breeding dogs whose parents had heart murmurs before 4 years of age was not permitted.[145]

In 2017, the program was further modified. Dogs must be a minimum of 3 years old for official certification. Dogs, whose parents did not have a cardiac health certificate at age 5 years, can be used for mating at 5 years of age or older so long as they have a valid cardiac health certificate. Dogs with murmurs before 5 years old are banned from breeding, and offspring of these dogs are banned from registration. Offspring of male dogs younger than 6 years old, which have already produced 5 litters, are banned from registration. Additional litters may be registered once the male dog has a renewed cardiac certification at 6 years of age. Male dogs that received a cardiac health certificate at 8 years of age are permitted to continue breeding if a murmur is identified at a later age.[144]

A comparison in the prevalence of heart murmurs in 6-year-old CKCS in the Swedish breed screening program was performed between dogs born in 2001 and dogs born in 2003. A heart murmur was evident in 52% of dogs born in 2001 and was evident in 55% of dogs born in 2003. There was no difference in murmur prevalence between the cohorts of dogs born in each year.[145] Although no improvement in heart murmur prevalence at 6 years of age was identified in dogs born over the first 2 years of this breeding program, it must be noted that this is a relatively short time period, and it is possible that there may be a much slower effect on disease prevalence that may be noted over a longer period. Furthermore, this assessment on the effect of breed screening on murmur prevalence was performed subsequent to the modifications made to this program in 2017, and it is also possible that these modifications may have also had an effect on murmur prevalence since then. More recent analyses of the effects of the Swedish breed screening program have not been performed.

Danish Kennel Club Cavalier King Charles Spaniel Breeding Scheme

In Denmark, there has been a mandatory breeding scheme for mitral valve disease in CKCS since 2001, which is a collaboration between the Danish Kennel Club Association, the Cavalier Club in Denmark, and the University of Copenhagen.[146] In this scheme, cardiac health is determined on both auscultatory and echocardiographic criteria. On echocardiographic examination, the degree of mitral valve prolapse is assessed from a right parasternal long-axis 4-chamber view and graded according to a 4-point scale from 0 to 3.[146] Dogs with mitral regurgitant murmurs grade 3/6 or greater or mitral valve prolapse grade 3 are automatically excluded from breeding. Furthermore, dogs with grade 2/6 murmurs are excluded from breeding if they also have mitral valve prolapse grades 2 or 3. Based on the aforementioned criteria, dogs with mitral regurgitant murmurs of less than or equal to 1/6 combined with a mitral valve prolapse grade 2 or less or murmurs of grade less than or equal to 2/6 combined with a mitral valve prolapse grade 1 or less are approved for breeding. Before 2007, before additional restrictions were added, dogs with a mitral valve prolapse of grade 3 were approved for breeding if their murmur grade was less than or equal to 1/6.[146] In this scheme, all dogs older than 1.5 years that fulfill the cardiac health criteria described are approved for breeding until 4 years of age, at which time they must undergo cardiac reevaluation and fulfill the cardiac health criteria to continue breeding. Since 2007, male dogs older than 6 years must also undergo cardiac reevaluation and fulfill the cardiac health criteria to continue breeding. Mitral regurgitant murmur grades and mitral valve prolapse grades are made freely available online via the Danish Kennel Club Association's Web site. Puppies can only be registered with the Danish Kennel Club Association if both the sire and dam meet the cardiac health criteria.[146]

An analysis of the breeding scheme's database was performed, in which comparisons were made between all dogs examined between 2002 and 2003, all dogs examined between 2010 and 2011 that were products of the breeding scheme (ie, both parents had fulfilled the cardiac health criteria of the scheme), and all dogs that were examined between 2010 and 2011 that were not products of the breeding scheme. Dogs examined during the time period 2010 to 2011 that were products of the scheme had a 73% reduced risk of having a mitral regurgitant murmur compared with dogs examined during time period 2002 to 2003, whereas dogs that were not products of the scheme in 2010 to 2011 had no difference in the odds of having a murmur compared with the 2002 to 2003 cohort. For all the dogs examined during the period 2010 to 2011, products of the breeding program also had a 69% risk reduction for having a mitral regurgitant murmur when compared with dogs that were not products of the breeding scheme.[146]

Furthermore, in the 2010 to 2011 cohorts, dogs that were products of the scheme also had a 36% reduced risk of having mitral valve prolapse grade greater than 1 when compared with dogs that were not products of the scheme. However, there was no difference in the odds of having mitral valve prolapse greater than 1 between 2010 to 2011 dogs and 2002 to 2003 dogs. These findings indicate a clear effect of this mandatory breeding scheme to reduce the prevalence of MMVD in CKCS.[146]

United Kingdom Cavalier Club Breed Screening Program

From 1991, the Cavalier Club in the UK began collecting breed screening data and in 1996 the club established guidelines for a voluntary breed screening program based on the presence or absence of a murmur suggestive of MVMD on cardiac auscultation. These guidelines recommended that dogs used for breeding should be at least 5 years of age without evidence of a murmur consistent with MMVD and that dogs older than two and a half years could be used for breeding if both parents had been older than 5 years before developing a murmur. Cardiac auscultation could be performed by either a veterinarian in general practice or by a certified veterinary cardiologist. Patient details including pedigree, auscultatory findings, and experience level of the veterinarian performing the examination were recorded on a central database. A list of dogs older than 5 years before development of a mitral murmur was published by the Cavalier Club. These guidelines were further refined in 2006 so that only dogs evaluated by a certified veterinary cardiologist would be included in the list of dogs older than 5 years at the time of murmur development.[87]

Analysis of submissions to this database between 1991 and 2010 was performed and identified a total of 16,887 examinations performed on a total of 8860 dogs over the time period assessed. Over the time period investigated, the proportion of dogs evaluated by a cardiologist increased from 24.9% in the first quartile of the study period to 77.6% in the fourth quartile of the study period. The median age at first detection of a murmur was 8.6 years for dogs examined by general practitioners versus 7.2 years for dogs examined by cardiologists. In female dogs examined by general practitioners, the age at initial murmur diagnosis was noted to increase from 8.6 years for the period 1991 to 1995 up to 9.2 years in the time period 2005 to 2010; however, similar changes over time were not noted for male dogs examined by general practitioners or for dogs of either sex examined by a cardiologist. Approximately 30% of dogs were older than 5 years at the time of presentation at each of the time quartiles of the study, with no change in age profile noted across the course of the study period.[87]

The increase in age at murmur diagnosis in female dogs assessed by general practitioners, although small, suggests that the guidelines for this breed screening program may be having an effect on the incidence of MMVD in CKCS in the UK.[87] It is also important to note that this is a voluntary breed screening program, and only 21% of CKCS puppies registered with the UK Kennel Club were bred by members of the Cavalier Club and indicates a significant number of dogs are bred by nonmembers of the club or those who did not take part in the scheme,[87] and so the findings of this study may not be reflective of the true incidence of MMVD, or any changes to this incidence over time, within the wider population of UK-bred CKCS.

DISCUSSION

Compared with the large amount of information regarding the etiopathogenesis, clinical consequences, and natural history of many heritable cardiac diseases in various dog breeds, information on the outcomes of breeding programs aimed to reduce the prevalence of these conditions is relatively limited. The limited amount of good epidemiological data makes assessment of the outcomes of breed screening difficult.[147] Based on the available data, breed screening programs for canine cardiac disease do seem to have overall positive effects in reducing the prevalence of certain conditions; however, the magnitude of the effects seems to be variable and depends on a variety of factors.

With regard to MMVD, mandatory breed screening programs seem to have a clearer effect on reducing the prevalence of this disease when compared with voluntary programs. The Danish Kennel Club's mandatory breed screening program for MMVD in CKCS demonstrated a 69% reduction in the risk of dogs produced in the program developing a mitral regurgitant murmur across the initial 8 years following establishment of the program[146]; this is in contrast to the UK Cavalier Club's voluntary MMVD breed screening program where no difference was noted between dogs that were products of the breeding program's guidelines and dogs that were not after 10 to 14 years of the breeding guidelines being implemented.[87] It is interesting to note that in the time period 10 to 14 years after establishment of breeding guidelines only 4% of the dogs examined had followed those breeding guidelines. Furthermore, only 21% of CKCS registered with the UK Kennel Club are bred by members of the Cavalier Club.[87] It is difficult to draw direct comparisons between the 2 programs; however, the voluntary nature of the UK breeding program may explain, at least in part, the much more modest effect in affecting the prevalence of MMVD in CKCS when compared with the mandatory Danish program. Nevertheless, an effect was still appreciated by way of an increase in the age of murmur detection over the course of the UK program.[87]

It is also important to consider the timeframes that may be necessary to result in significant phenotypic changes within a breed following implementation of breeding guidelines; this may explain why no significant effect in murmur prevalence at 6 years of age was detected in the Swedish CKCS breeding program after 2 years of implementation of that program's guidelines, which is mandatory for registration of CKCS puppies with the Swedish Kennel Club.[145] It is possible that evaluation of disease over a longer period following implementation of the program's guidelines may identify a positive effect on MMVD prevalence in Swedish CKCS; this would also seem to be supported by the Italian Boxer Club screening program where a significant reduction in the prevalence of PS was noted on analysis of data 20 years following implementation of the program guidelines versus analysis performed after 6 years of the program, which showed an increase in the PS prevalence. However, it is also important to note that the 2 populations of dogs assessed at the 6-year analysis were not identical so this also precludes direct comparison between the analyses.[15,141,143]

In addition, the effect of geographic location in the genetic variance and expression of traits should also be considered. Distinct differences in genetic traits and phenotypic manifestations of breed-associated cardiac disease have been noted between subpopulations of the same breed in different geographic locations,[31,32,89,110,113,135,136] and these may have implications for the development and implementation of breeding program guidelines for certain cohorts of dogs.

Unfortunately, many of the common hereditary cardiac diseases exhibit complex modes of inheritance, penetrance is often variable, and for some conditions the modes of inheritance have not been determined. Another confounding factor is that modes of inheritance for the same condition may differ between breeds (eg, aortic stenosis). Even for recessive traits, the variation in penetrance for some cardiac conditions is a significant limitation when selecting dogs for breeding because even mildly affected individuals may create severely affected offspring. In the author's practice, it is recommended to not breed dogs with definitive evidence of congenital disease regardless of severity. For dogs that are phenotypically equivocal it may be reasonable for them to be bred to a definitively normal individual so long as the breeder is aware of the risks that offspring with variable disease manifestation could result from the mating. Selection of suitable breeding animals is further complicated for acquired cardiac diseases, where the phenotype only manifests later in life, in some cases after the individuals have already been used for breeding. For acquired heart diseases, especially those with high penetrance (eg, MMVD, DCM), the main goal is to remove individuals that manifest the condition at a younger age from the breeding population. This approach necessitates repeated screening throughout an individual's lifetime. If early manifestation of acquired cardiac disease is identified after a dog has been used for breeding, then this warrants caution in selecting any offspring for breeding. Such offspring should also undergo similar screening throughout their lifetime if they are included in the breeding population. For conditions where parents do not have a disease phenotype but the offspring end up with a disease phenotype, it is recommended to avoid mating that breeding pair to each other again. It may be reasonable to breed the sire or dam to different individuals, but breeders should exercise caution in making this decision and closely evaluate resultant offspring.

Estimated breeding values (EBVs) are measures of the potential of an animal to pass a particular trait to its offspring and have been used in livestock breeding for decades, resulting in significant changes in various production traits, and more recently have also been calculated for health and welfare traits. These values are calculated using an individual's phenotype and those of relatives, combined with pedigree relationships and may be particularly in the selection of complex traits that may be influenced by multiple genes or environmental factors. Breeders can use EBVs to make breeding decisions even in the absence of phenotype information from the animal itself for example, calculating EBVs for dairy productivity traits in bulls from information in sired daughters. The UK Kennel Club recommends using EBVs for screening potential breeding candidates for diseases with complex inheritance or where the inheritance pattern is unknown. These EBVs have recently been introduced into screening of canine hip and elbow dysplasia in several countries.[1] Information on the use of EBVs in the setting of canine heart disease is currently lacking. Given the complex inheritance of several important cardiac diseases, EBVs would seem to have significant potential in reducing the prevalence of disease-associated traits within a breed while also minimizing the risk of concurrent inadvertent selection of other undesirable traits. Further studies on the outcomes and utility of using EBVs in selection of breeding candidates in canine breeds with high cardiac disease prevalence are warranted.

SUMMARY

Breed-associated cardiac diseases have a relatively high prevalence in dogs. Data are limited; however, breed screening programs do seem to have overall positive effects in reducing the prevalence of certain cardiac diseases. The magnitude and speed of these positive changes are variable and somewhat reflect complex modes of inheritance for certain conditions. Estimated breeding values may be beneficial in the selection of suitable breeding candidates to reduce the prevalence of breed-associated cardiac disease; however, further research in this area is warranted.

CLINICS CARE POINTS

- Phenotypic manifestation or clinical severity of inherited cardiac disease in offspring is not always reliably predicted by the phenotype or clinical severity expressed in the sire or dam.
- Absence of known associated genetic mutations does not preclude the development of any given cardiac condition in an individual or its offspring.
- Genetic testing alone is not sufficient for breed screening for cardiac disease.
- Breed screening for acquired cardiac diseases requires repeated screening throughout a breeding individual's lifetime, including beyond retirement from breeding; identification of acquired cardiac disease in an individual that has previously bred should prompt similar screening of offspring, especially those also intended for breeding.

DISCLOSURE

The author declares no conflicts of interest related to any of the topics presented in this article.

REFERENCES

1. Farrell LL, Schoenebeck JJ, Wiener P, et al. The challenges of pedigree dog health: approaches to combating inherited disease. Canine Genet Epidemiol 2015;2(1):1–14.
2. Axelsson E, Ljungvall I, Bhoumik P, et al. The Genetic Consequences of Dog Breed Formation - Accumulation of Deleterious Genetic Variation and Fixation of Mutations Associated with Myxomatous Mitral Valve Disease in Cavalier King Charles Spaniels. PLoS Genet 2021;17(9):e1009726.
3. Leppänen M, Paloheimo A, Saloniemi H. Attitudes of Finnish veterinarians about programs to control canine genetic diseases. Prev Vet Med 1999;38(4):239–57.
4. Fioretti M, Delli Carri E. Epidemiological survey of dilatative cardiomyopathy in dogs. Veterinaria 1988;2:81.
5. Buchanan JW. Prevalence of cardiovascular disorders. In: Fox PR, Sisson D, Moïse NS, editors. Textbook of canine and feline cardiology: principles and clinical practice. 2nd edition. Philadelphia: W.B. Saunders; 1999. p. 457–70.
6. Darke PGG. Congenital heart defects in small animals. Br Vet J 1986;142:203–9.
7. Patterson DF. Hereditary congenital heart defects in dogs. J Small Anim Pract 1989;30:153–65.

8. Bonagura JD, Lehmkuhl LB. Congenital heart disease. In: Fox PR, Sisson D, Moise NS, editors. Textbook of canine and feline cardiology: principles and clinical practice. 2nd edition. Philadelphia: W.B. Saunders; 1999. p. 471–535.

9. Aherne M, Beijerink NJ. Congenital heart disease : a case series of 135 dogs. Aust Vet Pract 2013;43(3):466–70.

10. Schrope DP. Prevalence of congenital heart disease in 76,301 mixed-breed dogs and 57,025 mixed-breed cats. J Vet Cardiol 2015;17(3):192–202.

11. Lucina SB, Sarraff AP, Wolf M, et al. Congenital Heart Disease in Dogs: A Retrospective Study of 95 Cases. Top Companion Anim Med 2021;43:100505.

12. Tidholm A. Retrospective study of congenital heart defects in 151 dogs. J Small Anim Pract 1995;38(3):94–138.

13. Baumgartner C, Glaus TM. Congenital cardiac defects in dogs: A retrospective analysis. Schweiz Arch Tierheilkd 2003;145(11):527–36.

14. Oliveira P, Domenech O, Silva J, et al. Retrospective review of congenital heart disease in 976 dogs. J Vet Intern Med 2011;25(3):477–83.

15. Brambilla PG, Polli M, Pradelli D, et al. Epidemiological study of congenital heart diseases in dogs: Prevalence, popularity, and volatility throughout twenty years of clinical practice. PLoS One 2020;15:1–17.

16. Fingland RB, Bonagura JD, Myer CW. Pulmonic stenosis in the dog: 29 cases (1975-1984). J Am Vet Med Assoc 1986;189(2):218–26.

17. Locatelli C, Spalla I, Domenech O, et al. Pulmonic stenosis in dogs: Survival and risk factors in a retrospective cohort of patients. J Small Anim Pract 2013;54(9):445–52.

18. Ontiveros ES, Fousse SL, Crofton AE, et al. Congenital cardiac outflow tract abnormalities in dogs: Prevalence and pattern of inheritance from 2008 to 2017. Front Vet Sci 2019;6:1–10.

19. Bussadori C, Amberger C, Le Bobinnec G, et al. Guidelines for the echocardiographic studies of suspected subaortic and pulmonic stenosis. J Vet Cardiol 2000;2(2):15–22.

20. Francis AJ, Johnson MJS, Culshaw GC, et al. Outcome in 55 dogs with pulmonic stenosis that did not undergo balloon valvuloplasty or surgery. J Small Anim Pract 2011;52(6):282–8.

21. Johnson MS, Martin M, Edwards D, et al. Pulmonic stenosis in dogs: balloon dilation improves clinical outcome. J Vet Intern Med 2004;18(5):656–62.

22. Stafford Johnson M, Martin M. Results of balloon valvuloplasty in 40 dogs with pulmonic stenosis. J Small Anim Pract 2004;45(3):148–53.

23. Pyle RL, Patterson DF, Chacko S. The genetics and pathology of discrete subaortic stenosis in the Newfoundland dog. Am Heart J 1976;92(3):324–34.

24. Kienle RD, Thomas WP, Pion PD. The natural clinical history of canine congenital subaortic stenosis. J Vet Intern Med 1994;8(6):423–31.

25. Ontiveros ES, Stern JA. Genetics of canine subvalvular aortic stenosis (SAS). Canine Med Genet 2021;8(1):1–9.

26. Thomas WP, Gaber CE, Jacobs GJ, et al. Recommendations for standards in transthoracic two-dimensional echocardiography in the dog and cat. J Vet Intern Med 1993;7(4):247–52.

27. Lehmkuhl LB, Bonagura JD. Comparison of transducer placement sites for Doppler echocardiography in dogs with subaortic stenosis. Am J Vet Res 1994;55(2):192–8.

28. Pradelli D, Quintavalla C, Crosta MC, et al. The influence of emotional stress on Doppler-derived aortic peak velocity in Boxer dogs. J Vet Intern Med 2014;28(6):1724–30.

29. Reist-Marti SB, Dolf G, Leeb T, et al. Genetic evidence of subaortic stenosis in the Newfoundland dog. Vet Rec 2012;170(23):597.
30. Ohad DG, Avrahami A, Waner T, et al. The occurrence and suspected mode of inheritance of congenital subaortic stenosis and tricuspid valve dysplasia in Dogue de Bordeaux dogs. Vet J 2013;197(2):351–7.
31. Stern JA, White SN, Lehmkuhl LB, et al. A single codon insertion in PICALM is associated with development of familial subvalvular aortic stenosis in Newfoundland dogs. Hum Genet 2014;133(9):1139–48.
32. Drögemüller M, Jagannathan V, Dolf G, et al. A single codon insertion in the PIC-ALM gene is not associated with subvalvular aortic stenosis in Newfoundland dogs. Hum Genet 2015;134(1):127–9.
33. Buchanan JW. Patent ductus arteriosus morphology, pathogenesis, types and treatment. J Vet Cardiol 2001;3(1):7–16.
34. Buchanan JW, Patterson DF. Etiology of patent ductus arteriosus in dogs. J Vet Intern Med 2003;17(2):167–71.
35. den Toom ML, Meiling AE, Thomas RE, et al. Epidemiology, presentation and population genetics of patent ductus arteriosus (PDA) in the Dutch Stabyhoun dog. BMC Vet Res 2016;12(1):1–7.
36. Bomassi E, Misbach C, Tissier R, et al. Signalment, clinical features, echocardiographic findings, and outcome of dogs and cats with ventricular septal defects: 109 cases (1992–2013). J Am Vet Med Assoc 2015;247(2):166–75.
37. Lopez L, Houyel L, Colan SD, et al. Classification of ventricular septal defects for the eleventh iteration of the international classification of diseases—Striving for consensus: A report from the International Society for Nomenclature of Paediatric and Congenital Heart Disease. Ann Thorac Surg 2018;106(5):1578–89.
38. Van Mierop LHS, Patterson DF, Schnarr WR. Hereditary conotruncal septal defects in Keeshond dogs: Embryologic studies. Am J Cardiol 1977;40(6):936–50.
39. Diez-Prieto I, García-Rodríguez B, Ríos-Granja A, et al. Cardiac conotruncal malformations in a family of beagle dogs. J Small Anim Pract 2009;50(11):597–603.
40. Brown WA. Ventricular septal defects in the English springer spaniel. In: Kirk RW, Bonagura JD, editors. Kirk's current veterinary therapy XII. Philadelphia: W.B. Saunders; 1995. p. 827–30.
41. Patterson DF, Pyle RL, Van Mierop L, et al. Hereditary defects of the conotruncal septum in keeshond dogs: Pathologic and genetic studies. Am J Cardiol 1974;34(2):187–205.
42. Patterson DF, Pexieder T, Schnarr WR, et al. A single major-gene defect underlying cardiac conotruncal malformations interferes with myocardial growth during embryonic development: Studies in the CTD line of keeshond dogs. Am J Hum Genet 1993;52(2):388–97.
43. Werner P, Raducha MG, Prociuk U, et al. The keeshond defect in cardiac conotruncal development is oligogenic. Hum Genet 2005;116(5):368–77.
44. Rausch WP, Keene BW. Spontaneous resolution of an isolated ventricular septal defect in a dog. J Am Vet Med Assoc 2003;223(2):219–20.
45. van de Watering A, Szatmári V. Spontaneous closure of an isolated congenital perimembranous ventricular septal defect in two dogs. BMC Vet Res 2022;18(1):4–9.
46. Hunt GB, Pearson MRB, Bellenger CR, et al. Ventricular septal defect repair in a small dog using cross-circulation. Aust Vet J 1995;72(10):379–82.

47. Fujii Y, Fukuda T, Machida N, et al. Transcatheter closure of congenital ventric-
    ular septal defects in 3 dogs with a detachable coil. J Vet Intern Med 2004;18:
    911–4.

48. Margiocco ML, Bulmer BJ, Sisson DD. Percutaneous occlusion of a muscular
    ventricular septal defect with an Amplatzer® Muscular VSD occluder. J Vet Car-
    diol 2008;10(1):61–6.

49. Chi IJB, Scansen BA, Potter BM, et al. Transcatheter closure of aneurysmal peri-
    membranous ventricular septal defect with the Canine Duct Occluder in two
    dogs. J Vet Cardiol 2022;43:61–9.

50. Chetboul V, Charles V, Nicolle A, et al. Retrospective study of 156 atrial septal
    defects in dogs and cats (2001-2005). J Vet Med Ser A Physiol Pathol Clin
    Med 2006;53(4):179–84.

51. Guglielmini C, Diana a, Pietra M, et al. Atrial septal defect in five dogs. J Small
    Anim Pract 2002;43(July):317–22.

52. Hamlin RL, Smith CR, Smetzer DL. Ostium secundum type interatrial septal de-
    fects in the dog. J Am Vet Med Assoc 1963;143:149–57.

53. Shelden A, Wesselowski S, Gordon SG, et al. Transcatheter closure of a small
    atrial septal defect with an Amplatzer™ patent foramen ovale occluder in a
    working dog with cyanosis and exercise intolerance at high altitude. J Vet Car-
    diol 2017;19(6):523–9.

54. Jeraj K, Ogburn PN, Johnston GR, et al. Atrial septal defect (sinus venosus type)
    in a dog. J Am Vet Med Assoc 1980;177(4):342–6.

55. Bellisario I, Barbisan D, Giancarlo T, et al. Unroofed coronary sinus: a rare expla-
    nation of right ventricular dilatation. Eur Hear J - Cardiovasc Imaging 2022;
    24(3):43.

56. Gordon SG, Nelson DA, Achen SE, et al. Open heart closure of an atrial septal
    defect by use of an atrial septal occluder in a dog. J Am Vet Med Assoc 2010;
    236(4):434–9.

57. Mizuno T, Mizuno M, Harada K, et al. Surgical correction for sinus venosus atrial
    septal defect with partial anomalous pulmonary venous connection in a dog.
    J Vet Cardiol 2020;28:23–30.

58. Liu S-K, Tilley LP. Malformation of the canine mitral valve complex. J Am Vet Med
    Assoc 1975;167(6):465–71.

59. Sudunagunta S, Hamilton-Elliott J, Dukes-McEwan J. Mitral valve dysplasia in
    eight English Springer Spaniels. J Vet Cardiol 2021;33:52–60.

60. Lehmkuhl LB, Ware WA, Bonagura JD. Mitral stenosis in 15 dogs. J Vet Intern
    Med 1994;8(1):2–17.

61. Otoni C, Abbott JA. Mitral valve dysplasia characterized by isolated cleft of the
    anterior leaflet resulting in fixed left ventricular outflow tract obstruction. J Vet
    Cardiol 2012;14(1):301–5.

62. Atwell RB, Sutton RH. Atrioventricular valve dysplasia in Dalmatians. Aust Vet J
    1998;76(1):31.

63. De Majo M, Britti D, Masucci M, et al. Hypertrophic obstructive cardiomyopathy
    associated to mitral valve dysplasia in the Dalmatian dog: two cases. Vet Res
    Commun 2003;27(Suppl 1):391–3.

64. Liu S-K, Tilley LP. Dysplasia of the Tricuspid Valve in the Dog and Cat. J Am Vet
    Med Assoc 1976;169(6):623–30.

65. Navarro-Cubas X, Palermo V, French A, et al. Tricuspid valve dysplasia: A retro-
    spective study of clinical features and outcome in dogs in the UK. Open Vet J
    2017;7(4):349–59.

66. Chetboul V, Tran D, Carlos C, et al. Congenital malformations of the tricuspid valve in domestic carnivores: A retrospective study of 50 cases. Schweiz Arch Tierheilkd 2004;146(6):265–75.

67. Lake-Bakaar GA, Griffiths LG, Kittleson MD. Balloon Valvuloplasty of Tricuspid Stenosis: A Retrospective Study of 5 Labrador Retriever Dogs. J Vet Intern Med 2017;31(2):311–5.

68. Chetboul V, Poissonnier C, Bomassi E, et al. Epidemiological, clinical, and echocardiographic features, and outcome of dogs with Ebstein's anomaly: 32 cases (2002–2016). J Vet Cardiol 2020;29:11–21.

69. Famula TR, Siemens LM, Davidson AP, et al. Evaluation of the genetic basis of tricuspid valve dysplasia in Labrador Retrievers. Am J Vet Res 2002;63(6):816–20.

70. Pasławska U, Noszczyk-Nowak A, Janiszewski A, et al. Tricuspid Dysplasia in Dogs. Bull Vet Inst Pulawy 2013;57(1):123–6.

71. Andelfinger G, Wright KN, Lee HS, et al. Canine tricuspid valve malformation, a model of human Ebstein anomaly, maps to dog chromosome 9. J Med Genet 2003;40(5):320–4.

72. Kornreich BG, Moïse NS. Right atrioventricular valve malformation in dogs and cats: an electrocardiographic survey with emphasis on splintered QRS complexes. J Vet Intern Med 1997;11(4):226–30.

73. de Madron E, Vet M, Kadish A, et al. Incessant atrial tachycardias in a dog with tricuspid dysplasia: clinical management and electrophysiology. J Vet Intern Med 1987;1(4):163–9.

74. Atkins CE, Kanter R, Wright K, et al. Orthodromic reciprocating tachycardia and heart failure in a dog with a concealed posteroseptal accessory pathway. J Vet Intern Med 1995;9(1):43–9.

75. Wright KN, Mehdirad AA, Giacobbe P, et al. Radiofrequency catheter ablation of atrioventricular accessory pathways in 3 dogs with subsequent resolution of tachycardia-induced cardiomyopathy. J Vet Intern Med 1999;13(4):361–71.

76. Santilli R a, Spadacini G, Moretti P, et al. Anatomic distribution and electrophysiologic properties of accessory atrioventricular pathways in dogs. J Am Vet Med Assoc 2007;231:393–8.

77. Keene BW, Atkins CE, Bonagura JD, et al. ACVIM consensus guidelines for the diagnosis and treatment of myxomatous mitral valve disease in dogs. J Vet Intern Med 2019;33(3):1127–40.

78. Borgarelli M, Haggstrom J. Canine degenerative myxomatous mitral valve disease: natural history, clinical presentation and therapy. Vet Clin North Am Small Anim Pract 2010;40(4):651–63.

79. Borgarelli M, Buchanan JW. Historical review, epidemiology and natural history of degenerative mitral valve disease. J Vet Cardiol 2012;14(1):93–101.

80. Lu C-C, Liu M-M, Culshaw G, et al. Gene network and canonical pathway analysis in canine myxomatous mitral valve disease: A microarray study. Vet J 2015;204(1):23–31.

81. O'Brien MJ, Beijerink NJ, Wade CM. Genetics of canine myxomatous mitral valve disease. Anim Genet 2021;52(4):409–21.

82. Borgarelli M, Zini E, D'Agnolo G, et al. Comparison of primary mitral valve disease in German Shepherd dogs and in small breeds. J Vet Cardiol 2004;6(2):27–34.

83. Sisson D, Kvart C, Darke PGG. Acquired valvular heart disease in dogs and cats. In: Fox PR, Sisson D, Moïse NS, editors. Textbook of canine and feline

cardiology: principles and clinical practice. 2nd edition. Philadelphia, PA, USA: W.B. Saunders; 1999. p. 536–65.

84. Mattin MJ, Boswood A, Church DB, et al. Prevalence of and risk factors for degenerative mitral valve disease in dogs attending primary-care veterinary practices in England. J Vet Intern Med 2015;29(3):847–54.

85. Stepien RL, Kellihan HB, Luis Fuentes V. Prevalence and diagnostic characteristics of non-clinical mitral regurgitation murmurs in North American Whippets. J Vet Cardiol 2017;19(4):317–24.

86. Lewis T, Swift S, Woolliams JA, et al. Heritability of premature mitral valve disease in Cavalier King Charles spaniels. Vet J 2011;188(1):73–6.

87. Swift S, Baldin A, Cripps P. Degenerative valvular disease in the Cavalier King Charles Spaniel: Results of the UK breed scheme 1991–2010. J Vet Intern Med 2017;31(1):9–14.

88. Madsen MB, Olsen LH, Häggström J, et al. Identification of 2 loci associated with development of myxomatous mitral valve disease in Cavalier King Charles Spaniels. J Hered 2011;102(Suppl):62–7.

89. Stern JA, Ueda Y. Inherited cardiomyopathies in veterinary medicine. Pflugers Arch Eur J Physiol 2019;471(5):745–53.

90. Dutton E, López-Alvarez J. An update on canine cardiomyopathies – is it all in the genes? J Small Anim Pract 2018;59(8):455–64.

91. Shen L, Estrada AH, Meurs KM, et al. A review of the underlying genetics and emerging therapies for canine cardiomyopathies. J Vet Cardiol 2022;40:2–14.

92. Wess G. Screening for dilated cardiomyopathy in dogs. J Vet Cardiol 2022;40: 51–68.

93. United States Food and Drug Administration. FDA investigating potential connection between diet and cases of canine heart disease. Available at: https://wayback.archive-it.org/7993/20201222194256/https://www.fda.gov/animal-veterinary/cvm-updates/fda-investigating-potential-connection-between-diet-and-cases-canine-heart-disease. Published 2018.

94. Jones J, Carey L, Palmer LA. FDA Update on dilated cardiomyopathy: Fully and partially recovered cases. In: Scientific forum exploring causes of dilated cardiomyopathy in dogs. 2020.

95. United States Food and Drug Administration. FDA investigation into potential link between certain diets and canine dilated cardiomyopathy - February 2019 update. Available at: https://www.fda.gov/animal-veterinary/news-events/fda-investigation-potential-link-between-certain-diets-and-canine-dilated-cardiomyopathy-february. Published 2019.

96. Kaplan JL, Stern JA, Fascetti AJ, et al. Taurine deficiency and dilated cardiomyopathy in golden retrievers fed commercial diets. PLoS One 2018;13(12):1–19.

97. Adin D, DeFrancesco TC, Keene B, et al. Echocardiographic phenotype of canine dilated cardiomyopathy differs based on diet type. J Vet Cardiol 2019; 21:1–9.

98. Freeman L, Rush J, Adin D, et al. Prospective study of dilated cardiomyopathy in dogs eating nontraditional or traditional diets and in dogs with subclinical cardiac abnormalities. J Vet Intern Med 2022;36(2):451–63.

99. Smith CE, Parnell LD, Lai CQ, et al. Metabolomic profiling in dogs with dilated cardiomyopathy eating non-traditional or traditional diets and in healthy controls. Sci Rep 2022;12(1):1–14.

100. Smith CE, Parnell LD, Lai CQ, et al. Investigation of diets associated with dilated cardiomyopathy in dogs using foodomics analysis. Sci Rep 2021;11(1):1–12.

101. Kittleson MD, Keene BW, Pion PD, et al. Results of the multicenter spaniel trial (MUST): taurine- and carnitine-responsive dilated cardiomyopathy in American Cocker Spaniels with decreased plasma taurine concentration. J Vet Intern Med 1997;11(4):204–11.

102. Backus RC, Cohen G, Pion PD, et al. Taurine deficiency in Newfoundlands fed commercially available complete and balanced diets. J Am Vet Med Assoc 2003;223(8):1130–6.

103. Fascetti AJ, Reed JR, Rogers QR, et al. Taurine deficiency in dogs with dilated cardiomyopathy: 12 cases (1997-2001). J Am Vet Med Assoc 2003;223(8):1137–41.

104. Bélanger MC, Ouellet M, Queney G, et al. Taurine-deficient dilated cardiomyopathy in a family of golden retrievers. J Am Anim Hosp Assoc 2005;41(5):284–91.

105. World Small Animal Veterinary Association. WSAVA Global Nutrition Committee: Guidelines on selecting pet foods. Available at: https://wsava.org/wp-content/uploads/2021/04/Selecting-a-pet-food-for-your-pet-updated-2021_WSAVA-Global-Nutrition-Toolkit.pdf. Published 2021.

106. Calvert CA, Jacobs GJ, Smith DD, et al. Association between results of ambulatory electrocardiography and development of cardiomyopathy during long-term follow-up of Doberman Pinschers. J Am Vet Med Assoc 2000;216(1):34–9.

107. Sisson DD, O'Grady MR, Calvert CA. Myocardial diseases of dogs. In: Fox PR, Sisson DD, Moïse NS, editors. Textbook of canine and feline cardiology: principles and clinical practice. 2nd edition. Philadelphia, PA, USA: WB Saunders; 1999. p. 581–620.

108. Dambach DM, Lannon A, Sleeper MM, et al. Familial dilated cardiomyopathy of young Portuguese water dogs. J Vet Intern Med 1999;13(1):65–71.

109. Wess G, Domenech O, Dukes-McEwan J, et al. European Society of Veterinary Cardiology screening guidelines for dilated cardiomyopathy in Doberman Pinschers. J Vet Cardiol 2017;19(5):405–15.

110. Meurs KM, Lahmers S, Keene BW, et al. A splice site mutation in a gene encoding for PDK4, a mitochondrial protein, is associated with the development of dilated cardiomyopathy in the Doberman pinscher. Hum Genet 2012;131(8):1319–25.

111. Meurs KM, Friedenberg SG, Kolb J, et al. A missense variant in the titin gene in Doberman pinscher dogs with familial dilated cardiomyopathy and sudden cardiac death. Hum Genet 2019;138(5):515–24.

112. Meurs KM, Stern JA, Adin DB, et al. Assessment of PDK4 and TTN gene variants in 48 Doberman Pinschers with dilatd cardiomyopathy. J Am Vet Med Assoc 2020;257(10):1401–4.

113. Mausberg TB, Wess G, Simak J, et al. A locus on chromosome 5 is associated with dilated cardiomyopathy in doberman pinschers. PLoS One 2011;6(5):5–10.

114. Owczarek-Lipska M, Mausberg TB, Stephenson H, et al. A 16-bp deletion in the canine PDK4 gene is not associated with dilated cardiomyopathy in a European cohort of Doberman Pinschers. Anim Genet 2013;44(2):239.

115. Harmon MW, Leach SB, Lamb KE. Dilated cardiomyopathy in standard schnauzers: Retrospective study of 15 cases. J Am Anim Hosp Assoc 2017;53(1):38–44.

116. Leach SB, Briggs M, Hansen L, et al. Prevalence, geographic distribution, and impact on lifespan of a dilated cardiomyopathy-associated RNA-binding motif protein 20 variant in genotyped dogs. J Vet Cardiol 2022;40:119–25.

117. Yost O, Friedenberg SG, Jesty SA, et al. The R9H phospholamban mutation is associated with highly penetrant dilated cardiomyopathy and sudden death in a spontaneous canine model. Gene 2019;697:118–22.

118. Meurs KM, Stern JA, Sisson DD, et al. Association of dilated cardiomyopathy with the striatin mutation genotype in boxer dogs. J Vet Intern Med 2013; 27(6):1437–40.

119. Meurs KM, Mauceli E, Lahmers S, et al. Genome-wide association identifies a deletion in the 3 untranslated region of Striatin in a canine model of arrhythmogenic right ventricular cardiomyopathy. Hum Genet 2010;128(3):315–24.

120. Philipp U, Vollmar A, Häggström J, et al. Multiple loci are associated with dilated cardiomyopathy in irish wolfhounds. PLoS One 2012;7(6):1–6.

121. Simpson S, Dunning MD, Brownlie S, et al. Multiple genetic associations with Irish Wolfhound dilated cardiomyopathy. BioMed Res Int 2016;2016:6374082.

122. Werner P, Raducha MG, Prociuk U, et al. A novel locus for dilated cardiomyopathy maps to canine chromosome 8. Genomics 2008;91(6):517–21.

123. Bonagura JD, Visser LC. Echocardiographic assessment of dilated cardiomyopathy in dogs. J Vet Cardiol 2022;40:15–50.

124. Dukes-McEwan J, Garven KE, Lopez Alvarez J, et al. Usefulness of cardiac biomarker screening to detect dilated cardiomyopathy in Dobermanns. J Small Anim Pract 2022;63(4):275–85.

125. Wess G, Butz V, Mahling M, et al. Evaluation of N-terminal pro-B-type natriuretic peptide as a diagnostic marker of various stages of cardiomyopathy in Doberman Pinschers. Am J Vet Res 2011;72(5):642–9.

126. Oyama MA, Boswood A, Connolly DJ, et al. Clinical usefulness of an assay for measurement of circulating N-terminal pro-B-type natriuretic peptide concentration in dogs and cats with heart disease. J Am Vet Med Assoc 2013;243(1): 71–82.

127. Wess G, Simak J, Mahling M, et al. Cardiac troponin I in Doberman pinschers with cardiomyopathy. J Vet Intern Med 2010;24:843–9.

128. Klüser L, Maier ET, Wess G. Evaluation of a high-sensitivity cardiac troponin I assay compared to a first-generation cardiac troponin I assay in Doberman Pinschers with and without dilated cardiomyopathy. J Vet Intern Med 2019; 33(1):54–63.

129. Summerfield NJ, Boswood A, O'Grady MR, et al. Efficacy of pimobendan in the prevention of congestive heart failure or sudden death in Doberman pinschers with preclinical dilated cardiomyopathy (The PROTECT Study). J Vet Intern Med 2012;26(6):1337–49.

130. Vollmar C, Vollmar A, Keene BW, et al. Dilated cardiomyopathy in 151 Irish Wolfhounds: Characteristic clinical findings, life expectancy and causes of death. Vet J 2019;245:15–21.

131. Friederich J, Seuß AC, Wess G. The role of atrial fibrillation as a prognostic factor in doberman pinschers with dilated cardiomyopathy and congestive heart failure. Vet J 2020;264:105535.

132. Eberhard J, Wess G. The prevalence of atrial premature complexes in healthy Doberman Pinschers and their role in the diagnosis of occult dilated cardiomyopathy. Vet J 2020;259-260:105475.

133. Basso C, Fox PR, Meurs KM, et al. Arrhythmogenic right ventricular cardiomyopathy causing sudden death in boxer dogs: a new animal model of human disease. Circulation 2004;109(9):1180–5.

134. Cunningham SM, Sweeney JT, MacGregor J, et al. Clinical Features of English Bulldogs with Presumed Arrhythmogenic Right Ventricular Cardiomyopathy: 31 Cases (2001–2013). J Am Anim Hosp Assoc 2018;54(2):95–102.

135. Meurs KM, Stern JA, Reina-Doreste Y, et al. Natural history of arrhythmogenic right ventricular cardiomyopathy in the boxer dog: a prospective study. J Vet Intern Med 2014;28(4):1214–20.

136. Palermo V, Stafford Johnson MJ, Sala E, et al. Cardiomyopathy in Boxer dogs: A retrospective study of the clinical presentation, diagnostic findings and survival. J Vet Cardiol 2011;13(1):45–55.

137. Oxford EM, Danko CG, Fox PR, et al. Change in β-Catenin localization suggests involvement of the canonical wnt pathway in boxer dogs with arrhythmogenic right ventricular cardiomyopathy. J Vet Intern Med 2014;28:92–101.

138. Keller GG. The use of health databases and selective breeding: a guide for dog and cat breeders and owners. 7th edition. OFA–The Canine Health Information Center; 2018.

139. CHIC Program. Orthopedic Foundation for Animals. Available at: https://ofa.org/chic-programs/. Published 2023.

140. Cardiac disease. Orthopedic Foundation for Animals; 2023. Available at: https://ofa.org/diseases/cardiac-disease/.

141. Bussadori C, Pradelli D, Borgarelli M, et al. Congenital heart disease in boxer dogs: Results of 6 years of breed screening. Vet J 2009;181(2):187–92.

142. Menegazzo L, Bussadori C, Chiavegato D, et al. The relevance of echocardiography heart measures for breeding against the risk of subaortic and pulmonic stenosis in Boxer dogs. J Anim Sci 2012;90(2):419–28.

143. Bussadori C, Quintavalla C, Capelli A. Prevalence of Congenital Heart Disease in Boxers in Italy. J Vet Cardiol 2001;3(2):7–11.

144. Health program and breeding recommendations. Swedish Kennel Club; 2023. Available at: https://www.cavaliersallskapet.net/avel-och-halsa/avelsrekommendationer/.

145. Lundin T, Kvart C. Evaluation of the Swedish breeding program for cavalier King Charles spaniels. Acta Vet Scand 2010;52(1):2–7.

146. Birkegård AC, Reimann MJ, Martinussen T, et al. Breeding Restrictions Decrease the Prevalence of Myxomatous Mitral Valve Disease in Cavalier King Charles Spaniels over an 8- to 10-Year Period. J Vet Intern Med 2016;30(1):63–8.

147. Häggström J, Luis-fuentes V. Cardiac disease in dogs and cats: Is breed screening the answer? Vet Rec 2013;172(17):440–1.

Common Orthopedic Traits and Screening for Breeding Programs

Jessica J. Hayward, PhD[a], Rory J. Todhunter, BVSc, MS, PhD, DACVS[b],*

KEYWORDS

• Orthopedic traits • Screening • Breeding • Dogs • Genetics

KEY POINTS

- Complex traits are controlled by many genes and environmental regulators that affect gene expression.
- Common orthopedic traits include hip and elbow dysplasia, rupture of the cranial cruciate ligament, patellar luxation, Legg-Calvé-Perthes disease, osteochondrosis, and osteosarcoma.
- Because they are inherited, registries for hip and elbow dysplasia are used to select breeding dogs, and thus to reduce the prevalence and severity of these traits, but they are either private or electively public, unlike some European registries in which all breeding dogs are included.
- Best current breeding practices rely on the application of deep pedigree information with orthopedic radiography and offspring follow-up, and, if available, estimated breeding values for hip and elbow dysplasia.
- Estimated breeding values for hip and elbow dysplasia measure the genetic orthopedic quality of a dog for transmission of its alleles to its offspring.

INTRODUCTION

Canine orthopedic traits (hip dysplasia, elbow dysplasia [ED], Legg-Calvé-Perthes disease [LCPD], patellar luxation, osteochondrosis [OCD], and rupture of the cranial cruciate ligament [CCL]) interrupt the structure or function of the articular surface of synovial joints, resulting in secondary osteoarthritis and joint-related pain and dysfunction. Osteoarthritis is a progressive disease of the entire synovial joint for which there is no specific antidote. Therefore, it seems prudent to take every opportunity to prevent these complex diseases. Complex diseases are the result of environmental risk factors

The authors have nothing to declare regarding this subject.
[a] Department of Biomedical Sciences, College of Veterinary Medicine, Cornell University, Ithaca, NY 14853, USA; [b] Department of Clinical Sciences, College of Veterinary Medicine, Cornell University, Ithaca, NY 14853, USA
* Corresponding author.
E-mail address: rjt2@cornell.edu

(eg, body weight, nutrition, growth rate) and a genetic component (multiple variants, each of which contribute to risk of developing the disease). One nongenetic factor that has been associated with increased risk of orthopedic disease, especially for hip dysplasia and rupture of the CCL, is early spay/neutering. The mechanism may be persistently elevated levels of luteinizing hormone affecting those tissues with luteinizing hormone receptors.[1] Body weight gain following neutering or spaying in large-breed dogs may also influence risk of orthopedic disease.[2] These effects seem less relevant in small-breed than in large-breed dogs and Hart and Hart[1] make the case for potential risk assessment for individual dogs. Nevertheless, without carrying the risk alleles or variants, no inherited trait can be expressed.

To prevent the transmission of disease-causing genetic variants from adults to puppies, one must first identify these genetic variants. Until they are discovered, we are left with visual inspection of pedigrees and radiographs of dogs in these pedigrees; progeny testing or at a minimum, interrogating owners about parental offspring orthopedic quality; application of estimated breeding values (EBVs) for hip dysplasia and ED; and/or genomic prediction of orthopedic genetic quality.

The public registry of the Orthopedic Foundation for Animals (OFA; https://ofa.org) is used to identify dogs seemingly free of hip dysplasia and ED. This approach to breeder selection, although useful, is inaccurate because a dog's genotype for a complex (polygenic) trait cannot be determined from its radiographic score (phenotype).[3] That is, a dog with an unaffected phenotype may carry trait-causing mutations but insufficient to cause overt trait expression. This characteristic of complex orthopedic traits, caused by the additive effects of many genetic variants, prevents the elimination of these traits from pure breed dogs and their hybrids.

The combination of pedigree relationships and radiographic scores of hips and elbows into a linear mixed statistical model is used to estimate the genetic quality of a dog in the form of EBVs for these orthopedic traits. A reference population, which has been genotyped and has EBVs for canine hip dysplasia (CHD) and ED, has been used to estimate genetic hip and/or elbow quality (genomic breeding values) of offspring based on the offspring genotypes in a research setting.[4] The prevalence and severity of CHD and ED is reduced when hip and elbow EBVs are used in closed breeding colonies.[5]

The OFA registry also includes records of less common complex orthopedic traits, such as LCPD, shoulder OCD, and patellar luxation. A common complex orthopedic trait, rupture of the CCL, is without a registry, yet Americans spend billions of dollars yearly having their dog's stifles stabilized following a CCL rupture. Here, we describe screening methods for orthopedic traits in registries that have been available to inform breeding decisions in the United States for decades, but these orthopedic traits persist because of their complex genetic underpinnings.

CANINE HIP DYSPLASIA

CHD is characterized by faulty conformation and laxity of the hip joint that often affects both hips. It is detected radiographically as subluxation between the femoral head and acetabulum and secondary osteoarthritis of the affected hip in older dogs (**Fig. 1**). The incipient synovitis, accompanied by effusion and perifoveal articular cartilage erosion, is not detectable radiographically. Additionally, subluxation of the femoral head from the acetabulum can be masked in the traditional extended-hip radiographic positioning used to image the hip for the OFA registry (see **Fig. 1**). Osteoarthritis is detected on a radiograph as osteophytes around the femoral head and enthesophytes at the capsular insertion on the femoral neck (Morgan's line) and acetabulum,

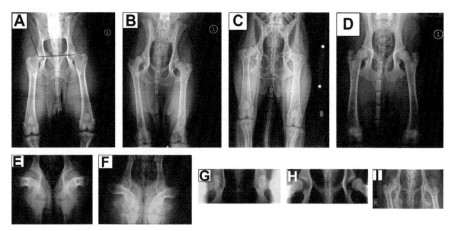

Fig. 1. (*A*) Ventrodorsal projection of the pelvis of a dog without evidence of hip dysplasia. The included angle drawn with the *black lines* is the Norberg angle. The higher the Norberg angle the better the hip conformation. (*B*) Ventrodorsal projection of the pelvis of a dog with bilateral hip subluxation, which is incontrovertible evidence of hip dysplasia. (*C*) Bilateral hip dysplasia and severe secondary osteoarthritis. All dogs were physically mature when the radiographs were taken. (*D*) Ventrodorsal projection of the pelvis of a 10-month-old dog with fair hip conformation. (*E*) The same dog as in *D* imaged in the dorsolateral subluxation ("kneeling") position. The femoral heads are subluxated bilaterally and therefore this dog has hip dysplasia, which is less evident in *D*. (*F*) Dog imaged in the dorsolateral subluxation position with normal hip conformation in which the femoral heads contact the medial acetabular wall at the fossa. (*G*) PennHIP distraction index radiographic projection of a dog with little maximum passive laxity. (*H*) PennHIP distraction index radiographic projection of a dog with passive laxity and likely hip dysplasia. I expect this dog and the dog represented in *E* to have positive Ortolani sign; a physical examination sign of an unstable and likely dysplastic hip in an adolescent or young dog and of which the OFA has no knowledge. (*I*) Ventrodorsal radiographic projection of an 11-month-old dog with right Legg-Calvé-Perthes disease.

accompanied by a flattening of the femoral head with a shallow acetabulum. Radiographic alterations are subtle in immature or mildly affected dogs.

Breed prevalence as estimated by the OFA varies from 1% to 75%, with the old English bulldog, pug, and bulldog the highest (worst) (https://ofa.org/diseases/disease_statistics/). The OFA does not receive all the normal or abnormal pelvic radiographs taken because the dog owner's veterinarian can evaluate them, nor are all those submitted for evaluation published in the OFA registry, likely resulting in a biased prevalence estimate. For the hip score based on the ventrodorsal, extended hip radiograph of the pelvis, heritability ranges between 0.2 and 0.3[6,7] and as high as 0.5 to 0.6 for the distraction index and dorsolateral subluxation (DLS) score[8,9] in closed populations.

Diagnosis

Reduction following manal coxofemoral subluxation may be palpable during physical examination in puppies and young dogs and is referred to as a positive Ortolani sign. Once the secondary osteoarthritis is established accompanied by fibrosis of the joint capsule, palpable hip laxity may be camouflaged. Any dog with a positive Ortolani sign has, or is susceptible to, CHD and breeding such a dog is ill advised. A negative Ortolani sign may mean that the hip is normal or the acetabulum is so shallow that the femoral head cannot be moved into or out of the acetabulum. Radiographic imaging is then necessary to confirm the hip conformation.

Since the 1960s, the OFA has provided a standard for radiographic evaluation of hips based on breed, age, and conformation. Similarities of the scores for the three major registries (OFA, European/Fédération Cynologique Internationale [FCI], and UK/Australasia) for scoring hip conformation in the ventrodorsal hip-extended position of the dog have been reported (**Tables 1** and **2**). In Switzerland, the numerical scoring system (see **Tables 1** and **2**) is only used within the dysplasia score group. The final numerical score per joint is then translated into the FCI scoring scheme A to E and it is this FCI score that is returned to the dog owner and the breed club (personal communication Mark Fluckiger, Zurich Switzerland, April 2023).

Under the OFA scheme, radiographs from dogs younger than 2 years of age are given a provisional assessment of hip status, whereas dogs 2 years or older are given a definitive hip evaluation. According to the OFA, the sensitivity of the OFA radiograph at 12 months of age for later development of osteoarthritis in affected hips ranges from 77% to 99% depending on the severity of the CHD at the earlier age, whereas 89% of hip evaluations between 4 and 23 months were the same as the 24-month-old or older age hip scores.[10] Others have shown that of all dogs developing hip osteoarthritis over their life span (assuming that hip osteoarthritis is the gold standard for antecedent CHD), only 55% had radiographic evidence of a CHD at 2 years of age.[11] Hip status is graded on a scale from "excellent" conformation to "severe" hip dysplasia; there are seven grades in all. If the focus is to control CHD, dogs with OFA hip scores of excellent, good, or fair hip conformation are the ones suitable for breeding and, even then, affected puppies can result because of the complex genetic underpinnings.

The PennHIP radiographic method measures the maximum amount of lateral passive hip joint laxity (distraction index).[12] There is a positive relationship between the distraction index and subsequent development of osteoarthritis. The PennHIP series of images entails an OFA-style ventrodorsal radiograph, a "compression" radiograph, and a "distraction" radiograph. The PennHIP registry reports back to the owner and the submitting veterinarian, an individual dog's distraction index relative to the average for the breed. Labrador retrievers with a low distraction index (less than 0.3) at 8 months of age have about a 90% chance of being normal, whereas those with a distraction index greater than 0.8 have about a 90% chance of being dysplastic (and succumbing to secondary hip osteoarthritis). Dogs with an index of 0.5 have about a 50% chance of being dysplastic. Therefore, when choosing between dogs for breeding, preferentially breed the dogs in the lower half of the distraction index range for the breed. The best age for PennHIP screening is at early maturity (6–8 months of age) and before breeding. A thorough comparison of the OFA and Penn-HIP methods is found in Reagan.[13]

The DLS score measures the proportion of the femoral head covered by the dorsal acetabular rim with the dog imaged in a "kneeling" and sternal position to mimic the normal standing position of the coxofemoral (hip) joints (see **Fig. 1**).[14] As the DLS score drops below 50% in young Labrador retrievers, they become positive for the Ortolani sign.[14] At 8 months of age, the sensitivity and specificity of the OFA-like radiograph was 38% and 96%, respectively, for the distraction index (values of >0.7 considered abnormal) was 50% and 89%, respectively, and for the DLS score (scores <55% were considered abnormal) was 83% and 84%, respectively, for secondary coxofemoral osteoarthritis.[15] For a single test, the DLS score is the most accurate in detection of affected and unaffected dogs.[16] In a closed dog colony, a combination of the DLS score and the Norberg angle gave the best estimate of a dog's likelihood of developing subsequent osteoarthritis.[16] The Norberg angle is a measure of femoral

Table 1
Hip screening methods based on the ventrodorsal, hip-extended projection across the major national registries using this system

FCI	Germany (Except Society for German Shepherd Dogs)	Germany (Society for German Shepherd Dogs)	United Kingdom, Australia, New Zealand (Worst Joint)	Switzerland (Worst Joint)	United States (OFA) Each Joint
A, Normal	A1	a, Normal	0	0	Excellent
	A2	a, Normal	1–3	1–2	Good
B, Borderline	B1	a, Fast normal	4–6	3–4	Good
	B2	a, Fast normal	7–8	5–6	Fair
C, Mild	C1	a, Noch zugelassen[a]	9–12	7–9	Borderline[b]
	C2	a, Noch zugelassen	13–18	10–12	Mild
D, Moderate	D1	D1	>18	13–15	Moderate
	D2	D2		16–18	Moderate
E, Severe	E1	E1		19–21	Severe
	E2	E2		22–24	Severe

[a] Noch zugelassen: German, but internationally understood expression "tolerated for breeding."
[b] Correct scoring not possible. Recheck after 6 months recommended.

From Fluckiger M: Scoring radiographs for canine hip dysplasia – the big three organizations in the world. Europ J Comp Anim Pract - Vol. 17 - Issue 2 October 2007 with permission.[72] Slight modifications have been made to the Swiss scoring system recently (https://www.fci.be/en/FCI-Scientific-Commission-71.html)

Table 2
Comparison of international hip scoring methods according to the orthopedic foundation for animals

OFA	FCI (Europe)	BVA/Kennel Club (UK/AU) (Score = Sum of Both Hips)	SV (Germany)
Excellent	A-1	0–4 (no >3/hip)	a, Normal
Good	A-2	5–10 (no >6/hip)	a, Normal
Fair	B-1	11–18	a, Near normal
Borderline	B-2	19–25	a, Noch zugelassen
Moderate	D	36–50	Moderate HD
Severe	E	51–106	Severe HD

From Fluckiger M: Scoring radiographs for canine hip dysplasia – the big three organizations in the world. Europ J Comp Anim Pract - Vol. 17 - Issue 2 October 2007 with permission.72

head coverage on the OFA-style extended hip radiograph. The Norberg angle ranges from 70° to 120° (see **Fig. 1**). An angle greater than 105° is preferable for breeding practices, but in one study was greater than 112° to be unequivocally phenotypically normal.[17]

ELBOW DYSPLASIA

Lameness localized to the elbow of young growing dogs, without history of trauma, is frequently a result of ED. This syndrome comprises ununited anconeal process, fragmented medial coronoid process (FCP), OCD of the medial humeral condyle, flexor enthesopathy or ununited medial epicondyle, and asynchronous growth between the radius and ulna.

Diagnosis

Examination of the dog shows a tendency toward a stiff, choppy gait characterized by external rotation of the distal forelimb. ED is bilateral in 20% to 50% of cases but usually one elbow is more affected than the other so that lameness in one limb may predominate or the lameness may shift from one forelimb to the other. In Labrador retrievers, heritability of elbow osteoarthritis secondary to OCD or FCP was estimated at 0.27.[18] A heritable basis for elbow OCD in rottweilers and golden retrievers has been reported. Other breeds that are at higher risk are the Bernese mountain dog, German shepherd, saint Bernard, great Dane, and the Newfoundland dog.[19–21] The OFA maintains an elbow registry similar to that for CHD and requires submission of a flexed lateral radiograph at 2 years of age, or older, for elbow morphologic certification.

On clinical examination, pain is elicited by internal and external rotation of the elbow with the carpus held in a flexed position or on elbow extension. Effusion may be present as an outpouching of the lateral elbow capsule, caudal to the lateral epicondyle, underneath the anconeus muscle. Detection of elbow pain in young dogs should be followed up with radiography, or preferably computed tomography, if surgical treatment is considered. FCP is difficult to directly identify on standard orthogonal radiographs (**Fig. 2**).

Juvenile large dogs, especially the German shepherd dog, are affected by ununited anconeal process (see **Fig. 2**). Etiologies include genetic, hormonal, metabolic, nutritional, traumatic, or OCD.[6,22,23] A separate center of anconeal ossification has been documented in some large breeds. The usual time of fusion of the anconeal process to the ulna is 4 to 5 months of age, or later in giant breeds.[24] The condition is bilateral in

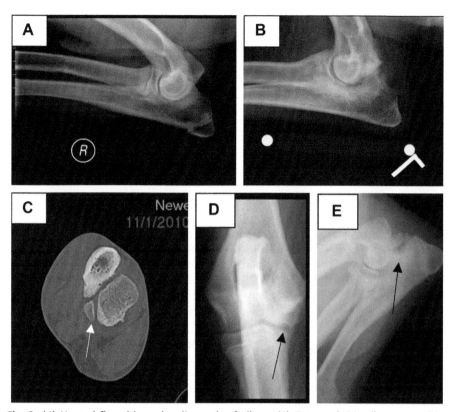

Fig. 2. (*A*) Normal flexed lateral radiograph of elbow. (*B*) Osteoarthritic elbow caused by elbow dysplasia. The *circular markers* are an internal size standard of 100 mm length. (*C*) Coronal computed tomography showing ununited medial coronoid process (the most common form of elbow dysplasia, *arrow*) and secondary osteoarthritis with osteophytosis and sclerosis of the medial coronoid bed and radial head. (*D*) OCD lesion (*arrow*) on articular surface of the medial humeral condyle. (*E*) Ununited anconeal process (*arrow*) on a flexed elbow radiograph.

approximately one-third of dogs. The flexed lateral radiographic view is helpful for diagnosis. Secondary osteoarthritis is evident radiographically if the animal is old enough.

FCP is the most common developmental condition affecting elbows of growing dogs, especially of retrievers, rottweilers, and German shepherd dogs (see **Fig. 2**). Heritability of ED (mostly attributable to FCP) seems to be approximately 0.2[25] but can be higher depending on the breed and pedigree used in the estimation. Cause of FCP is controversial[26]; it is more common in male dogs and often bilateral. Elbow incongruity from asynchronous growth between radius, ulna, and humerus that results in a shortened radius and longer ulna, or vice versa, may lead to FCP. The classic radiographic fingerprint signs of FCP are sclerosis of subchondral bone beneath the coronoid processes; osteophytes on the medial coronoid process and cranial radial head; and entheses along the dorsal olecranon, caudal to the anconeus, where the joint capsule attaches. Orthogonal radiographs of the elbow are preferable to a single projection to gain the clearest picture of articular bony anatomy.

The clinical signs of medial humeral OCD are similar to those of FCP and sometimes the two conditions occur in the same joint (see **Fig. 2**). The diagnosis is made radiographically based on subchondral lucency of the medial humeral condyle or, occasionally, a flap of articular cartilage with some mineralized tissue is seen with a separation from the subchondral bone on the cranial caudal radiographic projection.

As with CHD, because of the voluntary nature of reporting dogs affected with ED, the OFA registry is assumed to be biased. However, the breeds that have the highest disease frequency in the OFA database are the chow chow, followed by the American bully, rottweiler, bulldog, pug, and boerboel (https://ofa.org/).

MEDIAL PATELLAR LUXATION

Generally, medial patellar luxation occurs in small or miniature breeds. Lateral patellar luxation occurs more commonly in large breeds but large-breed dogs can also develop medial patellar luxation. Dogs present to veterinarians with intermittent lameness when the patella luxates spontaneously to chronic lameness and disability for irreducible patellar luxations. Radiographs are helpful to assess accompanying long bone deformities but the definitive diagnosis is made by palpation. The OFA maintains a database for medial patellar luxation based on physical examination. Heritability of patellar luxation (predominantly medial direction) was reported as 0.17 to 0.44 in three different dog breeds (Dutch kookier, flat-coated retriever, and Thai Pomeranian) across two continents.[27–29]

CRANIAL CRUCIATE LIGAMENT RUPTURE

Rupture of the CCL is a common cause of hind limb lameness in dogs. Most dogs with CCL rupture have a chronic course, without a distinct history of contact trauma. Diagnosis is made by direct palpation of instability and radiography of affected stifles. Breeds predisposed to CCL rupture include the Newfoundland, Labrador retriever, rottweiler, chow chow, and mastiff, but any breed and mixed breed dog can suffer a damaged CCL. The Newfoundland breed has a heritability of 0.27 for CCL rupture[30] and the Labrador retriever has a heritability estimate of 0.48 to 0.89.[31,32]

OSTEOCHONDROSIS (OTHER THAN OF THE MEDIAL HUMERAL CONDYLE)

OCD is a well-described, but incompletely understood, systemic disease of endochondral ossification. Dogs usually develop articular cartilage flap-like lesions with the caudal humeral head as the most common location. Various causes have been proposed including traumatic, vascular, genetic, endocrine/sex hormonal, conformational, and nutritional/environmental. Shoulder OCD has been estimated to have a heritability of 0.5 to 0.7 in Labrador retrievers.[33] In rottweilers and Bernese mountain dogs, heritability of OCD was reported as 0.1 and 0.45, respectively.[33–35] Males outnumber female dogs in incidence and the condition is bilateral in 20% to 85% of cases.

The diagnosis is based on clinical signs, palpation, and radiography (see **Fig. 1**). Plain lateral shoulder radiographs may reveal evidence of an osteochondritis dissecans flap or piece of cartilage. Computed tomography can provide the definitive diagnosis. Both the medial and lateral femoral condyles are affected by OCD but the lateral condyle may be affected more often. The talar ridges are affected by OCD in young growing dogs. Older dogs with enlarged hocks may have suffered from talar OCD at a young age and later, the secondary osteoarthritis results in large crepitant hocks with reduced range of motion.

LEGG-CALVÉ-PERTHES DISEASE

Hip pain in immature toy and small-breed dogs may be caused by LCPD, or aseptic necrosis of the femoral head (see **Fig. 1**). The clinical signs develop between 4 and 11 months of age and the condition is often unilateral and the diagnosis is confirmed radiographically. Histologic findings suggest that the disease is a result of infarction of epiphyseal and metaphyseal bone but the cause is still unknown. Compared with mixed-breed dogs, odds ratios for developing this trait range from 4.8 in dachshunds to 191.4 in Australian shepherds with odds ratios for the trait in cairn terriers, Chihuahua, Lhasa Apso, miniature pinscher, miniature poodle, toy poodle, West Highland white terrier, and Yorkshire terrier breeds lying between these odds.[35] The heritability of LCPD is approximately 0.8 in an experimental pedigree of Manchester terriers.[36] However, in this pedigree and a toy poodle pedigree,[37] neither a major locus with incomplete penetrance nor an autosomal-recessive mode of inheritance could be excluded.

COMPLEX TRAIT GENETICS

Complex orthopedic traits are controlled by mutations in at least several genes, called quantitative trait loci, and whose expression is affected by environmental regulators.[38] The interaction of these mutations with each other and nongenetic factors (eg, plane of nutrition, growth rate, neuter status, and exercise level) influence the final clinical (phenotypic) expression of each trait. Estimates suggest that 70% of the mutations responsible for these traits are not in coding (exonic) regions but are in regulatory regions, which affect gene expression. The entire genetic cause of complex orthopedic traits in dogs is unknown. One gene, *fibrillin 2*, has a deletion that segregates with CHD across several breeds.[39] These orthopedic traits are quantitative in nature, that is, they are expressed on a continuum from imperceptible to severe forms. They have heritabilities of about 0.2 to 0.7 depending on how and at what stage of development the trait is measured, and the size and extent of the pedigree where the heritability was estimated. A trait that was only caused by genetics would have a heritability of 1.

GENOME-WIDE ASSOCIATION STUDIES FOR COMPLEX ORTHOPEDIC TRAIT PHENOTYPES

Although the gold standard would be to sequence the entire genome of dogs of interest, a more cost-effective method is to genotype each case and control dog at single-nucleotide polymorphisms (SNPs) using a genotyping array. Current canine arrays include the canineHD 173k and 220k arrays (Illumina, San Diego, CA) and the Axiom 670k array (Affymetrix, Santa Clara, CA). These genotyping data from multiple phenotyped dogs are commonly used in a genome-wide association study (GWAS) to identify SNPs that are associated with the phenotype of interest. Significant associations point researchers to a region of the genome that harbors a variant that increases (or decreases) risk for the particular disease.

There have been many GWAS studies focusing on the genetics underlying CHD to identify the genes that affect hip conformation. Loci contributing to CHD have been identified on chromosomes 1, 3, 4, 7, 8, 9, 10, 12, 14, 15, 18, 19, 20, 21, 24, 26, 28, 34, 36, and 37, but there is poor overlap in the identified loci between independent studies.[40–47] Reasons why these studies have different results include the multiple ways to measure or score the CHD phenotype, inclusion of different breeds and populations, and use of some genotyping arrays that may not tag all causative variants.

However, some progress has been made to validate previously identified loci. Mikkola and colleagues[48] executed a validation study of 46 genetic markers in a cohort of nearly 1600 dogs from 10 different breeds comprised of Finnish Lapphund, golden retriever, Lagotto Romagnolo, Samoyed, Bernese mountain dog, Spanish water dog, great Dane, Labrador retriever, Karelian bear dog, and Finnish hound. Dogs were categorized into cases and control animals according to the hip scoring system defined by the FCI. Twenty-one different loci on 14 chromosomes were validated for their association. Twenty of these were associated with CHD in specific breeds, whereas one locus was unique to the across-breed study.

A GWAS of 174 Bernese mountain dogs identified four SNPs on CFA11 and 27 that were significantly associated with ED[40] and a later study identified significant loci for ED on CFA1 and 26, which affects risk in Labrador retrievers and German shepherds, and in golden retrievers and English setters, respectively.[41]

For CCL rupture, associated loci on chromosomes 1, 3, 4, 6, 7, 8, 9, 11, 18, 20, 21, 22, 23, 24, 26, 27, 29, 30, and 33 have been identified across many breeds in linear mixed single marker, multimarker, and Bayesian models[31,42,49–52] but the variants are not segregating in all breeds. For example, Huang and colleagues[42] identified three significantly associated SNPs segregating only in Labrador retriever, golden retriever, and German shepherd dogs. Most recently, the Comparative Orthopedic Research Lab at the University of Wisconsin has extended their genetic mapping associations into a multimarker genetic test to identify Labrador retrievers at risk of developing CCL (https://www.vetmed.wisc.edu/lab/corl/canine-genetic-testing/).

Three studies to discover variants associated with medial patellar luxation have been reported by the same group. A locus on CFA13 was associated with the trait in pomeranians,[29] on CFA7 in flat coated retrievers,[28] and on CFA3 in Dutch kooiker dogs.[27]

For canine LCPD, the gene *collagen type II alpha 1 chain* (COL2A1), which is reported to encode a mutation that segregates with LCPD in humans, has been excluded as a candidate gene,[53] but no other associations have yet been identified.

The major challenges facing successful GWAS for complex diseases are sample size and variant (marker) density. Simulations have shown that to detect moderate effect size loci for a canine complex trait, 500 to 1000 cases and 500 to 1000 control animals are needed, and power to detect an association increases with an increase in array density.[41]

More recently, GWAS studies have progressed to use imputed genotypes derived from a reference panel of whole genome sequences (WGS).[52,54–56] Imputation using a WGS reference panel has been performed for at least one orthopedic trait, CCL rupture.[52] The use of imputation allows an increase in the number of variants queried genome-wide, thus improving the likelihood that at least one variant is in linkage disequilibrium with the causal variant. A more cost-effective and accurate method for increasing variants to include in GWAS studies is to use low-pass WGS followed by imputation. This means the genome is sequenced to only about 1X coverage, allowing the inclusion of many more samples in a single sequencing run. This also means that all variants are directly queried and there is no genotyping array bias. This methodology of low-pass WGS followed by imputation has not yet been used for canine orthopedic traits.

Publicly available canine genomic resources have recently improved with more than 2000 whole genomes sequenced as part of the dog10k project[57] and new reference genome assemblies created using long-range sequencing technologies (canFam4, 5, 6).[58–60] The complexity of genetic mapping of the three most important canine spontaneous complex orthopedic diseases was recently extended to the use of breed-based statistics[61] for genetic mapping as an extension of fixed trait mapping for body size loci in dogs. For GWAS, individual unphenotyped dogs with high-coverage WGS data were assigned the breed prevalence of the trait and/or categorized into case and control based on high and low breed prevalence.[61] This approach circumvents the problem of combing public data for genotypes and phenotypes in that individual disease phenotypes are often lacking in repository data. Categorical GWAS was able to validate CHD candidate loci. Additionally, novel candidate loci and genes for CHD, ED, and CCL were discovered. These authors concluded that categorical GWAS of ancestral dog populations may contribute to the understanding of any disease for which breed epidemiologic risk data are available, including diseases for which GWAS has not been performed and candidate loci remain elusive.

ESTIMATED BREEDING VALUES FOR GENETIC QUALITY FOR COMPLEX ORTHOPEDIC TRAITS

In comparison with selecting breeding animals by phenotype, in which potentially deleterious alleles go undetected, its EBV provides an assessment of an individual dog's genetic risk for disease. In a UK study of 15 dog breeds, EBVs were shown to be 1.16 and 1.34 times more accurate for estimating the probability of CHD and ED, respectively, than selection using parental radiographs. More importantly, EBVs were 3 to 13 times more likely to be accurate for predicting CHD and ED, respectively, in immature animals when both parental phenotypes were available.[62]

In our most recent collaboration with the OFA, we used a bivariate (CHD and ED analyzed jointly) mixed linear model to derive hip and elbow EBVs of individual dogs in the OFA registry between 1974 and 2015 (Wagner, Packer, Todhunter, unpublished data 2018). CHD and ED EBVs for 1,796,711 dogs were obtained and compared with the public-only data of 1,055,270 unique dogs with 1,032,219 CHD records for 130 breeds and 243,147 ED records for 44 breeds. Bivariate CHD and ED model parameters were fitted using the same DMU software as in Hou and colleagues.[7] The heritability of hip and elbow scores was 0.42 and 0.22, respectively.

Over time, there was a trend showing decreased phenotypic scores for ED (**Fig. 3**). This decrease in phenotypic ED score is consistent with the decrease in mean EBV for ED score per year. Lower (better) breeding values implied that the random effect of the animal reduced (improved) predicted phenotypic scores. Despite reporting bias, the mean phenotypic score and EBVs steadily decreased, suggesting that elbow quality is slowly improving over time, reflecting genetic gain in the breeding of dogs in the United States. Similarly, the CHD EBVs steadily decreased, indicating slow genetic gain in the breeding of dogs for better hip quality (see **Fig. 3**). Inbreeding coefficients ranged from 0% to 1.83%. Thus, public registries can help control the prevalence and severity of complex orthopedic traits and the EBVs are only as accurate as the phenotypic and pedigree information provided to the model. The British Veterinary Association Canine Health Scheme provides publicly available EBVs for CHD and ED for all dogs in their Health Scheme registry (https://www.bva.co.uk/canine-health-schemes), a valuable service currently lacking in the United States.

GENOMIC PREDICTION OF CANINE HIP DYSPLASIA AND RUPTURE OF THE CRANIAL CRUCIATE LIGAMENT

Genomic prediction, in which many SNPs or variants are used to predict a phenotype, could be used to assist purchase and breeding decisions when accurate deep pedigree information and accompanying phenotypic data are not available. Previous empirical studies have indicated that the genomic prediction of CHD is feasible in a single purebred population[63] and a limited number of multiple breeds.[64] However, there are several limitations to the implementation of genomic prediction including sample size, multiple susceptible breeds, and unknown genetic relationships. The

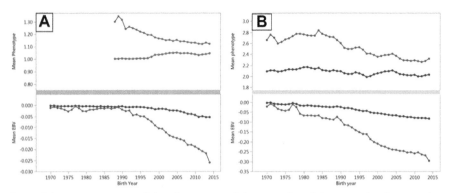

Fig. 3. (*A*) Trend over time of the elbow scores (phenotype) and their EBV for the complete (*blue*) and public-only (*red*) records of the Orthopedic Foundation for Animals. A decreasing mean indicates better elbow radiographic appearance and better genetic quality for this orthopedic trait is indicated by a decreasing EBV for ED. (*B*) Trend over time of the hip scores and their estimated breeding values for the complete (*blue*) and public-only (*red*) records of the Orthopedic Foundation for Animals. A decreasing mean indicates better hip radiographic appearance and better genetic quality for this orthopedic trait is indicated by a decreasing EBV for CHD. The entire data set shows stronger evidence for a reduction in hip and elbow dysplasia rather than the public-only data (Wagner, Packer, Todhunter, unpublished data 2018).

genetic relatedness among genotyped individuals may affect the accuracy of prediction, especially when models based on a genetic relationship matrix, such as the mixed linear model, are used for prediction.[65]

Genomic prediction of CCL rupture in the Labrador retriever has been investigated using a range of Bayesian models and machine learning.[66] Genotype data were used from a total of 622 dogs. The inclusion of covariates (sex, neuter status, body weight) improved prediction accuracy, and the Bayesian and machine learning models performed similarly.[66]

Recently, we investigated the accuracy of genomic prediction in 842 unique dogs from six breeds, with hip and stifle phenotypes genotyped on a customized Illumina high-density 183k SNP array[41] and also analyzed using an imputed dataset of 20,487,155 SNPs. To implement genomic prediction, two different statistical methods were used: Genomic Best Linear Unbiased Prediction and a Bayesian method called BayesC.[67] The cross-validation results showed that the two methods gave similar prediction accuracy (correlation coefficient of 0.3–0.4) for CHD (measured as the Norberg angle) and rupture of the CCL, in the multibreed population.

This report suggested that genomic prediction of CHD and rupture of the CCL with DNA array genotype data is feasible in a multiple breed population. Albeit these traits have heritability of about one-third, higher accuracy is needed to implement in a natural population and predicting a complex phenotype will require a much larger number of dogs within a breed and across breeds. It is possible that with higher accuracy, genomic prediction of these orthopedic traits could be implemented in the selection of dogs for breeding.

CURRENT RECOMMENDATIONS

Until the mutations conferring risk for these complex orthopedic traits are discovered and available for the public to test the breeding population, EBVs for CHD and ED when applied to make informed breeding decisions for individual breeds remain the

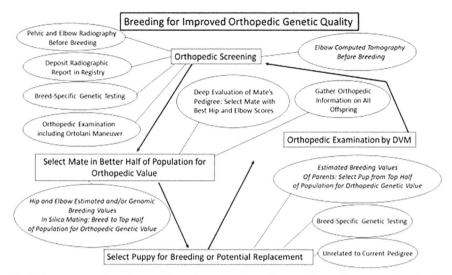

Fig. 4. Process to select dogs with optimum orthopedic genetic quality. At each cycle, the goal is to improve the orthopedic genetic value of the breeding dogs in a kennel and of the offspring. Boxes with nonitalicized lettering are available in the United States now. Boxes with italics are available in other countries, such as the United Kingdom, but could be available here with adequate funding.

most effective tool for breeder selection (**Fig. 4**). However, these are only available in the UK Kennel Club and in closed/private breeding colonies where dogs are bred for specific service work. No such tools are available for any other complex orthopedic trait. Genomic breeding values based on reference populations that have been genotyped and have EBVs has potential to revolutionize dog breeding. Higher selection response may be achieved using genomic breeding values compared with using EBVs[68–70] suggesting that genomic selection would therefore be the method of choice to improve hip conformation most efficiently. It would have special use in small breeding programs for which breeders do not have deep and extended pedigrees on which to estimate breeding values because the pool of reference individuals for a breed would house the genetic information needed for any dog of the same breed. Even after 60 years of controlled breeding in Sweden, a recent study suggests that further improvement in hip conformation is likely to rely on EBV and genomic selection.[71] Even when EBVs for hip conformation are applied in closed colonies, such as the Seeing Eye Foundation, CHD still occurs, leading the authors to suggest that genomic approaches are needed for maximum impact on trait severity and prevalence.[5] Nevertheless, until molecular genetic approaches like this are taken to reduce the incidence of these complex orthopedic traits, visual inspection of entire pedigrees to select breeders accompanied by follow-up to identify the results of all breeding pairs remains the only method to identify the dogs with the best genetic value, but it is fraught with errors because of the nature of complex trait genetics (see **Fig. 4**).

CLINICS CARE POINTS

- Gold standard for diagnosis is imaging: radiograph for CHD, LCPD, and osteochondrosis; computed tomography scan for ED; palpation for luxated patella.

- Because these are complex genetic traits, selection for breeding should include appropriate screening and removal of dogs exhibiting the more extreme versions of these traits from the breeding pool.
- Evaluation of orthopedic diseases in pedigrees by eye is an inexact science.
- Application of estimated breeding values for these orthopedic traits is ideal but likely will require the involvement of geneticists and regular updating of the genetic value of offspring.

REFERENCES

1. Hart LA, Hart BL. An ancient practice but a new paradigm: personal choice for the age to spay or neuter a dog. Front Vet Sci 2021;8:603257.
2. Oberbauer AM, Belanger JM, Famula TR. A review of the impact of neuter status on expression of inherited conditions in dogs. Front Vet Sci 2019;6:397.
3. Zhang Z, Zhu L, Sandler J, et al. Estimation of heritabilities, genetic correlations, and breeding values of four traits that collectively define hip dysplasia in dogs. Am J Vet Res 2009;70(4):483–92.
4. Leighton EA. Genetics of canine hip dysplasia. J Am Vet Med Assoc 1997; 210(10):1474–9.
5. Leighton EA, Holle D, Biery DN, et al. Genetic improvement of hip-extended scores in 3 breeds of guide dogs using estimated breeding values: notable progress but more improvement is needed. PLoS One 2019;14(2):e0212544.
6. Breur GJ, Lambrechts NE, Todhunter RJ. The genetics of canine orthopaedic traits. 2nd edition. Wallingford, UK: CABI; 2012. p. 136–60.
7. Hou Y, Wang Y, Lust G, et al. Retrospective analysis for genetic improvement of hip joints of cohort labrador retrievers in the United States: 1970-2007. PLoS One 2010;5(2):e9410.
8. Todhunter RJ, Bliss SP, Casella G, et al. Genetic structure of susceptibility traits for hip dysplasia and microsatellite informativeness of an outcrossed canine pedigree. J Hered 2003;94(1):39–48.
9. Tikekar A, Soo M, Lopez-Villalobos N, et al. Provisional heritability estimates of four distraction index traits in a breeding population of German Shepherd dogs. N Z Vet J 2018;66(6):319–24.
10. Corley EA. Role of the Orthopedic Foundation for Animals in the control of canine hip dysplasia. Vet Clin North Am Small Anim Pract 1992;22(3):579–93.
11. Smith GK, Lawler DF, Biery DN, et al. Chronology of hip dysplasia development in a cohort of 48 Labrador retrievers followed for life. Vet Surg 2012;41(1):20–33.
12. Runge JJ, Kelly SP, Gregor TP, et al. Distraction index as a risk factor for osteoarthritis associated with hip dysplasia in four large dog breeds. J Small Anim Pract 2010;51(5):264–9.
13. Reagan JK. Canine hip dysplasia screening within the United States: Pennsylvania Hip Improvement Program and Orthopedic Foundation for Animals Hip/Elbow Database. Vet Clin North Am Small Anim Pract 2017;47(4):795–805.
14. Farese JP, Todhunter RJ, Lust G, et al. Dorsolateral subluxation of hip joints in dogs measured in a weight-bearing position with radiography and computed tomography. Vet Surg 1998;27(5):393–405.
15. Lust G, Todhunter RJ, Erb HN, et al. Comparison of three radiographic methods for diagnosis of hip dysplasia in eight-month-old dogs. J Am Vet Med Assoc 2001;219(9):1242–6.

16. Todhunter RJ, Grohn YT, Bliss SP, et al. Evaluation of multiple radiographic predictors of cartilage lesions in the hip joints of eight-month-old dogs. Am J Vet Res 2003;64(12):1472–8.
17. Gaspar AR, Hayes G, Ginja C, et al. The Norberg angle is not an accurate predictor of canine hip conformation based on the distraction index and the dorsolateral subluxation score. Prev Vet Med 2016;135:47–52.
18. Studdert VP, Lavelle RB, Beilharz RG, et al. Clinical features and heritability of osteochondrosis of the elbow in labrador retrievers. J Small Anim Pract 1991; 32(11):557–63.
19. Ubbink GJ, Van De Broek J, Hazewinkel HAW, et al. Prediction of the genetic risk for fragmented coronoid process in Labrador retrievers. Vet Rec 2000;147(6): 149–52.
20. Mäki K, Liinamo AE, Ojala M. Estimates of genetic parameters for hip and elbow dysplasia in Finnish Rottweilers. J Anim Sci 2000;78(5):1141–8.
21. Janutta V, Hamann H, Klein S, et al. Genetic analysis of three different classification protocols for the evaluation of elbow dysplasia in German shepherd dogs. J Small Anim Pract 2006;47(2):75–82.
22. Breur G., Lust G., Todhunter R.J., Genetics of hip dysplasia and other orthopedic traits. In: The Genetics of the Dog. Ruvinsky A., Sampson J., eds CAB International: Wallingford, Oxon, UK, 2001, 267–298.
23. Vezzoni A, Benjamino K. Canine elbow dysplasia: ununited anconeal process, osteochondritis dissecans, and medial coronoid process disease. Vet Clin North Am Small Anim Pract 2021;51(2):439–74.
24. Breit S, Künzel W, Seiler S. Variation in the ossification process of the anconeal and medial coronoid processes of the canine ulna. Res Vet Sci 2004;77(1):9–16.
25. Lavrijsen ICM, Heuven HCM, Voorhout G, et al. Phenotypic and genetic evaluation of elbow dysplasia in Dutch Labrador retrievers, golden retrievers, and Bernese mountain dogs. Vet J 2012;193(2):486–92.
26. Michelsen J. Canine elbow dysplasia: aetiopathogenesis and current treatment recommendations. Vet J 2013;196(1):12–9.
27. Wangdee C, Leegwater PAJ, Heuven HCM, et al. Prevalence and genetics of patellar luxation in Kooiker dogs. Vet J 2014;201(3):333–7.
28. Lavrijsen ICM, Leegwater PAJ, Wangdee C, et al. Genome-wide survey indicates involvement of loci on canine chromosomes 7 and 31 in patellar luxation in flat-coated retrievers. BMC Genet 2014;15:64.
29. Wangdee C, Leegwater PAJ, Heuven HCM, et al. Population genetic analysis and genome-wide association study of patellar luxation in a Thai population of Pomeranian dogs. Res Vet Sci 2017;111:9–13.
30. Wilke VL, Conzemius MG, Kinghorn BP, et al. Inheritance of rupture of the cranial cruciate ligament in Newfoundlands. J Am Vet Med Assoc 2006;228(1):61–4.
31. Baker LA, Kirkpatrick B, Rosa GJM, et al. Genome-wide association analysis in dogs implicates 99 loci as risk variants for anterior cruciate ligament rupture. PLoS One 2017;12(4):e0173810, 1027.
32. Cook SR, Conzemius MG, McCue ME, et al. SNP-based heritability and genetic architecture of cranial cruciate ligament rupture in Labrador retrievers. Anim Genet 2020;51(5):824–8.
33. Guthrie S, Pidduck HG. Heritability of elbow osteochondrosis within a closed population of dogs. J Small Anim Pract 1990;31(2):93–6.
34. Thomson M, Robins G. Osteochondrosis of the elbow: a review of the pathogenesis and a new approach to treatment. Aust Vet J 1995;72(10):375–8.

35. LaFond E, Breur GJ, Austin CC. Breed susceptibility for developmental orthopedic diseases in dogs. J Am Anim Hosp Assoc 2002;38(5):467–77.
36. Vasseur PB, Foley P, Stevenson S, et al. Mode of inheritance of Perthes' disease in Manchester terriers. Clin Orthop Rel Res 1989;244:281–92.
37. Pidduck H, Webbon PM. The genetic control of Perthes' disease in toy poodles: a working hypothesis. J Small Anim Pract 1978;19(1–12):729–33.
38. Baker L, Muir P, Sample SJ. Genome-wide association studies and genetic testing: understanding the science, success, and future of a rapidly developing field. J Am Vet Med Assoc 2019;255(10):1126–36.
39. Friedenberg SG, Zhu L, Zhang Z, et al. Evaluation of a fibrillin 2 gene haplotype associated with hip dysplasia and incipient osteoarthritis in dogs. Am J Vet Res 2011;72(4):530–40.
40. Pfahler S, Distl O. Identification of quantitative trait loci (QTL) for canine hip dysplasia and canine elbow dysplasia in Bernese mountain dogs. PLoS One 2012;7(11):e49782.
41. Hayward JJ, Castelhano MG, Oliveira KC, et al. Complex disease and phenotype mapping in the domestic dog. Nat Commun 2016;7:10460.
42. Huang M, Hayward JJ, Corey E, et al. A novel iterative mixed model to remap three complex orthopedic traits in dogs. PLoS One 2017;12(6):e0176932.
43. Fels L, Distl O. Identification and validation of quantitative trait loci (QTL) for canine hip dysplasia (CHD) in German shepherd dogs. PLoS One 2014;9(5):e96618.
44. Sánchez-Molano E, Woolliams JA, Pong-Wong R, et al. Quantitative trait loci mapping for canine hip dysplasia and its related traits in UK Labrador Retrievers. BMC Genom 2014;15(1):833.
45. Bartolomé N, Segarra S, Artieda M, et al. A genetic predictive model for canine hip dysplasia: integration of genome wide association study (GWAS) and candidate gene approaches. PLoS One 2015;10(4):e0122558.
46. Mikkola L, Holopainen S, Pessa-Morikawa T, et al. Genetic dissection of canine hip dysplasia phenotypes and osteoarthritis reveals three novel loci. BMC Genom 2019;20(1):1027.
47. Kang JM, Seo D, Lee SH, et al. Genome-wide association study to identify canine hip dysplasia loci in dogs. J Anim Sci Technol 2020;62(3):306–12.
48. Mikkola L, Kyöstilä K, Donner J, et al. An across-breed validation study of 46 genetic markers in canine hip dysplasia. BMC Genom 2021;22(1).
49. Baird AEG, Carter SD, Innes JF, et al. Genome-wide association study identifies genomic regions of association for cruciate ligament rupture in Newfoundland dogs. Anim Genet 2014;45(4):542–9.
50. Baird AEG, Carter SD, Innes JF, et al. Genetic basis of cranial cruciate ligament rupture (CCLR) in dogs. Connect Tissue Res 2014;55(4):275–81.
51. Baker LA, Rosa GJM, Hao Z, et al. Multivariate genome-wide association analysis identifies novel and relevant variants associated with anterior cruciate ligament rupture risk in the dog model. BMC Genet 2018;19(1):39.
52. Hayward JJ, White ME, Boyle M, et al. Imputation of canine genotype array data using 365 whole-genome sequences improves power of genome-wide association studies. PLoS Genet 2019;15(9):e1008003.
53. Starr-Moss AN, Nowend KL, Alling KM, et al. Exclusion of COL2A1 in canine Legg-Calvé-Perthes disease. Anim Genet 2012;43(1):112–3.
54. Friedenberg SG, Meurs KM. Genotype imputation in the domestic dog. Mamm Genome 2016;27(9–10):485–94.

55. Piras IS, Perdigones N, Zismann V, et al. Identification of genetic susceptibility factors associated with canine gastric dilatation-volvulus. Genes 2020;11(11):1–19.
56. Srikanth K, von Pfeil DJF, Stanley BJ, et al. Genome wide association study with imputed whole genome sequence data identifies a 431 kb risk haplotype on CFA18 for congenital laryngeal paralysis in Alaskan sled dogs. Genes 2022; 13(10):1808.
57. Ostrander EA, Wang GD, Larson G, et al. Dog10K: an international sequencing effort to advance studies of canine domestication, phenotypes and health. Natl Sci Rev 2019;6(4):810–24.
58. Wang C, Wallerman O, Arendt ML, et al. A novel canine reference genome resolves genomic architecture and uncovers transcript complexity. Commun Biol 2021;4(1):185.
59. Halo JV, Pendleton AL, Shen F, et al. Long-read assembly of a Great Dane genome highlights the contribution of GC-rich sequence and mobile elements to canine genomes. Proc Natl Acad Sci U S A 2021;118(11). e2016274118.
60. Jagannathan V, Hitte C, Kidd JM, et al. Dog10K_Boxer_Tasha_1.0: a long-read assembly of the dog reference genome. Genes 2021;12(6):847.
61. Binversie EE, Momen M, Rosa GJM, et al. Across-breed genetic investigation of canine hip dysplasia, elbow dysplasia, and anterior cruciate ligament rupture using whole-genome sequencing. Front Genet 2022;13:913354.
62. Woolliams JA, Lewis TW, Blott SC. Canine hip and elbow dysplasia in UK Labrador retrievers. Vet J 2011;189(2):169–76.
63. Sánchez-Molano E, Pong-Wong R, Clements DN, et al. Genomic prediction of traits related to canine hip dysplasia. Front Genet 2015;6:97.
64. Guo G, Zhou Z, Wang Y, et al. Canine hip dysplasia is predictable by genotyping. Osteoarthr Cartil 2011;19(4):420–9.
65. Scutari M, Mackay I, Balding D. Using genetic distance to infer the accuracy of genomic prediction. PLoS Genet 2016;12(9).
66. Baker LA, Momen M, Chan K, et al. Bayesian and machine learning models for genomic prediction of anterior cruciate ligament rupture in the canine model. G3 (Bethesda) 2020;10(8):2619–28.
67. Jiang L, Li Z, Hayward JJ, et al. Genomic prediction of two complex orthopedic traits across multiple pure and mixed breed dogs. Front Genet 2021;12.
68. Hayes BJ, Bowman PJ, Chamberlain AJ, et al. Invited review: genomic selection in dairy cattle: progress and challenges. J Dairy Sci 2009;92(2):433–43.
69. VanRaden PM, Van Tassell CP, Wiggans GR, et al. Invited review: reliability of genomic predictions for North American Holstein bulls. J Dairy Sci 2009;92(1): 16–24.
70. Stock KF, Distl O. Simulation study on the effects of excluding offspring information for genetic evaluation versus using genomic markers for selection in dog breeding. J Anim Breed Genet 2010;127(1):42–52.
71. Hedhammar Å. Swedish experiences from 60 years of screening and breeding programs for hip dysplasia: research, success, and challenges. Front Vet Sci 2020;7:228.
72. Fluckiger M. Scoring radiographs for canine hip dysplasia: the big three organizations in the world. Eur J Comp Anim Pract 2007;17(2):135–40.

Body Condition and Fertility in Dogs

Jennifer Sones, DVM, PhD[a],*, Orsolya Balogh, DVM, PhD[b],*

KEYWORDS

- Obesity • Leptin • Reproduction • Pregnancy • Parturition • Semen

KEY POINTS

- Body condition and fat mass influences the onset of puberty in dogs.
- Gonadectomy and its timing in dogs has effects on body condition in adulthood.
- Male and female dog fertility is influenced by body condition.
- Obesity increases the risk of negative pregnancy and parturition outcomes.
- Balanced diet and regular exercise are recommended in male and female dogs.

INTRODUCTION OF BODY CONDITION SCORING IN DOGS

To obtain a numerical assessment of nutritional status in veterinary patients, a subjective scoring system is used (World Small Animal Veterinary Association). Based on visual inspection and palpation of subcutaneous fat, a dog can be assigned a body condition score (BCS) between 1 and 9 and categorized as very thin (1), thin (3), ideal (5), overweight (7), and obese (9) (**Fig. 1**).[1] Although this is helpful to both owners and veterinarians in managing the overall health of canines, it is only semiquantitative and does not reflect other aspects of nutritional and metabolic health, such as visceral fat accumulation and muscle atrophy. Whole body imaging would be more advantageous to determine lean versus fat mass. Studies using dual-energy-X-ray absorptiometry support the BCS scale as predictive for estimating body composition.[2] However, this is more challenging when a dog is overweight or obese.[3] According to the American Veterinary Medical Association, an adult dog is considered obese when it is 30% more than its ideal weight. However, this can be challenging to assign when breed differences exist in form and stature. Therefore, we group dogs based on body weight into size classes, toy (<5 kg), small (5 to <10 kg), medium (10 to <25 kg), large (25–40 kg), and giant (40+ kg), with breeds falling into one of these classes.[4] This has

a Veterinary Clinical Sciences, Louisiana State University School of Veterinary Medicine, Skip Bertman Drive, Baton Rouge, LA 70803, USA; b Department of Small Animal Clinical Sciences, Virginia-Maryland College of Veterinary Medicine, 215 Duck Pond Drive, Blacksburg, VA 24061, USA
* Corresponding authors.
E-mail addresses: jsones@lsu.edu (J.S.); obalogh@vt.edu (O.B.)

Vet Clin Small Anim 53 (2023) 1031–1045
https://doi.org/10.1016/j.cvsm.2023.04.005
0195-5616/23/© 2023 Elsevier Inc. All rights reserved.

vetsmall.theclinics.com

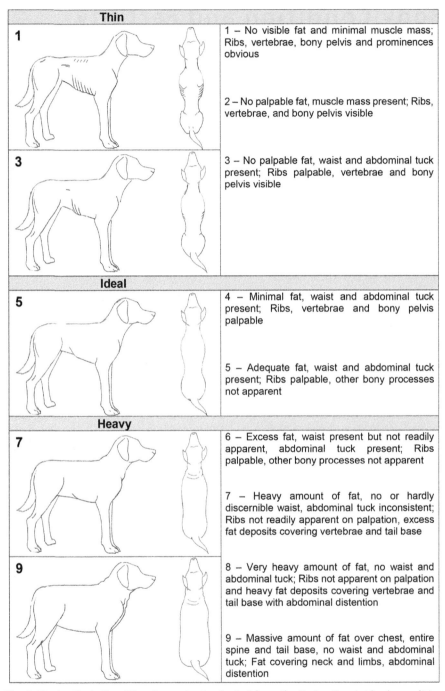

Fig. 1. Canine Body Condition Score chart, adapted from the Purina 9-point body condition scale. Illustrations by © Samantha J. McCarter.

recently been expanded to include 6 size categories (I–VI) that different breeds can be classified into based on body weight.[5] Modeling decades worth of body weight data from client owned dogs has allowed scientists to generate predictive models of ideal growth in dogs by breed and sex beginning as early as 12 weeks of age.

OBESITY IN ADULT DOGS

Obesity is a global health problem not only in humans but also in our dog population. One-third of Americans are overweight or obese and there is a correlation with increasing obesity in dogs. The canine incidence was 55.8% as reported by the Association for Pet Obesity Prevention in 2018 with 36.9% overweight and 18.9% obese (https://petobesityprevention.org). The close human–animal bond between dogs and their owners, and several of the environmental aspects they share explains why age, weight status, and physical activity of dog owners are associated with obesity risk of their pets.[6] Furthermore, body condition is also associated with the "job" of the animal such as actively performing dogs need muscle and lean body mass to perform their tasks. However, 26% of show dogs placed first to fifth in their class were overweight while none was underweight, and overweight status was more prevalent in certain breeds such as the Basset hound, Labrador retriever, or Pug.[7] Another study found 18.6% of dogs at a dog show being overweight and 1.1% obese with certain breeds and breed groups having generally higher BCS (eg, Molossoid breeds, Swiss Mountain and Cattle dogs, Retrievers, Water dogs, and so forth).[8] Many of the show dogs are considered to be exemplary of their breeds and are used for breeding, so discussing the reproductive consequences of overweight and obese status in affected individuals is important.

It is generally recognized that intact female dogs are more likely to be obese than intact males dogs. In Golden Retrievers, intact female dogs have a 43% increased risk of overweight/obesity compared with intact male dogs.[9] Among all gonadectomized dogs (males and females) in their study, spayed females had a 24% lower risk of becoming overweight/obese compared with neutered males. Furthermore, it was also observed in a large cohort of client-owned dogs in Denmark that adult male dogs have a propensity for increased body weight gain with castration.[10] In a study that analyzed the timing of gonadectomy and onset of an overweight/obesity BCS, nearly 3000 Golden Retrievers were assessed. They adjusted for age at study enrollment, owner-reported activity level, and sex of the dog, and separated into age cohorts (≤6 months, >6 months to ≤ 12 months, and >12 months). Gonadectomy was always associated with an increased risk of being overweight/obese.[9] Therefore, one might conclude that if gonadectomy is performed at any time, then being overweight/obese is inevitable in this breed. However, other data specific to Golden Retrievers suggest that delaying to postpubertal age would be advantageous for preventing certain neoplastic and musculoskeletal disorders.[11] Performing gonadectomy at 6 to 12 months of age increased the risk of becoming overweight/obese by 42% compared with delaying until after 12 months of age in Golden Retrievers.[9] Considered together, in this breed, delaying gonadectomy has beneficial effects on body condition and overall health. However, it is also noteworthy that increased energy expenditure, timing of feeding, and providing adequate rather than excessive macronutrients would also aid in preventing obesity after gonadectomy in dogs as well as in intact animals, and warrants consideration.

Obesity has negative impacts on various body systems and physiologic processes as well as shortening the dog's life span (see complete 2016 issue on Small Animal Obesity in this journal). With regards to the reproductive system, the consequences of obesity are not well documented in dogs. In humans, obesity negatively affects reproductive health both in women (eg, ovulatory dysfunction, infertility, miscarriage, pregnancy and parturition complications), and in men (eg, decreased semen quality).[12–17] On the other end, low body condition or undernutrition resulting in negative energy balance (NEB) also has severe consequences on fertility and reproductive performance. An example is the high-producing lactating dairy cow, where severe NEB postcalving is linked to impaired fertility through various mechanisms, for example, irregular cycles, delayed first ovulation, decreased oocyte quality, uterine inflammation/disease, impaired embryo development, and metabolic disorders, thus reduced conception and pregnancy rates.[18,19] In the dog, knowledge about the adverse outcomes of undernourishment is generally limited to the peripartum and postpartum periods.

THE INFLUENCE OF NUTRITION AND BODY CONDITION ON THE HYPOTHALAMO-PITUITARY-GONADAL AXIS

In mammalian species, including dogs, there is an inextricable link between body condition and the onset of puberty. Although BCS is determined subjectively with visual inspection of subcutaneous fat for the most part, internal obesity (visceral) also contributes to BCS. Leptin is an established biomarker of adiposity because its peripheral concentrations showed a significant, positive correlation with BCS and both subcutaneous and visceral fat areas in dogs.[20,21] The relationship between leptin and puberty will be discussed.

Similar to other mammals, the domestic dog relies on gonadotropin releasing hormone (GnRH) originating from the hypothalamus to stimulate pulsatility of gonadotropins, luteinizing hormone (LH), and follicle-stimulating hormone (FSH), which promote cyclicity in the bitch. GnRH regulates the onset of puberty and cyclicity with contributions from genetics (breed), nutrition, and perhaps even the circadian rhythm. The "critical-weight hypothesis" suggests body weight is a key indicator of pubertal onset. Using the Labrador and the Beagle dog, onset of puberty was achieved when they attained 71% and 81% of their adult body weight, respectively.[22,23] This is similar to what has been reported in cats where puberty has been reported at 80% adult body weight.[24] With adequate prepubertal energy intake, an appropriate body weight is achieved with the accumulation of fat mass. Leptin from adipose tissue will influence GnRH pulsatility and puberty onset. This is supported by the expression of leptin receptors on hypothalamic neurons, such as kisspeptin neurons, that synapse with GnRH neurons. Gonadectomy, including early (<6 months) and late (>12 months), likely influences the onset of becoming overweight/obese by several different mechanisms but potentially through the hypothalamic-pituitary-gonadal (HPG) axis via removing hypothalamic negative feedback and resulting in chronically increased LH[25], and perhaps the removal of estrogen, a known regulator of food intake in cats.[26] However, the precise mechanism is not fully understood.

The timing of puberty in female and male dogs varies by breed (earlier in small breeds than in large breeds) and individual animal, and occurs on average at 7 to 12 months of age (range 5 to >12 months).[27,28] In the female dog, the onset of puberty is defined as the first sign of proestrual bleeding. This would be associated with an increase in circulating estrogen and progesterone. Although fertile, puberty is different than sexual maturity (full reproductive potential), which is postulated to be after the second estrus.[28] This will depend on a number of factors including body condition, genetics, and breed. Puberty in the male dog is defined as the first appearance of spermatozoa in the ejaculate together with the attainment of libido and the ability to copulate, and it occurs slightly later than in the bitch.[27,28] Full reproductive potential and fertility is not reached until months later, closer to 2 years of age, with maximum ejaculate volume and total number of spermatozoa in the ejaculate.[27] The effect of body condition on the timing of female and male puberty in the dog is not fully known. In humans, being overweight or obese in childhood is associated with reaching pubertal milestones earlier in both boys and girls, whereas being underweight is related to delayed puberty onset.[29,30]

The canine estrous cycle is composed of 4 stages: proestrus, estrus, diestrus, and anestrus. The bitch cycles approximately twice a year; however, this is highly variable from animal to animal and cycle to cycle within the same animal. Some bitches, especially in certain breeds, may only cycle once per year. During proestrus, circulating levels of estradiol and testosterone increase before the LH surge that initiates ovulation. The LH surge demarcates the transition from proestrus to estrus. It is during estrus that the vaginal epithelium appears fully cornified due to estrogen exposure. Progesterone dominates during estrus increasing from basal levels even before ovulation is complete 2 to 3 days after the LH surge. Cytologic diestrus begins when the vaginal epithelium of the bitch is no longer 100% cornified. During this stage of the estrous cycle, progesterone reaches maximal concentrations because the corpora lutea are nourished by luteotropins, LH, and prolactin. Circulating levels of progesterone peak and then decline over several weeks. This occurs whether the bitch is experiencing a nonpregnant or pregnant diestrus with mammary development often occurring in either scenario. Anestrus is a variable length of time when the uterus undergoes involution and repair before entering into proestrus again. Circulating levels of FSH are high along with increasing LH pulsatility during late anestrus.[28,31]

BODY CONDITION AND FERTILITY IN THE BITCH
Ovarian Function and Cyclicity

In women, obesity, being underweight, or excessive exercise may have negative consequences on ovarian function and cyclicity.[17,32] Approximately 22% of body fat content is required to maintain ovulatory cyclicity in women.[33] Being over conditioned or under conditioned can influence reproductive performance in bitches, as well. Today, athletic lean hunting dogs as well as sedentary, overweight/obese dogs are being used in breeding programs. Bitches outside an ideal body condition may experience decreased fertility with irregular estrous cycles[34] in the form of split heats or anovulatory cycles, although the precise cause of inadequate HPG signaling in the bitch is unknown. Prolactin secretion is altered in obese dogs (hyperprolactinemia).[35] One might speculate this may contribute to irregular estrous cycle activity in bitches as dopamine agonism can increase plasma LH and promote folliculogenesis in the bitch.[36] In intact female Beagles, ad libitum feeding of a balanced commercial diet significantly increased plasma leptin levels and body condition from lean to obese over the 24 weeks transition period[37] but reproductive parameters such as cyclicity were not evaluated. Leptin excess as with obesity can be inhibitory to LH signaling to the female gonad. Furthermore, in addition to altering sex steroid hormone levels, chronic leptin production will also promote leptin resistance, hyperphagia, and weight gain in dogs. Obesity is associated not only with increased leptin but insulin-like growth factor 1 (IGF-1) levels.[38] Receptors for both hormones were found on canine ovarian follicular cells and in the corpus luteum,[39–41] and leptin receptors were also present in canine oocytes and cumulus cells.[42] As such, high circulating leptin and IGF-1 concentrations can exert direct effects on the ovary. A recent study in intact overweight and ideal-conditioned bitches did not find an association between serum leptin and progesterone levels, and no significant changes in peripheral leptin were noted by estrous cycle stage in either groups.[43] Until the metabolic regulation of fertility in the bitch is fully elucidated, increased body condition or being underweight cannot be excluded as potential causes for abnormal cyclicity and need to be considered during clinical diagnostic workup of anovulation and infertility. However, a healthy weight in dogs can be achieved through diet and exercise, as in people and other animals.

Pregnancy and Parturition

Current recommendations in breeding bitches include beginning pregnancy at an ideal BCS and only increasing body weight by 15% to 25% during pregnancy. This is for average-sized litters and therefore depends on litter size. After delivery, bitches would ideally weigh only 5% to 10% more than their preconception body weight.[44] Pregnant female dogs rely on ovarian progesterone for pregnancy maintenance the entire length of gestation. Pulsatility of LH along with prolactin is crucial during pregnancy for proper corpus luteum function in the bitch.[45] Circulating progesterone values alone are not good indicators of pregnancy status because they are not significantly different between pregnant and nonpregnant dogs, and only relaxin of placental origin is considered pregnancy-specific. Pregnancy termination can occur with either ovariectomy or hypophysectomy. Luteolysis, triggered by placental prostaglandin secretion from fetal trophoblasts at the end of gestation is necessary for the initiation of parturition.[28,31,46]

Low body condition and being underweight

Poorer fertility, reduced conception, and difficulties in maintaining pregnancy are concerns in underweight, underconditioned bitches.[34,47] In extreme cases, reducing the demand of pregnancy by decreasing litter size or abortion of the whole litter can occur.[48] Puppies born from underweight dams may have lower than normal birth weight and increased neonatal morbidity and mortality.[44] Maternal nutrition before and during conception and throughout pregnancy is therefore crucial, not only for energy but also for macronutrient and micronutrient requirements.

The counterregulatory responses of glucagon and norepinephrine are suppressed in pregnant bitches,[49] making hypoglycemia more difficult to cope with. If fetal nutrient demands are too high, or the nutrient supply of the dam is insufficient such as with underweight and undernourished dams, pregnancy toxemia (ketosis) can develop during late gestation, which is characterized by persistent hypoglycemia, ketonemia and ketonuria, with associated clinical signs, for example, weakness, ataxia, collapse, seizures, and coma.[28,50] Ketosis is a life-threatening condition both for the dam and the puppies. In a recent study in dogs undergoing Cesarean section electively at term or due to dystocia, higher maternal serum nonesterified fatty acids and β-hydroxybutyrate concentrations were found in small size bitches and in bitches where the proportion of the total litter weight (combined weight of all puppies) by maternal pregnant body weight was larger than 10%.[51] Although none of these bitches showed clinical signs of pregnancy toxemia, this finding underlines the high metabolic demand of pregnancy, especially if bitches are carrying a large litter compared with their body size.

Finally, although hypoglycemia and hypocalcemia have not been consistently found in parturient eutocic or dystocic bitches,[52,53] low glucose and ionized calcium levels may occur more frequently in undernourished bitches, and this, along with decreased muscle mass, can predispose them to dystocia.

Being overweight and obesity

Being overweight and obese were noted to result in poorer conception and smaller litter size in the bitch.[34,47] Besides the metabolic and endocrine alterations, obesity is associated with chronic, low-grade systemic inflammation where concentrations of proinflammatory cytokines are increased.[54] This inflammatory milieu may interfere with implantation and establishment of pregnancy, which is characterized by delicately balanced immune events at the embryo–maternal interface.[55,56] The canine uterus expresses IGF1 and its receptor,[57] and leptin and leptin receptor were also found in the uterus and placenta of the bitch with potential role in implantation and parturition,[58] providing another link where nutrition can interact with reproduction. Of note is that peripheral leptin increases during canine pregnancy with a tendency for higher concentrations with larger litter size,[59,60] and this gestational increase is likely physiologic due to placental contribution[58] and perhaps also by greater adipose tissue secretion.

During canine pregnancy, fetal nutrient demands are met by maternal endocrine and metabolic adaptation. One of the mechanisms of nutrition partitioning is the development of maternal insulin resistance to provide glucose to the developing fetus. In dogs, signs of diabetes mellitus can be observed during diestrus because altered carbohydrate metabolism occurs in dogs under the influence of progesterone; growth hormone is stimulated by progesterone, and insulin antagonism can result in hyperglycemia. Although canine pregnancy is normally associated with decreased insulin sensitivity from midgestation onward and it is usually more profound than during the nonpregnant diestrus,[31,50,61] it rarely progresses to gestational diabetes mellitus (GDM). Obesity in dogs has been associated with insulin resistance,[38] and obese women are at an increased risk of metabolic disorders and other complications during pregnancy, which also affect neonatal outcomes, for example, GDM, preeclampsia, preterm birth, macrosomia, stillbirth, and increased risk of infant mortality.[14–16,62] Macrosomia is observed in diabetic bitches,[28] similar to babies born to women with GDM. It is plausible therefore to assume that overweight and obese bitches could be at a higher risk to develop GDM, but the extent to which obesity may exacerbate insulin resistance during pregnancy resulting in GDM in the dog is so far unknown.

Bitches that are obese or overweight have a higher risk of dystocia,[47,63,64] including uterine inertia.[28,65] Dystocia may result from increased adipose tissue within and around the birth canal[63] or from postulated fat infiltration of the uterine musculature predisposing to diminished contractions[34]; however, the exact mechanisms are still unknown and are probably more complex than we know. Obese women are prone to having postdated pregnancies, prolonged labor, oxytocin augmentation for labor, and are at a higher risk for labor induction and Cesarean section delivery.[12,14–16] Leptin, the main adipokine, may be one of the contributing factors, because it negatively affects human myometrial contractility in vitro.[66] A recent study in nonobese dogs showed that the presence of leptin receptors in interplacental uterine sites and thus leptin signaling was linked to primary uterine inertia in more than half of the bitches diagnosed with this condition.[67] Therefore, high circulating leptin levels and other physiologic, metabolic, or endocrine alterations of obesity could predispose to dystocia and decreased uterine contractions. As obese bitches are generally less active, the impact of exercise, physical fitness and general muscle strength on the course of parturition and dystocia risk needs to be weighed in as well. Some of the basic management principles laid out to reduce the incidence of dystocia/uterine inertia in the bitch were described several decades ago[65] and are still valid, for example, a well-balanced diet, not allowing the bitch to become overweight and providing exercise, maintaining general good health, providing a familiar and comfortable environment for the whelping with supervision that is not distracting and efficient, and avoiding breeding bitches with highly excitable and neurotic temperament.

Obese dogs have compromised cardiopulmonary function due to the physical effects of increased fat mass, inflammatory mediators, and neurohormonal influence,[68] such as moderate increases in blood pressure, increased heart rate, cardiac remodeling, increased respiratory rate, reduced tidal volume, and lower blood oxygen saturation. Because pregnancy itself alters respiratory, cardiovascular, neurologic, hepatic, renal, and gastrointestinal physiology, and there is also the mechanical effect of a distended uterus,[69] obese bitches have an increased risk for cardiopulmonary complications during pregnancy or anesthesia for Cesarean section. These effects may be more pronounced in brachycephalic breeds due to their airway conformation. Adiposity may predispose to osteoarthritis,[70] and even 15% to 25% body weight gain during normal pregnancy could have added negative impacts, although short term, by increasing the mechanical stress on the joints and the skeletal system.

Postpartum and Neonatal Health

As the nutritional and energy requirements of lactation are much higher than those of pregnancy,[44,71] underweight bitches in low body condition are at risk of further weight loss after parturition and inadequate milk production (hypogalactia),[47,64] which can negatively impact the health of their puppies. In these bitches, provision of adequate calories from a complete and balanced, high-quality, highly digestible commercial diet with 28% to 32% animal-based protein, minimum 18% to 20% fat, and 20% to 30% carbohydrate content (eg, all life stages or puppy food) that is supported by research and feeding studies[44,48] is especially important, together with monitoring the bitch's weight and body condition (See article "Nutrition for the Pregnant Bitch and Puppies" by Kim and Wakshlag of this issue). The puppies' daily weight gain should be closely monitored because this is the most important indicator of adequate milk production in a healthy dam that nurses her pups. If hypogalactia is expected or confirmed, galactogogues (metoclopramide at 0.1–0.2 mg/kg subcutaneously or orally q 6–12 hours or domperidone at 2.2 mg/kg orally q 8–12 hours) alone or in combination with oxytocin (0.25–1 IU/animal subcutaneously q 2–4 hours for 1-2 days) can be given to increase milk production through increasing prolactin secretion and stimulation of milk let-down.[72,73] Proactively addressing the risk of failure of passive immune transfer in the puppies may be necessary by providing previously banked canine colostrum or serum/plasma, or fostering neonates on a surrogate dam that is producing colostrum. Supplemental feeding of puppies with a canine milk replacer may also be indicated.

The metabolite profile of human milk is influenced by maternal obesity, alters offspring gastrointestinal microbiome and increases the risk of offspring obesity.[74–76] The composition of milk from obese versus lean bitches is unknown. Maternal obesity was implicated in contributing to dystocia and increased neonatal mortality in dogs,[47] perhaps also through inadequate milk production.[64] Recommendations on managing hypogalactia in obese bitches are similar to those outlined above. The extent of which maternal obesity during pregnancy and lactation affects puppies both short-term and long-term is not known.

BODY CONDITION AND FERTILITY IN THE STUD DOG
Low Body Condition and Being Underweight

Although a previous study found no alterations in the spermiogram of thin compared with normal weight men,[77] a meta-analysis concluded that low body mass index (BMI) is associated with decreased semen volume and total sperm count, whereas no significant difference in sperm concentration or motility was found.[78] More recently, a systematic review and meta-analysis of human studies showed that being underweight was linked to decreased sperm normal morphology with no other parameters of the spermiogram being affected.[79] We do not know how low body condition affects reproductive function in male dogs, but it is reasonable to assume that similar to men, semen quality may be negatively affected.

Obesity and Being Overweight

In men, with regards to obesity, a 12% increased risk of infertility was found for every 3 units of BMI beyond 25 (BMI category 18.5–24.9 considered normal weight). Obesity is associated with dysregulation of the HPG axis, changes in adipokines, reproductive and metabolic hormones, increased production of reactive oxygen species and inflammatory mediators that affect spermatogenesis, and with epigenetic changes. Inhibin B, total testosterone, and sex hormone-binding globulin are reduced, whereas increased adipose tissue aromatization leads to high estradiol concentrations exerting a negative feedback on the HPG axis and consequently on Leydig cell testosterone secretion and spermatogenesis.[17,79] Being overweight or obese was found to be associated with lower semen volume, sperm concentration and total sperm count, % sperm vitality, total motility, and normal morphology compared with normal weight in men according to a recent large review and meta-analysis.[79]

Thermoregulation of the testes might be defective in obese males due to periscrotal fat deposition, which can lead to increased intrascrotal temperatures and spermiogram abnormalities (oligospermia, teratospermia, and asthenozoospermia) in dogs[28,80] and men.[17] Leptin, IGF-1 and their receptors were found on germ and Leydig cells of the canine testis,[81] so these hormones may directly modulate spermatogenesis and Leydig cell function during obesity. There are only a few studies that investigated the relationship between semen quality and body condition in dogs. A recent small study found that obese dogs had lower ejaculate volumes and reduction in some of the sperm kinematic parameters but no difference in DNA fragmentation compared with controls. Additionally, lectin histochemistry revealed changes in the glycosylation status of ejaculated spermatozoa surface in the obese group.[82] Another study in 28 healthy show-type male Labrador retrievers found no difference in serum levels of testosterone and Anti-Müllerian hormone (AMH), a biomarker of Sertoli cell function,[83] between lean (BCS 4–5/9) and overweight (BCS 6–8/9) dogs.[84] Semen collection and evaluation were not performed in that study. Based on information from the human literature and the very limited canine studies, it is prudent to assume that being overweight or obese could also result in reduced semen quality in the dog.

ENDOCRINE DISORDERS AND CANINE OBESITY

One of the clinical signs of canine hyperadrenocorticism and hypothyroidism is weight gain and obesity or fat redistribution, and both conditions have been reported in association with female and male reproductive dysfunction.[28,85] Hyperadrenocorticism is usually diagnosed in middle-age to older dogs that are likely not in breeding programs. Anestrus and testicular atrophy are the main clinical symptoms in affected dogs, which is the result of negative feedback from hypercortisolism on the pituitary gonadotrophins and perhaps also from hyperprolactinemia in females.[85] The reproductive consequences of hypothyroidism have been evaluated in a few prospective studies. In experimentally induced hypothyroid female Beagles, clinical hypothyroidism was associated with weaker and longer uterine contractions during parturition, increased neonatal mortality, decreased birth weight, and on the long-term also with decreased pregnancy rates, whereas other reproductive parameters (eg, interestrus interval, serum progesterone levels, and so forth) were unaffected. These reproductive abnormalities could be reversed by levothyroxine supplementation along with other clinical symptoms including returning to normal weight.[86,87] In male Beagles, where hypothyroidism was induced by oral administration of ^{131}I, obesity developed in all animals with typical clinical and laboratory signs associated with this condition; however, reproductive function, that is, libido, total scrotal width, semen quality (daily sperm output, motility, morphology), and testicular biopsy did not differ between hypothyroid obese and normal control dogs. Interestingly, hypothyroid dogs had a prolonged testosterone response to GnRH stimulation test.[88] Weight gain was reported in these studies, and although thyroid dysfunction is the most likely cause of the reproductive abnormalities observed, a role for obesity cannot be completely ruled out. Because normal thyroid function is crucial for general health and normal reproductive processes, screening for lymphocytic (autoimmune) thyroiditis is recommended by the Orthopedic Foundation for Animals and parent clubs of several breeds where the prevalence of this condition is high and thought to be hereditary.

RECOMMENDATIONS FOR THE BROOD BITCH AND STUD

It is beyond the scope of this article to discuss all aspects of nutritional management including questions on dietary supplements. We refer to relevant journal articles (See article "Nutrition for the Pregnant Bitch and Puppies" by Kim and Wakshlag of this issue) and books focusing on small animal nutrition aspects.

Proper nutrition for dogs starts during their growth and development, and continues through all their reproductive stages.[44] Weight and body condition should be regularly monitored and nutrition adjusted to keep them in ideal condition. Bitches that are intended to be bred should be at peak health to have the best chance of a successful pregnancy and parturition, and to raise healthy puppies. A complete and balanced diet approved by the Association of American Feed Control Officials and supported by feeding trials is recommended at all times, with specific recommendations during pregnancy and lactation to incorporate the needs of the developing fetus(es) and lactation. Moderate, regular exercise is important to keep bitches in optimal shape and prepare them for an easier, smooth whelping. Ideally, obesity should be addressed and managed before breeding plans are made; however, this is not always the real-life situation. There are no standardized weight-management programs in place for overweight and obese dogs while they actively reproduce. The provision of adequate amounts of nutrients to the developing conceptuses and later through milk to the neonates is of high importance. Weight loss during these times can disrupt this balance and is therefore not recommended. The same basic principles apply for the stud dog for maximizing health and semen quality. Although a healthy weight and ideal body condition should be promoted in our breeding bitches and stud dogs, there is need for more research to fully understand the consequences of obesity on canine fertility and reproductive performance, including epigenetic effects of maternal weight during pregnancy and lactation on the future reproduction of female and male offspring.

CLINICS CARE POINTS

- Consideration should be given for time of gonadectomy in dogs and plan for ensuring ideal body condition long term.

- Body condition should be well monitored post-pubertal to ensure ideal prior to breeding.
- Body condition outside of ideal should be a differential in case of adverse reproductive outcome.
- Not all under- or overconditioned dogs will present with fertility/reproductive problems despite having an increased risk.
- Reversal of obesity in breeding bitches is best before conception.
- Besides monitored caloric intake, an exercise plan can also help maintain an ideal body condition in dogs.

DISCLOSURE

The authors have nothing to disclose.

ACKNOWLEDGEMENT

The authors would like to thank Dr. Samantha J. McCarter from the Virginia-Maryland College of Veterinary Medicine for the beautiful illustrations in Figure 1.

REFERENCES

1. Laflamme D. Development and validation of a body condition score system for dogs. Canine Pract 1997;22(4):10–5.
2. Speakman J, Booles D, Butterwick R. Validation of dual energy X-ray absorptiometry (DXA) by comparison with chemical analysis of dogs and cats. Int J Obes Relat Metab Disord 2001;25(3):439–47.
3. Zanghi B, Cupp C, Pan Y, et al. Noninvasive measurements of body composition and body water via quantitative magnetic resonance, deuterium water, and dual-energy x-ray absorptiometry in awake and sedated dogs. Am J Vet Res 2013; 74(5):733–43.
4. Hawthorne A, Booles D, Nugent P, et al. Body-weight changes during growth in puppies of different breeds. J Nutr 2004;134(8 Suppl):2027S–30S.
5. Salt C, Morris P, German A, et al. Growth standard charts for monitoring body-weight in dogs of different sizes. PLoS One 2017;12(9):e0182064.
6. Suarez L, Bautista-Castaño I, Peña Romera C, et al. Is Dog Owner Obesity a Risk Factor for Canine Obesity? A "One-Health" Study on Human-Animal Interaction in a Region with a High Prevalence of Obesity. Vet Sci 2022;9(5):243.
7. Such Z, German A. Best in show but not best shape: a photographic assessment of show dog body condition. Vet Rec 2015;177(5):125.
8. Corbee R. Obesity in show dogs. J Anim Physiol Anim Nutr 2013;97(5):904–10.
9. Simpson M, Albright S, Wolfe B, et al. Age at gonadectomy and risk of over-weight/obesity and orthopedic injury in a cohort of Golden Retrievers. PLoS One 2019;14(7):e0209131.
10. Bjørnvad C, Gloor S, Johansen S, et al. Neutering increases the risk of obesity in male dogs but not in bitches - A cross-sectional study of dog- and owner-related risk factors for obesity in Danish companion dogs. Prev Vet Med 2019;170: 104730.
11. Torres de la Riva G, Hart B, Farver T, et al. Neutering dogs: effects on joint disorders and cancers in golden retrievers. PLoS One 2013;8(2):e55937.
12. Zhang J, Bricker L, Wray S, et al. Poor uterine contractility in obese women. BJOG An Int J Obstet Gynaecol 2007;114(3):343–8.

13. Metwally M, Li T, Ledger W. The impact of obesity on female reproductive function. Obes Rev 2007;8(6):515–23.
14. Carlson N, Hernandez T, Hurt K. Parturition dysfunction in obesity: time to target the pathobiology. Reprod Biol Endocrinol 2015;13:135.
15. Denison F, Price J, Graham C, et al. Maternal obesity, length of gestation, risk of postdates pregnancy and spontaneous onset of labour at term. BJOG An Int J Obstet Gynaecol 2008;115(6):720–5.
16. Krishnamoorthy U, Schram C, Hill S. Maternal obesity in pregnancy: Is it time for meaningful research to inform preventive and management strategies? BJOG An Int J Obstet Gynaecol 2006;113(10):1134–40.
17. Practice Committee of the American Society for Reproductive Medicine. Obesity and reproduction: a committee opinion. Fertil Steril 2021;116(5):1266–85.
18. Wathes D, Fenwick M, Cheng Z, et al. Influence of negative energy balance on cyclicity and fertility in the high producing dairy cow. Theriogenology 2007;68(Suppl 1):S232–41.
19. Pascottini O, Leroy J, Opsomer G. Maladaptation to the transition period and consequences on fertility of dairy cows. Reprod Domest Anim 2022;57(Suppl 4):21–32.
20. Müller L, Kollár E, Balogh L, et al. Body fat distribution and metabolic consequences - Examination opportunities in dogs. Acta Vet Hung 2014;62(2):169–79.
21. Ishioka K, Hosoya K, Kitagawa H, et al. Plasma leptin concentration in dogs: effects of body condition score, age, gender and breeds. Res Vet Sci 2007;82(1):11–5.
22. Taha M, Noakes D, Allen W. Some aspects of reproductive function in the male beagle at puberty. J Small Anim Pr 1981;22(10):663–7.
23. Wildt D, Seager S, Chakraborty P. Behavioral, ovarian and endocrine relationships in the pubertal bitch. J Anim Sci 1981;53(1):182–91.
24. Little S. Female Reproduction. In: Little S, editor. *The Cat: Clinical Medicine and Management.* 1st ed. St. Louis, MO, USA: Elsevier Saunders; 2012. p. 1195–227. https://doi.org/10.1016/B978-1-4377-0660-4.00040-5.
25. Kutzler M. Possible Relationship between Long-Term Adverse Health Effects of Gonad-Removing Surgical Sterilization and Luteinizing Hormone in Dogs. Anim 2020;10(4):599.
26. Oberbauer A, Belanger J, Famula T. A Review of the Impact of Neuter Status on Expression of Inherited Conditions in Dogs. Front Vet Sci 2019;6:397.
27. England GCW. Physiology and endocrinology of the male. In: England GCW, von Heimendahl A, editors. *BSAVA manual of canine and Feline reproduction and neonatology.* 2nd edition. Gloucester, UK: BSAVA, Quedgeley; 2010. p. 13–22.
28. Johnston SD, Root Kustritz MV, Olson PNS. *Canine and Feline Theriogenology.* 1st ed. Philadelphia, PA, USA: Saunders; 2001.
29. Brix N, Ernst A, Lauridsen L, et al. Childhood overweight and obesity and timing of puberty in boys and girls: cohort and sibling-matched analyses. Int J Epidemiol 2020;49(3):834–44.
30. Aghaee S, Deardorff J, Quesenberry C, et al. Associations between childhood obesity and pubertal timing stratified by sex and race/ethnicity. Am J Epidemiol 2022;191(12):2026–36.
31. Concannon PW. Canine pregnancy and parturition. Vet Clin North Am Small Anim Pract 1986;16(3):453–75.
32. Carson S, Kallen A. Diagnosis and management of infertility: A review. J Am Med Assoc 2021;326(1):65–76.

33. Van der Spuy Z. Nutrition and reproduction. Clinincs Obstet Gynaecol 1985; 12(3):579–604.
34. Barstow C, Wilborn R, Johnson A. Breeding soundness examination of the bitch. Vet Clin North Am Small Anim Pr 2018;48(4):547–66.
35. Martin L, Siliart B, Dumon H, et al. Hormonal disturbances associated with obesity in dogs. J Anim Physiol Anim Nutr 2006;90(9–10):355–60.
36. Spattini G, Borghi V, Thuróczy J, et al. Follicular development and plasma concentrations of LH and prolactin in anestrous female dogs treated with the dopamine agonist cabergoline. Theriogenology 2007;68(6):826–33.
37. Grant RW, Vester Boler BM, Ridge TK, et al. Adipose tissue transcriptome changes during obesity development in female dogs. Physiol Genomics 2011; 43(6):295–307.
38. Gayet C, Bailhache E, Dumon H, et al. Insulin resistance and changes in plasma concentration of TNFalpha, IGF1, and NEFA in dogs during weight gain and obesity. J Anim Physiol Anim Nutr 2004;88(3–4):157–65.
39. Balogh O, Kowalewski M, Reichler I. Leptin and leptin receptor gene expression in the canine corpus luteum during diestrus, pregnancy and after aglepristone-induced luteolysis. Reprod Domest Anim 2012;47(Suppl 6):40–2.
40. Balogh O, Müller L, Boos A, et al. Expression of insulin-like growth factor 1 and its receptor in preovulatory follicles and in the corpus luteum in the bitch. Gen Comp Endocrinol 2018;269:68–74.
41. Müller L. Interactions between nutritional status, metabolic biomarkers and reproductive function in dogs. PhD thesis. Published online 2021.
42. Maltana A, Podda A, Falchi L, et al. Immunodetection of leptin receptor in canine oocytes in two different stages of the oestrus cycle. In: Proceedings of the 19th International Congress on Animal Reproduction. Bologna, Italy, 26-30 June 2022:78.
43. Müller L, Kok E, Kollár E, et al. Changes in serum leptin concentrations in relation to the oestrous cycle and body fat content in female dogs. Literature review and own data. Magy Állato Lapja 2019;141:411–24.
44. Case LP, Daristotle L, Hayek MG, et al. *Canine and Feline Nutrition: A Resource for Companion Animal Professionals*. 3rd edition. Maryland Heights, MO, USA: Mosby Elsevier; 2011. https://doi.org/10.1016/C2009-0-39175-8.
45. Papa P, Kowalewski M. Factors affecting the fate of the canine corpus luteum: Potential contributors to pregnancy and non-pregnancy. Theriogenology 2020;150: 339–46.
46. Kowalewski M, Beceriklisoy H, Pfarrer C, et al. Canine placenta: a source of prepartal prostaglandins during normal and antiprogestin-induced parturition. Reproduction 2010;139(3):655–64.
47. Johnson C. Pregnancy management in the bitch. Theriogenology 2008;70(9): 1412–7.
48. Kelley R. Canine reproductive management: Factors influencing litter size. In: Proceedings of the Society for Theriogenology Annual Meeting, August 7-11, 2002, Colorado Springs (CO). 2002:291-301.
49. Connolly C, Aglione L, Smith M, et al. Pregnancy impairs the counterregulatory response to insulin-induced hypoglycemia in the dog. Am J Physiol Endocrinol Metab 2004;287(3):E480–8.
50. Johnson C. Glucose homeostasis during canine pregnancy: Insulin resistance, ketosis, and hypoglycemia. Theriogenology 2008;70(9):1418–23.
51. Balogh O, Bruckmaier R, Keller S, et al. Effect of maternal metabolism on fetal supply: Glucose, non-esterified fatty acids and beta-hydroxybutyrate

concentrations in canine maternal serum and fetal fluids at term pregnancy. Anim Reprod Sci 2018;193:209–16.

52. Hollinshead F, Hanlon D, Gilbert R, et al. Calcium, parathyroid hormone, oxytocin and pH profiles in the whelping bitch. Theriogenology 2010;73(9):1276–83.

53. Frehner B, Reichler I, Keller S, et al. Blood calcium, glucose and haematology profiles of parturient bitches diagnosed with uterine inertia or obstructive dystocia. Reprod Domest Anim 2018;53(3):680–7.

54. Cortese L, Terrazzano G, Pelagalli A. Leptin and immunological profile in obesity and its associated diseases in dogs. Int J Mol Sci 2019;20(10):2392.

55. Schäfer-Somi S, Beceriklisoy H, Budik S, et al. Expression of genes in the canine pre-implantation uterus and embryo: implications for an active role of the embryo before and during invasion. Reprod Domest Anim 2008;43(6):656–63.

56. Tavares Pereira M, Nowaczyk R, Payan-Carreira R, et al. Selected uterine immune events associated with the establishment of pregnancy in the dog. Front Vet Sci 2021;7:625921.

57. Kautz E, Gram A, Aslan S, et al. Expression of genes involved in the embryo-maternal interaction in the early-pregnant canine uterus. Reproduction 2014; 147(5):703–17.

58. Balogh O, Staub LP, Gram A, et al. Leptin in the canine uterus and placenta: possible implications in pregnancy. Reprod Biol Endocrinol 2015;13:13.

59. Cardinali L, Troisi A, Verstegen J, et al. Serum concentration dynamic of energy homeostasis hormones, leptin, insulin, thyroid hormones, and cortisol throughout canine pregnancy and lactation. Theriogenology 2017;97:154–8.

60. Troisi A, Cardinali L, Menchetti L, et al. Serum concentrations of leptin in pregnant and non-pregnant bitches. Reprod Domest Anim 2020;55(4):454–9.

61. Connolly CC, Papa T, Smith MS, et al. Hepatic and muscle insulin action during late pregnancy in the dog. Am J Physiol Regul Integr Comp Physiol 2007;292(1): R447–52.

62. Johansson S, Villamor E, Altman M, et al. Maternal overweight and obesity in early pregnancy and risk of infant mortality: a population based cohort study in Sweden. BMJ 2014;349:g6572.

63. German AJ. The growing problem of obesity in dogs and cats. J Nutr 2006;136(7 Suppl):1940S–6S.

64. Bebiak D, Lawler D, Reutzel L. Nutrition and management of the dog. Vet Clin North Am Small Anim Pr 1987;17(3):505–33.

65. Bennett D. Canine dystocia–a review of the literature. J Small Anim Pract 1974; 15(2):101–17.

66. Moynihan AT, Hehir MP, Glavey SV, et al. Inhibitory effect of leptin on human uterine contractility in vitro. Am J Obstet Gynecol 2006;195(2):504–9.

67. Frehner BL, Reichler IM, Kowalewski MP, et al. Implications of the RhoA/Rho associated kinase pathway and leptin in primary uterine inertia in the dog. J Reprod Dev 2021;67:3207–15.

68. Chandler M. Impact of obesity on cardiopulmonary disease. Vet Clin North Am Small Anim Pr 2016;46(5):817–30.

69. Pascoe P, Moon P. Periparturient and neonatal anesthesia. Vet Clin North Am Small Anim Pr 2001;31(2):315–40.

70. Frye C, Shmalberg J, Wakshlag J. Obesity, exercise and orthopedic disease. Vet Clin North Am Small Anim Pr 2016;46(5):831–41.

71. Ramsey JJ. Determining energy requirements. In: Fascetti AJ, Delaney SJ, editors. *Applied veterinary clinical nutrition.* 1st edition. Chichester, West Sussex, UK: Wiley-Blackwell; 2012. p. 23–45.

72. Keller SR, Abonyi-Tóth Z, Sprenger N, et al. Effect of metoclopramide treatment of bitches during the first week of lactation on serum prolactin concentration, milk composition, and milk yield and on weight gain of their puppies. Am J Vet Res 2018;79(2):233–41.
73. Gonzales K. Periparturient diseases in the dam. Vet Clin North Am Small Anim Pr 2018;48(4):663–81.
74. Isganaitis E, Venditti S, Matthews TJ, et al. Maternal obesity and the human milk metabolome: associations with infant body composition and postnatal weight gain. Am J Clin Nutr 2019;110(1):111–20.
75. Prentice PM, Schoemaker MH, Vervoort J, et al. Human milk short-chain fatty acid composition is associated with adiposity outcomes in infants. J Nutr 2019;149(5): 716–22.
76. Lemas DJ, Young BE, Baker PR, et al. Alterations in human milk leptin and insulin are associated with early changes in the infant intestinal microbiome. Am J Clin Nutr 2016;103(5):1291–300.
77. Belloc S, Cohen-Bacrie M, Amar E, et al. High body mass index has a deleterious effect on semen parameters except morphology: results from a large cohort study. Fertil Steril 2014;102(5):1268–73.
78. Guo D, Xu M, Zhou Q, et al. Is low body mass index a risk factor for semen quality? A PRISMA-compliant meta-analysis. Med 2019;98(32):e16677.
79. Salas-Huetos A, Maghsoumi-Norouzabad L, James E, et al. Male adiposity, sperm parameters and reproductive hormones: An updated systematic review and collaborative meta-analysis. Obes Rev 2021;22(1):e13082.
80. Oettlé E. Sperm abnormalities in the dog: a light and electron microscopic study. PhD thesis. Published online 1990.
81. Müller L, Kowalewski M, Reichler I, et al. Different expression of leptin and IGF1 in the adult and prepubertal testis in dogs. Reprod Domest Anim 2017;52(Suppl 2): 187–92.
82. Desantis S, Albrizio M, Santamaria N, Cinone M. Can obesity affect the glycocalyx of dog sperm? In: Proceedings of the 19th International Congress on Animal Reproduction. Bologna, Italy, 26-30 June 2022:75.
83. Holst B. Diagnostic possibilities from a serum sample-Clinical value of new methods within small animal reproduction, with focus on anti-Müllerian hormone. Reprod Domest Anim 2017;52(Suppl 2):303–9.
84. Andersson E. Testosterone and Anti-Müllerian Hormone (AMH) in lean and overweight Labrador retrievers. Degree Thesis in Veterinary Medicine Programme. Published online 2016.
85. Feldman EC, Nelson RW. *Canine and Feline Endocrinology and Reproduction.* 3rd edition. St. Louis, MO, USA: Saunders; 2004.
86. Panciera D, Purswell B, Kolster K, et al. Reproductive effects of prolonged experimentally induced hypothyroidism in bitches. J Vet Intern Med 2012;26(2): 326–33.
87. Panciera D, Purswell B, Kolster K. Effect of short-term hypothyroidism on reproduction in the bitch. Theriogenology 2007;68(3):316–21.
88. Johnson C, Olivier N, Nachreiner R, et al. Effect of 131I-induced hypothyroidism on indices of reproductive function in adult male dogs. J Vet Intern Med 1999; 13(2):104–10.

Update on Brucella canis

Understanding the Past and Preparing for the Future

Mary K. Sebzda, DVM[a,b,1], Lin K. Kauffman, DVM[c],*

KEYWORDS

• Abortion • *Brucella* • Infertility • Dog importation • Zoonosis

KEY POINTS

• *Brucella canis* causes canine brucellosis, an emerging zoonosis.
• Antimicrobial treatment is not curative and recrudescence of the disease is common.
• Seroprevalence in most locales and worldwide has not been established.
• Importation of dogs from areas where brucellosis is endemic increases the risk of spreading the disease to both dogs and humans.

ETIOLOGY

Brucella species currently include: *B canis, abortus, suis, mellitensis, ovis, ceti, microti, neotomae, pinnipedialis, papionis, vulpis,* and *inopinata.*[1–8] Two novel and distinct strains found in amphibians are yet to be named, but appear to be similar to *Brucella inopinata.*[9]

Though varied in hosts, genetic sequencing studies indicated that there is much homology across the *Brucella* genus, although small sequence differences between species exist.[10,11] Some authors propose a "one species" theory that states all *Brucella spp.* are the same.[2,10] Each species has a preferred reservoir host, yet most *Brucella* species can infect numerous mammalian hosts, hence its propensity as a zoonotic infection.[12–14]

EPIDEMIOLOGY OF CANINE BRUCELLOSIS

Globally, brucellosis remains an important zoonotic disease with the highest rates of prevalence in animals and humans currently found in the Middle East, Africa, Asia

[a] Newport Harbor Animal Hospital, 125 Mesa Drive, Costa Mesa, CA 92627, USA; [b] Western University of Health Sciences, Pomona, CA 91766, USA; [c] Prairie View Animal Hospital, 1830 Southeast Princeton Drive Suite A, Grimes, IA 50111, USA
[1] Present address: 266 Woodcrest Lane, Aliso Viejo, CA 92656.
* Corresponding author. Prairie View Animal Hospital, 1830 Southeast Princeton Drive, Suite A, Grimes, IA 50111.
E-mail address: linkauf@yahoo.com

Vet Clin Small Anim 53 (2023) 1047–1062
https://doi.org/10.1016/j.cvsm.2023.05.002
0195-5616/23/© 2023 Elsevier Inc. All rights reserved.

vetsmall.theclinics.com

and Latin America.[2] An estimated 500,000 new human infections occur annually, usually due to *Brucella abortus*, *suis* or *mellitensis*.[15] Canine brucellosis is similarly found worldwide (**Fig. 1**).[16] True seroprevalence, although not known across North America, has been reported in various serosurveys in the United States in shelter animals, as somewhere around 0% to 9%, with occasional outbreaks at higher rates [17–22] and there are no consistent studies determining its seroprevalence worldwide.[16–18,22,23] The reported rates are likely an underestimate owing to the underreporting of the disease,[18] inconsistency in the test[23] used and rising interstate and international adoptions and movement of dogs. The market for dog ownership has been steadily increasing since 2000[24] with growth of supply in dogs from shelter/rescue groups outmatching supply from breeders within the United States.[24,25] The inability to track the number of dogs imported annually for adoption from a multitude of countries, along with no required screening prior to their movement, compromises the ability to know the true seroprevalence and risk for dissemination.[26,27] Reports include solitary cases in Germany,[28] the United Kingdom,[29] Egypt[30] sudden increase in rates of cases as in the Netherlands[31] Sweden,[32] Hungary,[15] Columbia,[15] Israel,[33] and Costa Rica,[34] and serosurveys of the canine population in Argentina.[35] These cases stress the link between international movement of breeding dogs and outbreaks of this disease.[16,27,34,35]

B.CANIS PATHOGENESIS

B.canis, like other *Brucella spp.*, has a strong tropism for the lymphoendoreticular & reproductive systems.[36] *Brucellae* enter the host by penetrating mucosal epithelium,

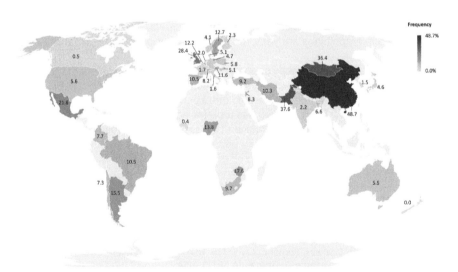

Fig. 1. Global map depicting *Brucella canis* seropositivity. (Image: Courtesy of Dr. R.L. Santos Worldwide distribution of the frequency of *B. canis* infected dogs by country. The frequency of each country was obtained by the weighted average of the frequency reported in each study available on PubMed and Google Scholar. The map was generated using Microsoft Excel software. Regions in gray indicate countries without epidemiological surveys while countries showing patterns with black lines indicate countries with reports of dogs infected with *B. canis* but without studies of disease frequency.)

usually of the reproductive tract after sexual or reproductive transmission, or through oral transmission. Afterward, the bacteria achieve the colonization of reproductive tissue, mammary glands and the spleen, as demonstrated by bacterial culture, The proposed infectious dose of a virulent *Brucella spp.* can be as low as 10^3 to 10^4 colony-forming units.[2,37]

CLINICAL PRESENTATION OF *B CANIS* INFECTION AND ROUTES OF TRANSMISSION
Clinics Care Points

General presentation
Non-specific general signs of *B canis* infection can include vague signs of lethargy, poor hair coat, fever, fatigue, weight loss, exercise intolerance, and lymphadenopathy early on in the disease process.[13,37–42] The disease may progress to splenomegaly and uveitis. Additionally, orthopedic issues such as lameness, muscle weakness, spinal pain related to vertebral osteomyelitis and intervertebral disc infection (diskospondylitis) caused by the bacteria are found in infected dogs.[38,39,41] Veterinarians should always have *B canis* on their differential list when dealing with cases that include these signs especially if the dog is intact or adopted/rescued.

Any sexually mature, reproductively active, dog is susceptible to *B canis.* Even dogs not reproductively active can contract the disease if exposed to infected bodily fluid (including milk) or aborted materials.[15,40,43] Puppies can be infected *in utero*, while nursing, or while being housed with an infected bitch. Puppies not aborted and born to an infected bitch may die shortly after birth and show similar lesions to the aborted fetuses, or they may survive and shed bacteria in their environment for several months and can also develop clinical disease after puberty.[15,41]

Canine blood would represent a less common route of transmission. In one Canadian study, approximately 0.033% of over 6000 canine blood units were positive for *B canis.*[44] An interesting potential new route of infection for *Brucella spp.* may exist via blood-sucking parasites, from which *B canis* can be isolated, although direct transmission of *B canis* from ticks to dogs has not yet been confirmed.[45] However, ticks carrying other *Brucella spp.* are widely distributed in China and can promote spread of disease.[46]

Male-specific presentation
Clinical signs seen in the stud dog mainly involve the testicles, epididymides, and prostate. The most common signs seen are acute epididymitis and prostatitis with orchitis seen less frequently.[2,27,38,40,41] Initial presentation can start as moist scrotal dermatitis secondary to licking from epididymitis or orchitis and progress to testicular atrophy, which is permanent. Any disease involving the testicles will lead to changes with the sperm and with *B canis* one can see sperm agglutination, sperm morphological abnormalities and inflammatory cells.[39–41] Experimentally abnormal sperm have been noted as soon as 2 weeks postinfection and by 20 weeks postinfection 90% of the sperm can become affected.[2]

Infertility of a stud dog can be another presentation of *B canis.* The stud may have a history of infertility documented as a series of failures to achieve pregnancies with different proven females. A semen analysis may give crucial clues since several abnormalities of the sperm can be seen; specifically head-to-head sperm agglutination along with bent tails, double tails, swollen midpieces, retained protoplasmic droplets, and deformed acrosomes[2,39,40] (**Fig. 2**). *B canis* testing needs to be part of any infertility workup even if one thinks there is minimal chance for this disease. Neutering only prevents bacteria in semen and bacteria are commonly shed in prostatic fluid and urine, as well.

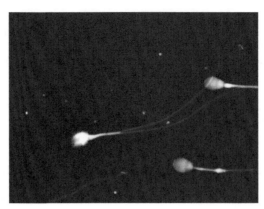

Fig. 2. Abnormal sperm due to *B. canis* infection: Note the double tails, retained protoplasmic droplets, and swollen midpiece. (Image: Courtesy of Dr. L. Kauffman.)

Female-specific presentation

The most common presenting clinical sign of *B canis* in the bitch is late-term abortion after Day 45 gestation.[15,38–40] Aborted fetuses from these cases are usually partially autolyzed with subcutaneous edema, hemorrhage, and congestion (**Fig. 3**). These aborting bitches have a prolonged vaginal discharge that is dark and fetid, which can last for 1 to 6 weeks postabortion.[15,39] Gross pathology of the uterus postabortion commonly reveals endometritis and placentitis.[2,47] The bitch may have a history of chronic infertility issues or she may have a history of an abortion but then go on to have several successful litters only to have issues with infertility or abortion again later in life.[41]

Human presentation

Most human cases report clinical signs involving "flu-like" symptoms and lymphadenopathy. Physicians rarely have brucellosis of any species on their differential list when seeing patients with the aforementioned clinical signs and with unreliable diagnostic tools to confirm human cases this low number is not surprising. Diagnosis of human cases mostly relies on blood culture. Though most cases respond to antibiotic therapy, re-emergence of disease is common and no approved human vaccine is available.

Disease in humans caused by *B canis* must be reported to the National Notifiable Disease Surveillance System in the United States,[15] though not all states follow this protocol. Though only recognized with *Brucella mellitensis*, a single case of sexual transmission of brucellosis has been documented in China in a couple where only one partner had previously been exposed to the organism through contact with livestock.[48]

Human infections are reported to be uncommon though actual case numbers are seldom known due to rare reporting of the disease and misdiagnosis, both within and outside of the United States.[19,37,49,50] Multiple studies have been done around the world in an attempt to identify the incidence of human disease caused by *B canis* but results vary greatly, most likely due to the type of test used to identify the disease along with the population studied.[2,15] *B canis* as a zoonotic disease may soon be seen in higher frequency in the human population spreading outward into pet owning homes as rates of international adoptions of infected dogs continue.

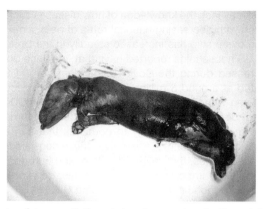

Fig. 3. Aborted canine fetus, partially autolyzed, secondary to *B. canis* infection at Day 48 gestation. (Image: Courtesy of Dr. L. Kauffman.)

HIGH-RISK POPULATIONS FOR CANINE BRUCELLOSIS

Feral and stray dogs are predominant reservoirs for *B canis* and these dogs are more likely to be intact than pet dogs.[16,37,51–55] Secondarily, prevalence can be high in large commercial breeding kennels.[18,37] Unrestricted movement of infected dogs and puppies risks spreading this disease. Spilling over into the human population, veterinarians, laboratory personnel, animal caretakers, dog breeders, and pet owners would certainly be in jeopardy of exposure to brucellosis.[16,37,49,50] Even though the dog may be spayed or neutered, it still can shed bacteria in its saliva, nasal secretions, genital secretions and urine.[15,43,56] In the United States ~30% of pet dogs are adopted from shelters and this number is growing.[15] Many pet owners report sleeping with their dogs and yet testing for *B canis* is not standard procedure before adopting these dogs out to their new owners.

REGULATIONS AND GUIDELINES SURROUNDING *B CANIS*

Currently, there are no federal regulations in the United States for mandatory *B canis* testing prior to interstate or international movement of a dog. Positive dogs are being shipped within countries and internationally.[15] Few countries have *B canis*-specific regulation and there seems to be a lack of regulatory interest in this disease at a federal level.

A trend in the importation of dogs internationally has continued to increase over the past decade.[26] Relocation of these dogs can occur for a variety of reasons such as natural disasters (Hurricane Katrina 2005); perceived poor quality of life for dogs that live in third world countries from increasing international animal welfare awareness (dog meat trade in Asia); mass dog cull prior to international sporting events (2014 Winter Olympics), and war (Ukraine 2022). Many underdeveloped countries, through rapid population growth and poor rates of responsible pet ownership, have increasing stray dog populations.[26] International adoptions represent a way to decrease stray dog populations without resorting to mass culling, which is perceived by some as inhumane. Shelters importing dogs often do not test for *B.canis*, can become overcrowded, and may not have suitable facilities for the isolation of positive dogs.

Rescue personnel may lack the knowledge of how diseases such as brucellosis are spread.[26] In contrast, with decreasing national rates of pets surrendered to shelters, the demand for dog ownership has increased steadily in the United States. An estimated 89.7 million US households reported having at least one dog in 2017 and this number further increased during the Covid-19 pandemic.[25,57] Current demand for pet dogs is estimated at around 8 million per annum and projected to grow to 9.2 million by 2036.[58] Even with the Centers for Disease Control (CDC) imposing a ban on the importation of dogs from 113 countries considered high risk for rabies since 2021, dogs are still moved internationally to countries that can accept them for a period of quarantine (usually 6 months). Eventually, these dogs are transported to destinations like the United States, the United Kingdom, and Europe.[26,59] While quarantine may reduce the risk of importing dogs with rabies, dogs are still not screened for other pathogens of zoonotic importance including *B canis*.

In the United States, *B canis* is a reportable disease in some states, like any other *Brucella* species, and several states along with the Center for Disease Control & Prevention (CDC) have protocols in place when positive cases are reported.[15,60,61]

DIAGNOSIS OF DISEASE

- Case History
  - Diagnosing canine brucellosis based on case history alone is unlikely; additional diagnostics are required to confirm the suspicion of infection. Not all *B canis* clinical signs are present in every case, and infertility may be the only presenting clinical sign in bitches or stud dogs. A history of adoption, importation, or being a breeding animal puts dogs at higher risk.
- Physical Exam
  - A thorough physical examination is essential for all cases presenting for pre-breeding examinations and any type of reproductive problem plus annual exams. In most cases, physical examination findings are unremarkable, but occasionally abnormalities associated with *B canis* infection are identified and warrant further investigation.
- Laboratory Testing
  - Blood Culture
    - Though listed as the earliest (2 weeks post-infection) and most accurate method for diagnosis, challenges to the successful isolation of *B canis* include finding a laboratory with proper biosafety conditions (BL3).[23] It is important to have knowledge of factors that may limit successful culture such as the use of EDTA as an anticoagulant in place of preferred heparin or sodium citrate that can inhibit bacterial growth as they can lead to inadequate conditions for storage or transport.[23] Negative cultures do not rule out the possibility of this disease.[41]
- Other fluids for culture:
  - Positive cultures can be obtained from urine even when blood cultures are negative.[16] Diagnostic samples collected by cystocentesis are best since they prevent bacterial overgrowth by unwanted urethral contaminants.[16,39] However, diagnostic samples collected by catheterization may have greater levels of semen in the sample, which can be a predominant source of *B canis* organisms. Postabortion vaginal discharge, aborted placenta as well as aborted fetal tissue contain large numbers of *B.canis* organisms (10^{10} bacteria/mL)[2] and are excellent samples for culture. Semen and seminal fluid

(prostatic portion of the ejaculate) are good fluid samples to culture, especially during the first 3 months of infection.[37]

o If only excised tissues are available such as in the case of postmortem samples in a kennel depopulation, or a suspect animal was spayed/neutered, then the best tissues to collect for culture would include male reproductive organs such as prostatic, testicular, and epididymal tissue. Semen and seminal fluid may be collected from the epididymis, which may contain higher numbers of *B canis* organisms. The best tissues for culture in the female reproductive organs include swabs of the vagina and uterus along with submission of any fluid found within these structures.

- Serology
  - Serologic testing for *B canis* utilizes a reaction between *B canis* antibodies in the host to either rough *B canis* bacteria cell wall antigen or cytoplasmic protein antigen used in the test.[39] Test results utilizing serology may be positive 2 to 4 weeks after the onset of infection.
  - Serum antibody titers can be delayed as long as 12+ weeks after exposure to the disease.[41] These antibody titers can fluctuate even with a persistent bacteremia and the magnitude of the titer does not reflect the stage of this disease.[39] Truly positive dogs may test negative initially. Chronically infected dogs may also falsely test negative on serology, due to low circulating antibody titers.[38] Treatment with antimicrobial drugs can affect test results by eliminating bacteremia, thereby reducing antibody production, and so should be avoided during the testing period.[15] Clinicians should note that serologic tests designed to detect infections with smooth *Brucella spp.* (eg, *B abortus*) will NOT detect infection with rough *B canis* due to the lack of the O-lipopolysaccharide side chain used as the antigen in smooth coat *Brucella* tests.[15]

- Rapid Slide Agglutination Test (RSAT or card test)
  - RSAT was first developed in 1974 as a simple in-house card test, available as D-Tec CB manufactured by Zoetis (Kalamazoo, MI, USA). It is no longer available commercially.

- Modified RSAT (ME-RSAT & M-RSAT)
  - The ME-RSAT test incorporates 2-mercaptoethanol (2 ME) into the traditional RSAT test to inactivate the IgM on the *Brucella ovis* bacteria, which stops the cross-reaction (and consequent false positive test) with the large capsule organisms and certain gram-negative bacteria.[39] Similarly, it is not currently available commercially.

- Tube Agglutination Test (TAT)
  - TAT is a serodiagnostic procedure done to confirm infection dogs after a positive result with other assays.[37] The solution contains heat-killed and washed *B canis* bacteria.[39] Availability of this solution for testing purposes is erratic. Cross-reactions between other infectious agents may occur, so 2 ME clarification is needed with this test[37] and false-positive test results are still possible.[38] Test results are semi-quantitative with a 1:200 titer considered evidence of an active infection.[39] When titers are low, those dogs should be considered suspect positive and need to be retested 2 weeks later, when *B canis* diagnosis will likely be confirmed.[41] Hemolyzed sera samples should not be used for testing due to increased risk for cross-reaction.[41] Positive test results often correlate with positive blood cultures. Due to a lack of standardized reagents or testing methods, it

is difficult to compare ME-TAT titers from one case to another for diagnostic purposes. No commercial tests for TAT are currently available on the market.[41]

- Agar Gel Immunodiffusion Test (AGIDcpa & AGIDcwa)
  - AGIDcpa is considered a confirmation test for suspected *B canis* cases. The AGIDcpa utilizes cytoplasmic protein antigens (cpa) extracted from the *B canis* cytoplasm. This test is highly specific for the genus *Brucella* and is useful in distinguishing between infected and non-infected dogs.[40] The AGIDcwa (cell wall antigen) is a less specific test that may incur more positive cross-reactions seen with aforementioned bacteria.[39,41] The test is comprised of seven wells cut into agarose gel, which is used to test multiple "suspect" sera samples. There are six peripheral wells to hold the "suspect" sera samples and a central well that contains *B canis* antigen. Antibodies from the "suspect" sera diffuse inward to meet outbound antigen. Distinct smooth precipitin arcs are formed where the positive sera and *B canis* antigen meet, which indicates a positive result.[39] Positive test results using AGIDcpa can be expected 8 to 12 weeks postinfection and test results usually become negative 3 to 4 years later.[39] Unfortunately, there are a limited number of diagnostic laboratories that perform *B canis* testing via AGIDcpa. Special media is needed for this test along with trained personnel, making cost for this test higher than most *B canis* diagnostic testing. Additionally, this test should not be used as a "screening test" since other tests such as TAT, ELISA, and culture are more sensitive in picking up *B canis* infections earlier in the course of disease where AGID test results would likely be negative[39]

- Enzyme-linked immunoassay (ELISA)
  - ELISA testing can utilize either *Brucella* surface antigens or cytoplasmic protein, meaning that this test can serve as both a screening and/or confirmatory test for *B canis*. ELISA testing is considered less sensitive than TAT as a screening test, but more sensitive than the agglutination tests or AGID. This type of testing can detect antibodies as early as 30 days postinfection, but also in chronically infected dogs. Sensitivity and specificity will vary according to the antigen used.[16,23] Cornell University's Animal Health Diagnostic Center offers an ELISA-like test on a Luminex bead platform (Multiplex *Brucella canis* screening test) with an estimated sensitivity of 95.3%.[62]

- Immunochromatographic Assay (ICA)
  - The current lack of production of the Witness D-Tec CB test has left a gap in available in-house screening tests for the small animal clinical practitioner. A few websites have popped up offering immunochromatographic test kits; however, these tests do not have current USDA or FDA approval (Bionote USA, personal communication, January 8, 2023). The technology has now been widely used for in-home COVID-19 testing. Certainly, its low cost, lack of need for specialized laboratory equipment, ease of use, and rapid execution makes them attractive as a potential screening test for *B canis*. There is a high association between traditional 2ME-RSAT and ICA assay test results.[63] Unfortunately ICA assays showed 10.41% false negative results in dogs confirmed by culture to be infected with *B canis*, and are felt to be lacking in sensitivity, making them an inadequate screening test option.[64]

- Genetic Detection of *B canis*
  - The entire genome of *B canis* has been successfully sequenced so that the genetic exploration of this organism can move forward.[65,66]

- Polymerase Chain Reaction (PCR)
  - PCR primers have been designed to detect *B canis* DNA in whole blood, vaginal secretions, urine and semen targeting gene sequences that are conserved among *Brucella spp* such as *bcsp*31, 16S ribosomal subunit, and *recap*.[15,16,56,67,68] Genetic detection of bacterial DNA is more sensitive and specific than blood cultures and serology in detecting infection.[38] Quantitative PCR can give insight into the amount of DNA within a particular diagnostic sample. PCR is a useful confirmatory test for seropositive dogs, but also has the potential to rapidly screen kennel populations for the presence of disease.[15] PCR also allows for species as well biovar identification, which opens the window to genetic fingerprinting, assisting with both disease control and epidemiological study.[38] There is minimal biological containment required for this type of testing and relatively short test turn-around time for results, certainly shorter than culture, and it is not affected by viability of the organism (organism can be detected live or dead). However, the sensitivity of the technique can be lowered by the use of serum in place of whole blood, antibiotic use and the use of PCR inhibitors such as heparin.[16] Unfortunately, this type of testing is not available at most diagnostic laboratories and costs related to PCR testing makes testing cost prohibitive for most kennels at this time.

- Clustered Regularly Interspaced Short Palindromic Repeats (CRISPR-Cas systems)
  - CRISPR-Cas is a relatively newly discovered defense system that protects bacteria against invasion by mobile genetic elements such as viruses and plasmids. The utilization of CRISPR-Cas systems to detect pathogens via CRISPR-based biosensors has attracted more attention by utilizing sensing strategies that can be coupled with electrochemistry, fluorescence colorimetry, or other detection methods to detect disease. Based on the detection of the conserved genetic sequence of omp2a, both a fluorescent CRISPR (F-CRISPR) and electrochemical CRISPR (E-CRISPR) have been used to detect the infection of *Brucella spp*. in blood and milk samples.[69] RPA-based F-CRISPR has the distinct advantage that it can quickly detect *Brucella* without the need for complex instruments. The test shows good specificity in the detection of *Brucella* from other pathogenic bacteria, but overall sensitivity and comparison to other methods were not mentioned.[69] It is not currently available for clinical use.

See Addendum for more information on the availability of *B canis* testing.

Medical Treatment Versus Sterilization for Clinical Cases

Medical treatment for this disease is not recommended even though there are published protocols listed in many textbooks and journals. *B canis* bacteria hide from the host immune system inside cells for extended periods of time and bacteremia can be episodic; making effective treatment problematic.[37,41]

As such, long durations of therapy, often for several months are required, and even then antibiotic therapy does not guarantee clearance from these sites with relapse or reinfection common. Because of this potential for antimicrobial resistance, combination antibiotic therapy may be warranted.[37,39] Several studies have indicated that combination therapy with doxycycline, enrofloxacin, and streptomycin can lead to loss of seropositivity indicating possible cure, but this has yet to be proven.[70,71]

Sterilization by removal of some of the reproductive organs of the dog certainly is a means to reduce the shedding of bacteria, both by excision of infected tissue and prevention of mating, but does not completely eliminate risk. Vaginal secretions, urine, and prostatic fluid are still potential sources of bacterial shredding into the environment. Normal dog behaviors such as sniffing and licking at each other and these secretions provide access to infected secretions.

Prevention and Owner Education

Currently, prevention is focused on limiting kennel exposure to infection, coupled with the identification and elimination of infected dogs, both from kennels as well as from the public sector. This requires yearly testing of all breeding stock as well as testing of imported dogs. Biosecurity of the kennel is of the utmost importance once a negative *B canis* status has been obtained for the kennel.[38] The USDA and the Georgia Department of Agriculture have websites with strategies for breeding facilities to follow to help prevent disease caused by *B canis*.[38] In the United States, if an owner has a positive dog there are published recommendations to follow for case management.[15] Owner education by their veterinarian is an important part of this disease so owners understand the disease process and how to avoid bringing *B canis* into their home or kennel.

Future Possibilities

- Nanotechnology or other drug formulation changes

There are ongoing research efforts to facilitate better tissue penetration to treat *B canis* infection. Among these new technologies are liposomal formulations[72] and the use of micro or nanoparticle to release drugs that target monocytes and macrophages, frequent host cells of this infection.[72–75] Ideally, nano particles are bound to a drug, are biodegradable, non-toxic, can protect the drug from cellular injury and then deliver the drug to its target site. This can include liposomes, micelles, dendrimers, nanotubules, and polymeric nanoparticles such as solid lipid nanoparticles (SLN).[75] To date, although liposomal formulations are in use for anti-fungal and anti-parasitic drugs, there has not been considerable market desire for the development of these formulations for antibiotics to treat *B canis*. More interest currently exists in nano drug delivery to treat *B abortus* and *Brucella melitensis* in developing countries.

- Vaccine Possibilities

Although a *B canis* vaccine is not currently available, its development could drastically decrease the incidence of infection in a population of dogs, which then reduces the risk of transmission of disease to humans. There are concerns that a vaccine for *B canis* would invoke an antibody response that would interfere with diagnostic testing. However, there are other vaccines on the market such as *B abortus* (RB51) that utilize vaccine modifications allowing for the identification of vaccinated versus infected animals.[40,76] On the horizon, two new vaccine candidates, *B.ovis* abcBA and *B.canis* RM6/66 vjbR have been studied in the mouse model and shown to offer protection against experimental challenges. The latter was noted to not be shed in urine or semen when administered subcutaneously to dogs.[16,20]

Legislative and Bureaucratic Challenges

Many countries do not have rules or regulations related to *B canis* testing or control. This attitude is predominantly because there is a lack of awareness of the emotional and financial devastation this disease can cause.[23,39,49,56]

Few serological studies have been performed to track this disease, especially in humans, so this disease has been able to spread unchecked for a number of years internationally.[15] There is a need for required testing of imported and breeding dogs and their offspring at a national and international level, mandated before interstate and international movement of dogs. Only with such regulations in place can we hope to fully understand and reduce the risk of transmission of *B canis* between dogs and from dogs to humans.[15]

At the time of this writing, the Healthy Dog Importation Act HR 4239 is a bill to be brought before the United States Congress to amend the Animal Health Protection Act with respect to the importation of live dogs. It would require an imported dog to be permanently identified (microchip or tattoo) and deemed to be in good health prior to entry. Additionally, a complete vaccine history and negative infectious disease test results would be mandated for entry into the US. A certificate would accompany the dog attesting to its vaccination status and negative test results along with endorsement by the veterinarian issuing the certificate. The exceptions to this requirement include: dogs imported for research purposes and dogs imported to seek veterinary treatment (dog is taken directly to the veterinary facility with appropriate quarantine observed and then exported back to its country of origin). Finally, if a puppy is less than 6 months of age it can be imported into the state of Hawaii as long as it is in compliance with that state's regulations and is not transported out of Hawaii prior to 6 months of age.[77] Considering some puppies may be infected and have the potential to shed *B canis*, this last exception is concerning. This proposed bill represents a much-needed start to tackling the problem of the international movement of dogs and monitoring for zoonotic disease.

The CDC's temporary suspension of dogs imported from high-risk countries endemic for rabies has been extended through July 31, 2023. This means if a dog's country of origin can be determined as a country where rabies is considered high risk it may enter the United States with the proper paperwork. The dog must be older than 6 months of age with permanent identification by ISO-compatible microchip. It has to have a valid US-issued rabies vaccination certificate, a valid CDC record that includes the vaccination history and microchip information plus rabies serology test results showing adequate titers drawn within 45 days and 1 year of arrival.[78] Rabies is currently the only vaccination and testing required for entry into the United States even though it is not the only disease of zoonotic concern. The hope is that required testing for *B canis* and other zoonotic diseases (Leishmaniasis, intestinal parasites, and so forth) will be implemented for entry of dogs into the United States, especially in light of the increased number of dogs being imported for adoption/rescue.

SUMMARY

Brucella canis is a disease that is becoming a more prominent problem in dogs. General practitioners need to have heightened awareness of this disease. Practitioners need to be able to identify presenting clinical signs, as well as how to diagnose it effectively and manage the disease in household pets and kennels. Advising owners on proper screening for this disease, treatment recommendations, and kennel management is paramount. This disease is enzootic in dogs in many parts of the world and these dogs are now being imported without prior infectious disease screening. This disease will remain an underrecognized threat to animal welfare and human health until there are international guidelines for infection control and management of it. A good first step in this process would be requiring mandatory *B canis* testing of any dog before international movement in addition to interstate movement. With this simple step, the movement of infected dogs could be stopped and the spread of this disease reduced.

CLINICS CARE POINTS

Clinical signs of disease
- General
  Lethargy, poor hair coat, fatigue, weight loss, exercise intolerance, lymphadenopathy, splenomegaly, recurrent uveitis, lameness, muscle weakness, spinal pain, neurological dysfunction, discospondylitis, osteomyelitis.
- Female
  Infertility, late-term abortion after Day 45 to 59 gestation, endometritis, placentitis along with a dark fetid vaginal discharge.
- Male
  Infertility, acute epididymitis, prostatitis, orchitis, moist scrotal dermatitis, testicular atrophy, sperm agglutination, sperm abnormalities, and inflammatory cells in ejaculate.

DISCLOSURE

The authors have no commercial or financial conflicts of interest and any funding sources to disclose.

SUPPLEMENTARY DATA

Supplementary data related to this article can be found online at https://doi.org/10.1016/j.cvsm.2023.05.002.

REFERENCES

1. Kauffman LK, Petersen CA. Canine brucellosis: Old foe and reemerging scourge. Vet Clin North Am Small Anim Pract 2019;49(4):763–79.
2. Olsen SC, Palmer MV. Advancement of knowledge of *Brucella* over the past 50 years. Vet Pathol 2014;51:1076–80.
3. Xavier MN, Costa EA, Paixão TA, et al. The genus *Brucella* and clinical manifestations of brucellosis. Cienc Rural 2009;39:2252–60.
4. Whatmore AM, Dawson CE, Groussaud P, et al. Marine mammal *Brucella* genotype associated with zoonotic infection. Emerg Infect Dis 2008;14:517–8.
5. Scholz HC, Hubalek Z, Sedlacek I, et al. *Brucella microti* sp. nov., isolated from the common vole Microtus arvalis. Int J Syst Evol Microbiol 2008;58:375–82.
6. Whatmore AM, Davison N, Cloeckaert A, et al. *Brucella papionis* sp. nov., isolated from baboons (*Papio spp.* Int J Syst Evol Microbiol 2014;64:4120–8.
7. Scholz HC, Revilla-Fernandez S, Dahouk S, et al. *Brucella vulpis* sp. nov., isolated from mandibular lymph nodes of red foxes (*Vulpes vulpes*). Int J Syst Evol Microbiol 2016;66:2090–8.
8. De BK, Stauffer L, Koylass MS, et al. Novel *Brucella* strain (BO1) associated with a prosthetic breast implant infection. J Clin Microbiol 2008;46:43–9.
9. Helmick KE, Garner MM, Ryan J, et al. Clinicopathologic features of infection with novel *Brucella* organisms in captive waxy tree frogs *(Phyllomedusa sauvagii)* and Colorado River toads (*Incilius alvarius*). J Zoo Wildl Med 2017;49:153–61.
10. Hoyer BH, McCullough NB. Homologies of deoxyribonucleic acids from *Brucella ovis*, canine abortion organisms, and other *Brucella* species. J Bacteriol 1968;96:1783–90.
11. Foster JT, Okinaka RT, Svensson R, et al. Real-time PCR assays of single-nucleotide polymorphisms defining the major *Brucella* clades. J Clin Microbiol 2008;46:296–301.

12. Schoenemann J, Lutticken R, Scheibner E. [*Brucella canis* infection in man]. Dtsch Med Wochenschr 1986;111:20–2.

13. Rumley RL, Chapman SW. *Brucella canis*: an infectious cause of prolonged fever of undetermined origin. South Med J 1986;79:626–8.

14. Lum MK, Pien FD, Sasaki DM. Human *Brucella* canis infection in Hawaii. Hawaii Med J 1985;44:66–8.

15. Hensel ME, Negron M, Arenas-Gamboa AM. Brucellosis in dogs and public health risk. Emerg Infect Dis 2018;24:1401–6.

16. Santos RL. Souza,TD, Mol JPS, Eckstein C, Paixão TA. Canine brucellosis: an update. Fronti Vet Sci 2021;8(594291):1–17.

17. Whitten TV, Brayshaw G, Patnayak D, et al. Seroprevalence of *Brucella canis* antibodies in dogs entering a Minnesota humane society, Minnesota, 2016-2017. Prev Vet Med 2019;168:90–4.

18. Daly R, Willis KC, Wood J, et al. Seroprevalence of *Brucella canis* in dogs rescued from South Dakota indian reservations, 2015-2019. Prev Vet Med 2020;184(105157):1–5. https://doi.org/10.1016/j.prevetmed.2020.105157.

19. Dentinger CM, Jacob K, Lee LV, et al. Human *Brucella canis* infection and subsequent laboratory exposures associated with a puppy, New York City, 2012. Zoonoses Public Hlth 2015;62(5):407–14.

20. Stranahan LW, Sankar PC, Garcia-Gonzalez DG, et al. Evaluation of the efficacy of the *Brucella canis* RM6/66 △vjbR vaccine candidate for protection against *B.canis* infection in mice. mSphere 2020;5:e00172.

21. Brower A, Okwumabua O, Massengill C, et al. Investigation of the spread of *Brucella canis* via the U.S. interstate dog trade. Int J Infect Dis 2007;11(5):454–8.

22. Hubbard K, Wang M, Smith DR. Seroprevalence of brucellosis in Mississippi shelter dogs. Prev Vet Med 2018;159:82–6.

23. Mol JPS, Guedes ACB, Eckstein C, et al. Diagnosis of canine brucellosis: comparison of various serologic tests and PCR. J Vet Diagn Invest 2020;32:77–86.

24. Strand P, Smith F, New J, et al. How outdated perceptions have reshaped the dog marketplace. Clin Theriogenology 2019;11(3):225–33.

25. Pieracci EG, Williams CE, Wallace RM, et al. U.S. dog importations during the COVID-19 pandemic. Do we have an erupting problem? PLoS One 2021;16(9): e0254287.

26. Polak K. Dog transport and infectious disease risk. Vet Clin North Am Small Anim Pract 2019;49:599–613.

27. Egloff S, Schneeberger M, Gobeli S, et al. *Brucella canis* infection in a young dog with epididymitis and orchitis. Schweiz Arch Tierheilkd 2018;160(12):743–8.

28. Schnelle A, Korber H, Goericke-Pesch S. Brucella canis- a potentially underestimated infection in Germany. In: ISCFR-EVSSAR Proceedings. 2022. Available at: http://www.ivis.org/library/iscfr/iscfr-evssar-symposium-italy-2022. Accessed Jan 19, 2023.

29. Morgan JVP, Rys H, Wake T, et al. *Brucella canis* in a dog in the UK. Vet Rec 2017; 180(15):384–5.

30. Hamdy MER, Abdel-Haleem MH, Dawod RE, et al. First seroprevalence and molecular identification report of *Brucella canis* among dogs in Greater Cairo region and Damietta Governorate of Egypt. Vet World 2023;16(1):229–38.

31. van Dijk MAM, Engelsma MY, Visser VXN, et al. Transboundary spread of *Brucella canis* through import of infected dogs, the Netherlands, November 2016-December 2018. Emerg Infect Dis 2021;27(7):1783–8.

32. Kaden R, Agren J, Baverud V, et al. Brucellosis outbreak in a Swedish kennel in 2013; determination of genetic markers for course tracing. Vet Microbiol 2014; 174(3–4):523–30.

33. Bardenstein S, Waner T, Etinger M, et al. First diagnosis of *Brucella canis* infection in dogs in Israel. Isr J Vet Med 2021;2021(76):12–5.

34. Suarez-Esquivel M, Ruiz-Villalobos N, Hidalgo-Jara W, et al. Canine brucellosis in Costa Rica reveals widespread *Brucella canis* infection and the recent introduction of foreign strains. Vet Microbiol 2021;257(109072):1–8.

35. Boeri EJ, Madariaga MJ, Dominguez ML, et al. *Brucella canis* group 2 isolated in Argentina. Rev Argent Microbiol 2021;53:98–103.

36. de Souza TD, de Carvalho TF, Mol J, et al. Tissue distribution and cell tropism of *Brucella canis* in naturally infected canine foetuses and neonates. Sci Rep 2018; 8:7203.

37. Greene CE, Carmichael LE. Canine Brucellosis. In: Greene CE, editor. Infectious Diseases of the Dog and cat. 4th edition. Athens, GA: Elsevier; 2012. p. 398–411.

38. Cosford KL. *Brucella canis*: An update on research and clinical management. Can Vet J 2018;59:74–81.

39. Hollett RB. Canine brucellosis: outbreaks and compliance. Theriogenology 2006; 66:575–87.

40. Carmichael LE, Shin SJ. Canine brucellosis: a diagnostician's dilemma. Semin Vet Med Surg (Small Anim) 1996;11:161–5.

41. Wanke MM. Canine brucellosis. Anim Reprod Sci 2004;82-83:195–207.

42. Blankenship RM, Sanford JP. *Brucella canis*. A cause of undulant fever. Am J Med 1975;59:424–6.

43. Serikawa T, Muraguchi T. Significance of urine in transmission of canine brucellosis. Jpn J Vet Sci 1979;41:607–16.

44. Nury C, Blais MC, Arsenault J. Risk of transmittable blood-borne pathogens in blood units from blood donor dogs in Canada. J Vet Intern Med 2021;35:1316–24.

45. Peres JN, Godoy AM, Barg L, et al. Isolamento de *Brucella canis* de carrapatos (*Rhipicephalus sanguíneus*). Arquivos da Escola de Veterinaria da UFMG 1981; 83:51–5.

46. Jia W, Chen S, Chi S, et al. Recent progress on tick-borne animal diseases of veterinary and public health significance in China. Viruses 2022;14(355):1–14 v14020355. .

47. Dillon AR, Henderson RA. *Brucella canis* in a uterine stump abscess in a bitch. J Am Vet Med Assoc 1981;178:987–8.

48. Li N, Yu F, Peng F, et al. Probable sexual transmission of brucellosis. IDCases 2020;21(e00871):1–3.

49. Krueger WS, Lucero NE, Brower A, et al. Evidence for unapparent *Brucella canis* infections among adults with occupational exposure to dogs. Zoonoses Public Hlth 2014;61(7):509–18.

50. Marzetti S, Carranza C, Roncall M, et al. Recent trends in human *Brucella canis* infection. Comp Immunol Microbiol Infect Dis 2012;36:55–61.

51. Boebel FW, Ehrenford FA, Brown GM, et al. Agglutinins to *Brucella canis* in stray dogs from certain counties in Illinois and Wisconsin. J Am Vet Med Assoc 1979; 175:276–7.

52. Brown J, Blue JL, Wooley RE, et al. *Brucella canis* infectivity rates in stray and pet dog populations. Am J Public Health 1976a;66:889–91.

53. Brown J, Blue JL, Wooley RE, et al. A serologic survey of a population of Georgia dogs for *Brucella canis* and an evaluation of the slide agglutination test. J Am Vet Med Assoc 1976b;169:1214–6.

54. Lovejoy GS, Carver HD, Moseley IK, et al. Serosurvey of dogs for *Brucella canis* infection in Memphis, Tennessee. Am J Public Health 1976;1976(66):175–6.
55. Myers DM, Varela-Diaz VM. Serological and bacteriological detection of *Brucella canis* infection of stray dogs in Moreno, Argentina. Cornell Vet 1980;70:258–65.
56. Kauffman LK, Bjork JK, Gallup JM, et al. Early detection of *Brucella canis* via quantitative polymerase chain reaction analysis. Zoonoses Public Hlth 2014; 61(1):48–54.
57. Bedford E. Number of dogs in the United States from 2000 to 2017 (in millions). Statista 2022;. https://www.statista.com/statistics/198100/dogs-in-the-united-states-since-2000/. Accessed April 9, 2023.
58. Kavin K. Does America have enough dogs for all the people that want one? The Washington Post. February 8, 2017 https://Washingtonpost.com/news/animalia/wp/2017/02/08/does-Amerioca-have-enough-dogs-for-all-the   people-who-want-one?utm_term=.ed2c1ba72c07d. Accessed April 9, 2023.
59. Hobart E. Morocco has 3 million stray dogs. Meet the people trying to help them. Natl Geogr 2021;. http://nationalgeographic.com/animals/article/meet-the-peopel-helping-morocco-stray-dogs/. Accessed January 18, 2023.
60. Georgia Department of Agriculture, Animal Industry Division. Chapter 40-13-4: Infectious and Contagious Diseases. Revised May 21, 2008. http://agr.georgia.gov/vgn/images/portal/cit_1210/9/34/4124608640-13-4%20Chapter%20Infectious%20and%20Contagious%20Diseases.pdf. Accessed Jan 18, 2003.
61. Centers for Disease Control and Prevention (CDC). Public Health Emergency Preparedness and Response. Brucellosis. Revised May 1, 2018. http://www.bt.cdc.gov/agent/brucellosis/index.asp. Accessed Jan 18, 2023.
62. Cornell University Animal Health Diagnostic Center Website. Changes to Brucella canis Serology Testing. May 11, 2022. https://vet.cornell.edu/animal-health-diagnostic-center/news/changes-brucella–canis-serology-testing. Accessed January 19, 2023.
63. Kim JW, Lee YJ, Han MY, et al. Evaluation of immunochromatographic assay for serodiagnosis of Brucella canis. J Vet Med Sci 2007;69:1103–7.
64. Keid LB, Diniz JA, Oliveira TMFS, et al. Evaluation of an immunochromatographic test to the diagnosis of canine brucellosis caused by Brucella canis. Reprod Domest Anim 2015;50:939–44.
65. Ferreira VA, Girault G, Corde Y, et al. New insights into phylogeography of worldwide Brucella canis isolates by comparative genomics-based approaches: focus on Brazil. BMC Genom 2018;19:636.
66. Wang L, Cui J, Misner MB, et al. Sequencing and phylogenetic characterization of *Brucella canis* isolates, Ohio, 2016. Transbound Emerg Dis 2018;65(4):944–8.
67. Keid LB, Soares RM, Vasconcellos SA, et al. A polymerase chain reaction for detection of *Brucella canis* in vaginal swabs of naturally infected bitches. Theriogenology 2007;68(9):1260–70.
68. Keid LB, Soares RM, Vasconcellos SA, et al. A polymerase chain reaction for the detection of *Brucella canis* in semen of naturally infected dogs. Theriogenology 2007;67(7):1203–10.
69. Xu J, Ma J, Li Y, et al. A general RPA-CRISPR/Cas12a sensing platform for *Brucella spp.* detection in blood and milk samples. Sens. Actuators B Chem 2022; 364(131864):1–9.
70. Wanke MM, Delpino MV, Baldi PC. Use of enrofloxacin in the treatment of canine brucellosis in a dog kennel (clinical trial). Theriogenology 2006;66(6–7):1573–8.
71. Vitas AI, Diaz R, Gamazo C. Protective effect of liposomal gentamicin against systemic acute murine brucellosis. Chemotherapy 1997;43:204–10.

72. Bodaghabadi N, Hajigholami S, Vaise Malekshahi Z, et al. Preparation and evaluation of rifampicin and co-trimoxazole-loaded nanocarrier against *Brucella melitensis* infection. Iran Biomed J 2018;22:275–82.

73. Lecaroz C, Gamazo C, Blanco-Prieto MJ. Nanocarriers with gentamicin to treat intracellular pathogens. J Nanosci Nanotechnol 2006;6:3296–302.

74. Phanse Y, Lueth P, Ramer-Tait AE, et al. Cellular internalization mechanisms of polyanhydride particles: implications for rational design of drug delivery vehicles. J Biomed Nanotechnol 2016;12:1544–52.

75. Hosseini SM, Taheri M, Nouri F, et al. Nano drug delivery in intracellular bacterial infection treatments. Biomed Pharmacother 2022;146(112609):1–13.

76. Dorneles EM, Sriranganathan N, Lage AP. Recent advances in *Brucella abortus* vaccines. Vet Res 2015;46:76.

77. H.R. 4239 Healthy Dog importation Act 117th Congress (2021-2022). Available at: https://www.congress.gov/bill/117th-congress/house-bill/4239/text?r=82&s=1/. Accessed January 28, 2023.

78. High Risk Countries for Dog Rabies. CDC >Importation > Bringing an Animal into the United States > Dogs. Available at: https://www.cdc.gov/importation/bringing-an-animal-into-the-united-states/high-risk.html. Accessed March 17, 2023.

An Update on Male Canine Infertility

Stuart J. Mason, BVSc (Hons) MANZCVS DACT

KEYWORDS

- Male infertility • hCG • Semen alkaline phosphatase • Testicular biopsy
- Phytoestrogen • Azoospermia • Oligozoospermia

KEY POINTS

- Male infertility is half of the equation in respect of breeding dogs.
- Alkaline phosphatase measurement in semen is an indicator of completeness of ejaculation.
- Human chorionic gonadotropin response testing allows for hormone assessment in male dogs.
- Early testicular biopsy may allow for treatment to improve fertility before irreversible changes occur in the testicles.
- Spermatozoa production and fertility are sensitive to dietary constituents, the environment, and age of the animal.

INTRODUCTION

Male dogs presenting for fertility assessment are commonplace in small animal reproduction clinics. It is common to find articles outlining semen and prostate fluid analysis for infertility investigations in male dogs[1-3]; however, there are few articles discussing in detail what to do after obtaining results from spermiograms in dogs.[4-7] This article aims to outline processes involved in working up fertility issues of male dogs that are normal on clinical examination; however, their spermiograms contain suboptimal motility values and or percentage of morphologically normal spermatozoa. The minimum recommended criterion for optimally fertile fresh semen is 70% progressively motile spermatozoa[8] and 60% morphologically normal spermatozoa.[9] In bulls, it is recommended to have a maximum of 15% (noncompensable) to 25%(compensable) of any one morphological abnormality[10]; however, to the author's knowledge, there is no specific study related to this in dogs, yet it would be prudent to still follow these guidelines. Spermatogenesis in the dog is a protracted process, 62 days plus 14 days epididymal transit time, so a "wait and see approach" will not suit all cases because spermatogenesis may cease in this time period. It is important to understand

Monash Veterinary Clinic, 1662 Dandenong Road, Oakleigh East, Victoria 3166, Australia
E-mail address: drstuartmason@gmail.com

Vet Clin Small Anim 53 (2023) 1063–1081
https://doi.org/10.1016/j.cvsm.2023.04.006
0195-5616/23/© 2023 Elsevier Inc. All rights reserved.

when assessing morphological abnormalities in the spermiogram where in the production process the abnormalities are produced in order to have an idea of when next to test the semen and expect an improvement in the quality of the spermiogram. Spermiograms are often classified as azoospermic (complete absence of spermatozoa in the ejaculate), oligozoospermic (reduced numbers of spermatozoa in the ejaculate), and teratozoospermic (increased number of abnormal spermatozoa in the ejaculate). Causative processes of all 3 of these classifications overlap as does the advanced investigation.

ALKALINE PHOSPHATASE ANALYSIS IN SEMINAL FLUID

Within the canine reproductive tract, alkaline phosphatase (AP) has been shown to be secreted mainly from the epididymis in dogs; primarily the cauda epididymis.[11] Levels of AP in the canine ejaculate are greatest in the second, semen-rich fraction, compared with the first or third prostate fluid fractions.[4,5,11] The measurement of AP levels in the ejaculate of dogs has been recommended to differentiate azoospermia due to obstructive causes from azoospermia due to secretory issues from the testes.[2–5,12–15] Carnitine has also been shown to be produced by the epididymis of dogs; however, assays for carnitine are not readily available.[13] Specific levels of AP in the canine ejaculate indicating complete ejaculation, partial ejaculation, and absence of bilateral outflow obstructions from the epididymis are commonly quoted as being more than 5000 IU/L,[2,3,13–15] and if the level is less than 5000 IU/L, then ejaculation is considered incomplete or a bilateral epididymal outflow obstruction is present.[2,12] Review of the referenced literature by Frenette,[11] indicates that no studies have been performed to come up with the cutoff of 5000 IU/L AP[11]; however, they do indicate levels of AP activity in the units of micromole per hour per milligram protein, which to the author's knowledge is not able to be converted to the commonly used units for measuring AP of international units per liter. Johnston first made mention of the 5000 IU/L AP level[4]; however, review of that article shows that they were indicating that in most dogs, AP is very high and so very low levels would indicate incomplete ejaculation or bilateral outflow obstruction, and a cutoff number for complete or incomplete ejaculation was not intended (personal communication with author, S. Johnston, 2022). What should be ascertained from the references is that in a good, complete ejaculate, the level of AP in the fluid will be very high, and if there is an obstruction or incomplete ejaculation, the level will be low. Therefore, azoospermia with a high AP level indicates a problem of testicular origin, whereas azoospermia with a low AP level does not identify the source of the problem because it could be due to obstructive disease, psychosomatic issues, or failure of adequate ejaculation. It is the author's recommendation to not use a numerical cutoff for complete or incomplete ejaculation in future.

Obstructive azoospermia in dogs seems to be not a well-documented issue through analysis of the literature. It is suspected but difficult to prove in the dog because in many cases, the male dog may not ejaculate well for the person collecting the semen, resulting in low AP levels.[6] To the author's knowledge, there is no publication of a case of obstructive azoospermia in the dog.

If the AP level in the canine ejaculate is high, then it is recommended to progress to human chorionic gonadotropin (hCG) response testing as the next step in infertility investigation. If the AP level is low, then collection again may be attempted in different situations, that is, with or without a teaser bitch, different breeds or sizes of teaser bitches, making sure the teaser is at the peak of estrus, trying the semen collection outside in nature rather than in a veterinary consulting room, with the prior use in the male of anxiolytic medications such as trazadone, or through the use of natural prostaglandin F2α, which has been shown to increase sperm numbers in the ejaculate.[16] The author has been presented with one case of a male dog for semen collection and semen freezing on multiple occasions wherein the male seems to ejaculate normally; however, the ejaculate was clear, azoospermic, and the AP level was less than 5000 IU/mL. This male dog both before, during and after the attempted semen collection techniques continued to get bitches pregnant with good litter size. The male was subsequently collected via electroejaculation under general anesthesia; however, a semen sample good enough to freeze was not attained. Therefore, the presence of azoospermia with low AP levels may not always indicate a problem with the testicles or ejaculation process as a source of infertility and electroejaculation or test matings to known fertile bitches may be attempted to ascertain if the male dog in question is in fact infertile. If though the AP level is low with azoospermia in a male dog, which has failed to get multiple known fertile bitches pregnant, then the next step in investigation is ultrasound of the reproductive tract.

RETROGRADE EJACULATION

In cases of azoospermia and oligozoospermia, it is important to analyze a urine sample via cystocentesis for the presence of spermatozoa after semen collection. In both dogs with normal fertility and those with azoospermia and oligozoospermia, spermatozoa will be found in urine samples after semen collection.[17] In some male dogs, they may undergo retrograde ejaculation, which occurs as a result of seminal fluid passing from the proximal urethra into the bladder rather than out through the distal urethra as would occur in antegrade ejaculation.[18,19] Retrograde ejaculation occurs when there is the presence of spermatozoa in the urine of azoospermic dogs, or subjectively large numbers of sperm in the urine of oligospermic dogs. If retrograde ejaculation is confirmed, treatment is in most cases successful through the use of phenylpropanolamine at 4 mg/kg once daily for 5 days before semen collection.[17] This dose of phenylpropanolamine is higher than the labeled dose rate for urinary incontinence.

ULTRASOUND OF THE TESTES AND PROSTATE

Testicular and prostate ultrasounds are well documented in the literature.[2,20,21] Testicles should undergo ultrasound examination in a way to show both testes at once to compare the architecture between testes. The use of a linear probe aids in this process. The normal testes are homogenous in appearance, with the presence of hypoechoic lesions indicating fluid of some sort, and hyperechoic areas suggesting increased cellular density such as inflammation, granulomas, or tumors. These are the most common changes seen on ultrasound of the testis. The presence of isolated hyperechoic lesions will allow for ultrasound-guided fine needle aspiration (FNA) under sedation.

Chronic prostate inflammation and disease will result in poor-quality semen samples due to inflammation extending through the whole reproductive tract.[2] Prostate ultrasound allows for the objective assessment of size and texture of the prostate gland.[20] Ultrasound of the canine prostate is simple to perform, and can be done either standing, lateral, or dorsal recumbency, with no clipping needed as the ultrasound can be easily performed using alcohol and acoustic gel in the groin.[20] Three ultrasound views in each of the transverse and sagittal (longitudinal) planes should be taken using the hypoechoic urethra as a landmark to ensure the image of the prostate is complete.[20] The average of the width (W, centimeter) seen in the transverse and sagittal images, height (H, centimeter) from the transverse images and the length (L, centimeter) from the sagittal images are inserted into the following formula to calculate the prostatic volume (V, cubic centimeter). The volume of the prostate is calculated using the following formula: $V = L \times H \times W \times 0.523$. As a guide, a calculation for normal prostate volume (V, cubic centimeter) is obtained using the following formula considering variations in body weight (BW) in kilogram and age in years (A)[21]: $V = (0.087 \times BW) + (1.885 \times A) + 15.88$; values obtained in excess of this calculated volume indicates an enlargement of the prostate. Digital palpation of the prostate is purported by many to assess for size, texture, and pain; however, in the author's experience, the prostate gland is difficult to palpate digitally except for the caudo-dorsal border in glands that have not fallen cranially over the pelvic brim. Pain is also difficult to assess because most dogs resent digital rectal palpation and this resistance may be misinterpreted as pain.

Chronically inflamed canine prostate glands will invariably show small (<2 mm) hyperechoic cystic lesions scattered throughout the enlarged prostate gland. In the author's experience, prostate ultrasound is best interpreted in conjunction with cytological analysis of the third fraction of the ejaculate (the prostate fluid). With evidence of inflammation of this third fraction, indicated by increased numbers of lymphocytes or macrophages and red blood cells on cytology, a presumptive diagnosis of benign prostatic hyperplasia (BPH) is most often made[2] and the presence of large numbers gram-negative rods (rarely gram-positive) in conjunction with increased numbers of neutrophils with or without intracellular bacteria indicates overlying prostatitis.[20] *Escherichia coli* is the most common pathogen found on culture of prostatic fluid in animals with prostatitis.[20] Serum canine prostate-specific arginine esterase, an enzyme produced by the canine prostate, increases in cases of BPH and may aid in its diagnosis; however, availability of testing is limited currently to the United Kingdom and Europe, with many countries not offering the test.[20] If the animal is not intended to be used further for breeding, castration is curative; however, in breeding animals, BPH may be treated with the use of finasteride (a 5α-reductase inhibitor) or osaterone acetate (a progestin and antiandrogen)[22–24] enabling treatment of the BPH while having no negative effects on fertility. At the time of writing this article, osaterone acetate is only available in Europe and the United Kingdom. Both of these treatments result in transient improvement in semen quality, peaking in effect at 4 months after treatment with osaterone acetate[22,24] or 4 months after beginning treatment with finasteride (observed unpublished data by author S. Mason, 2023). It is not recommended to use the dog for stud duties in the first 4 months of treatment as semen quality will not improve and may transiently decline in this period with the use of osaterone acetate.[22,24] Deslorelin (a GnRH agonist) may too be used for successful treatment of BPH; however, due to the variable length of action, up to 2.7 years with a single dose of deslorelin,[25] deslorelin is best reserved for nonbreeding animals, or animals in which semen has been preserved previously to the diagnosis of BPH because its use will result in azoospermia from continued suppression of the hypothalamic pituitary axis. A full discussion of workup of disease of the prostate including treatments is discussed in a previous issue.[20]

SEMEN CULTURE

Semen collection in the dog is not a sterile process; however, the presence of an overgrowth of one bacterial species may indicate the presence of bacterial orchitis, requiring treatment with appropriate antibiotics based on culture and sensitivity results. Semen samples should be cultured aerobically, and for mycoplasma and ureoplasma. Bacteria commonly cultured in canine semen comprise bacteria of the normal flora of dogs; these include but are not limited to *Streptococcus canis*, *Staphylococcus pseudointermedius, Pasteurella multocida,* and *Moraxella species.*[6] The author recommends culture of both the second, sperm-rich fraction, and third, prostate fraction separately. The growth of mixed flora or low-grade growth of one species of bacteria is not thought significant. In countries where *Brucella canis* is endemic animals should undergo regular testing to ensure the breeding animals are free of this disease. *B canis* is a difficult bacteria to culture, and serology tests sometimes yield false positive results, therefore the use of more specific polymerase chain reaction testing may be recommended[6,26–28] (See article "Canine Brucellosis Update" by Kauffman and Sebdza of this issue).

Low-grade chronic orchitis or epididymitis may give rise to autoimmune orchitis or epididymitis through the continued chronic inflammatory process from a low-grade infection as diagnosed by testicular biopsy, as discussed later.[6] Some animals with orchitis may be unwilling to provide semen samples due to pain, wherein FNA or biopsy of the testis and epididymis may be required (see later discussion). Autoimmune orchitis and epididymitis are diagnosed via testicular biopsy (see later discussion) with treatments including appropriate antibiotics and anecdotally corticosteroids for autoimmune disease, although it must be remembered that the use of corticosteroids may control the inflammation and immune reaction in the testes, it may too be detrimental to fertility because cortisol opposes the action of luteinizing hormone (LH).

HUMAN CHORIONIC GONADOTROPIN/GONADOTROPIN RELEASING HORMONE RESPONSE TESTING

Spermatogenesis in all mammalian species is controlled by the hypothalamic pituitary gonadal axis, and an understanding of this process is important because aberrations in normal hormone profiles will affect the quantity and morphology of spermatozoa produced by the testicles.

Normal Hypothalamic Pituitary Gonadal Axis Function

Gonadotropin releasing hormone (GnRH) is a neuropeptide released from neurons in the hypothalamus, which in turn stimulates the release of glycoproteins follicle stimulating hormone (FSH) and LH from the gonadotroph cells of the anterior lobe of the pituitary into the blood stream. In male mammals, LH stimulates testosterone production from the interstitial cells of Leydig, which diffuses across into the seminiferous tubules and the blood stream.[29] In the seminiferous tubules testosterone binds to receptors on the Sertoli cells, and with FSH, testosterone acts on the Sertoli cells of the testes to stimulate follicular development (and subsequent spermatocyte production and development to spermatids and spermatozoa), and estradiol synthesis.[29,30] GnRH secretion is controlled via negative feedback of testosterone and estradiol produced from the testes. The Sertoli cells also produce inhibin and activin, with activin stimulating FSH production and inhibin having an inhibitory effect on FSH secretion once spermatids are produced.[30,31]

Estrogens also affect the production of testosterone through negative feedback on the hypothalamic pituitary axis and stimulate resorption of 96% of the rete testis fluid in the efferent ductules of the epididymis.[32] Additionally, estrogens control the osmolarity and pH of the fluid in the epididymis to minimize damage to sperm plasma membranes, and help maximize the number of morphologically normal motile spermatozoa in the ejaculate.[32] Estrogens are produced in the testes by cytochrome P450 aromatase in the germ cells, epithelial cells of the efferent ducts and epididymis, and interstitial cells of the epididymis.[32]

Prolactin is secreted from lactotroph cells in the anterior pituitary and is well known for its effect to stimulate milk production in bitches. Hyperprolactinemia has been shown in males to cause hypogonadism and affect fertility in species other than canines.[33,34] Prolactin reduces the production of testosterone by Leydig cells by increasing the number and affinity of LH receptors,[34] insinuating that low levels of prolactin are required to create enough functional LH receptors but if levels are excessive, they will block the LH receptors. This is important to understand because when prolactin-reducing drugs are used in the dog, severe depression of prolactin may inhibit testosterone function. From review of the literature, unlike other species, induced hyperprolactinemia and hypoprolactinemia does not seem to affect the motility or morphology of semen samples in the dog[33,34]; however, treatment times with dopamine agonists (prolactin antagonists) were quite short, 6 weeks[33] and 9 weeks,[35] and may not be long enough to present an effect on spermatogenesis considering the spermatogenic cycle of the dog is much longer than this time frame. The use of dopamine agonists in male dogs is purported by some to improve semen quality[16]; however, there is no published evidence to support this at this time.

Human Chorionic Gonadotropin Response Testing Purpose

In order to assess a male dog with an abnormal spermiogram for issues related to hormone levels, an hCG or GnRH stimulation test is performed. The reason for performing an hCG or GnRH stimulation test is due to the fact that the reported normal laboratory values for LH, FSH, testosterone, estrogen, and prolactin in dogs are quite varied[6] and results will vary dramatically with the method used for analysis.[36] The published methodology for hCG and GnRH stimulation testing is varied in the literature[37–42] with most measuring LH, FSH, testosterone, and estrogen frequently during a short period following stimulation; from 1 hour[40] to 7 days[43] and others perform just one off samples.[6]

In clinical practice, LH and FSH are not evaluated because there are no known diseases related purely to LH or FSH levels; however, assays for testosterone, estrogen (estradiol), and prolactin are performed because their abnormal levels will affect sperm production. Due to the lack of native GnRH availability, hCG is the preferred stimulant to assess the hypothalamic-pituitary-gonadal axis of male dogs because it is a chorionic glycoprotein with largely LH stimulatory effects, allowing assessment of stimulation of the interstitial cells of Leydig to produce testosterone, and how in turn the testosterone affects estrogen levels, and the involvement of prolactin. Gonadorelin, a GnRH analog can also be used; however, gonadorelin has less specificity on stimulating LH (it will stimulate both LH and FSH production) and, in the author's opinion, is inferior in use to assess hormone production from stimulation of the LH receptors of the testicles. If hCG is unavailable, then gonadorelin may be used.

Protocol

Collect a resting serum sample. Inject the animal with 500 IU of hCG (Chorulon, MSD Animal Health Australia) IM under 10 kg body weight (BW) and 1000 IU of Chorulon IM over 10 kg BW. Collect further serum samples at 30 minutes, 60 minutes, 120 minutes, 24 hours, and 48 hours after stimulation with hCG.

If using Gonadorelin, replace the above dose of hCG with 1 µg/kg of gonadorelin (Fertagyl, MSD Animal Health, Australia) IM or IV.[44]

Interpretation of Results

Testosterone

In a normal dog, it is expected for testosterone at 60 minutes after stimulation to be twice the baseline level, and by 2 hours after stimulation, testosterone remains elevated[45] or is back to basal levels.[46] In the initial 2-hour window after stimulation, there is a stimulation of LH receptors causing a release of testosterone stored in the testes (Leydig cells). By 24 hours after stimulation, it is expected that testosterone be again twice baseline levels and then either stay high or drop down to basal levels by 48 hours.[47] These later 2 tests are assessing the dogs ability to synthesize new testosterone when stimulated.[47]

Estradiol
In a normal dog, estradiol levels will remain lower than testosterone throughout the testing process. Testosterone is aromatized to estrogen in the normal dog at low levels through aromatase produced by the germ cells in the testes, and epithelial cells of the efferent ductules and interstitium of the epididymis.[32] The estrogen produced has some negative feedback to control testosterone secretion.

Prolactin
In a normal dog, prolactin levels will be low. High prolactin levels at any point can have deleterious effects on fertility as discussed earlier. Prolactin levels can fluctuate and while its production is not in any way stimulated by hCG or GnRH analogs, repetitive sampling will increase the chances of revealing an elevated level.

Results
Interpretation of hormone levels obtained from hCG/GnRH response testing is shown in **Table 1**.

Table 1	
Results of human chorionic gonadotropin response tests and possible treatments	
Low testosterone throughout	Suggests a primary problem of the HPA pituitary axis or receptor issue in the testes
High estrogen throughout	Suggests exogenous estrogen source, testicular tumor, diet phytoestrogen or exposure to hormone replacement therapy (HRT) medications from owners
Estrogen behaving like testosterone	Suggests increased conversion of testosterone to estrogen and trial therapy with an aromatase inhibitor, anastrazole at 0.1 mg/kg/d. Although not shown to improve semen quality, treatment was stopped short of a full sperm cycle.[48] Previously administration of other aromatase inhibitors that are no longer available (Formestane) showed improvement in semen quality in dogs[49]
Prolactin elevated	Trial response to prolactin antagonist cabergoline 5 μg/kg once daily[16,35]
Low testosterone on day 1 but elevated on days 2 and/or 3	Issue of poor storage of testosterone, but testes can make it when stimulated. Trial treatment with gonadorelin (Fertagyl, MSD Animal Health, Australia; 0.33 μg/kg once weekly for 16 week[16])
Low estrogen and testosterone	Suggests a primary problem of the HPA pituitary axis or receptor issue in the testes
Normal estrogen, testosterone, and prolactin profile	Indicates not an HPA issue or hormonal problem

NUTRIENT CONTENT OF DOG FOODS, AGE OF STUD DOGS, AND ENVIRONMENTAL TOXINS

Phytoestrogens in Dog Foods

Phytoestrogens are plant-derived compounds with estrogenic activity; they are sub-classified into 3 groups: isoflavones, coumestans, and lignans.[50] Both commercial and homemade canine diets can be high in phytoestrogens, depending on their ingredients. Soy bean and its by-products are commonly used in dog foods and have been shown have high levels of all 3 subgroups of phytoestrogen.[50] In addition to soy bean, other ingredients of commercial dog foods that are high in phytoestrogens include, but are not limited to, flaxseed (linseed), sesame seeds, legumes (alfalfa, chickpeas, peas, lima beans), apples, and corn.[51] In 1946, it was published that ewes fed on high subterranean clover-containing pastures had reduced lambing rates due to reduced fertilization rates, increased cystic uterine disease, and increased dystocia.[52] Subsequently, in 1969 phytoestrogens that were estrogenic in mice were also shown to be estrogenic in ewes.[53] Phytoestrogens have been more recently shown to affect the fertility of male dogs by reducing the number of tubules in the testes, reducing the spermatogenic epithelium and increasing the numbers of abnormal spermatozoa and reducing the sperm concentration in ejaculates.[54] There is very little research work done on the effects of phytoestrogens on the fertility of male dogs, with some indication that the effect is short term and may be reversible; dogs having evidence of reduced spermatogenesis after 4 weeks of exposure to soy bean diet seemed to revert to normal spermatogenesis after 52 weeks of chronic exposure to soy bean, suggesting an adaption to continued phytoestrogen exposure[55]; however, the number of male dogs in the study was small. The author has observed 2 cases of high exposure to phytoestrogen compounds (flaxseed) to previously fertile dogs that has resulted in irreversible azoospermia (observed unpublished data from author, S Mason, 2016). For this reason, in any animal with poor fertility, it is prudent to obtain a full dietary analysis of ingredients and avoidance of any high phytoestrogen ingredients.

Phytoestrogens are compounds that bind to and exert effects on estrogen receptors[50] and so will not be detected through estrogen assays in an hCG response test. Additionally, testing of serum samples from dogs fed high-phytoestrogen diets for the presence of isoflavones, coumestans, and lignans is neither practical nor feasible due to difficulties in testing.

It is recommended to not feed a diet containing high levels of phytoestrogens to stud dogs due to potential effects on fertility. Although not all dogs may be affected equally,[55] it is not possible to predict the ones that may or may not be affected by the phytoestrogens, so it is best to avoid them for all stud dogs.

Effects of Age of Stud Dogs

Anecdotally it is thought that male dogs are most fertile after puberty, between 2 and 5 years of age (observed, unpublished data by author, S Mason, 2006-2023). Although reductions in progressive sperm motility and percentage of morphologically normal sperm and increased production of reactive oxygen species (ROS) in semen has been shown to change with age in the equine,[56] the same cannot be said for the dog.[57] Although some smaller studies[58] have shown an increase in ROS negatively correlates with progressive motility and percentage normal morphology values in canine semen, more recent studies show a trend to this with age but the results were not significant,[57] and others have shown that there is a balance between enough ROS to maximize progressively motile sperm in dogs and too much ROS, which negatively affects the number or morphologically normal spermatozoa in semen samples, suggesting that the balance of ROS may change with age and help explain why a decline in semen quality is seen with age in dogs[59]; however, more research needs to be undertaken in this area.

Endocrine Disruptors (Environmental Contaminants)

The effects of environmental contaminants contributing to increasing frequencies of infertility in man and other species are an emerging and important area of research.[60,61] Within the environment high levels of anthropogenic chemicals such as polychlorinated biphenyls (PCB) are still found today, despite their use in plastic production being banned in the 1970s.[62] Phthalates (most importantly bisphenol A and PCB) have been identified as endocrine disruptors and interfere with normal hormonal actions.[61,63] These chemicals concentrate in pastures either through the application of contaminated fertilizers and seem to concentrate in herbivorous species that graze these pastures or through carnivores and omnivores fed meat grown from these pastures. Omnivorous species seem to concentrate less of these chemicals in their bodies. These same environmental contaminants are also found in water sources, with heated bottled water appearing to have the highest levels.[64] Once concentrated in the body, these chemicals will then be concentrated into the developing fetuses of pregnant females, potentially increasing the risk of birth defects or loss of the fetus.[62] In male dogs with increasing levels of environmental chemicals there seems to be an increase in testicular dysgenesis[65] and cryptorchidism in male pups from animals with reduced sperm quality.[60]

Environmental Temperature

The testicles sit separate to the body as spermatogenesis requires a lower temperature in which to occur than normal body temperature, by 2°C to 4°C.[66] The pampiniform plexus provides a countercurrent heat exchange mechanism to reduce testicular temperature from body temperature, and in conjunction with the tunica dartos muscle regulates the testicles at an appropriate temperature.[67] When environmental temperatures become high, the maintenance of the appropriate testicular temperature would be expected to become difficult. When environmental temperatures get extreme (>35°C/95°F) the motility and percentage of morphologically normal spermatozoa reduces, even in animals housed in air-conditioned environments because they still go outside in the heat to urinate and defecate (observed unpublished data by author, S Mason 2006-2023). The effect of temperature on sperm quality should also be considered in show dogs, which may spend extended periods in small crates or show trolleys, with a reduced ability to thermoregulate adequately, or those whose grooming involves prolonged exposure to hot air dryers. In the author's experience, animals exposed to persistent chronic high, seasonal environmental temperatures may adapt to the higher temperatures and the quality of the canine ejaculate may improve by the end of the summer period. However, it would be expected that the exposure to extreme heat will result in changes to the testicular spermatogenic cells as is seen in other species, resulting in permanent changes to sperm quality and output.[66,68]

TESTICULAR BIOPSY

It is the author's opinion to reserve testicular biopsies for cases where the less invasive testing processes for infertility have been exhausted. Traditionally, it has been recommended to avoid testicular biopsies as the risk of performing FNA, core, or incisional biopsies breaching the blood–testes barrier and inducing the formation of antisperm antibodies must be weighed against the benefits of the testing results.[7] However, recent studies have shown no effects on sperm production via FNA[69,70] or core biopsy of the testes using a Trucut (Baxter Healthcare Corporation, Valencia, CA) needle,[71,72] possibly due to less tissue trauma when compared with incisional biopsy.[72] Although serum antisperm antibodies are produced in a proportion of dogs undergoing testicular biopsy, the antibodies seem short lived, with antibodies being produced for a longer period (approximately 4 weeks) when an FNA is performed compared with core biopsy (2 weeks).[71] This difference in longevity of antisperm antibodies may be due to a higher level of trauma and poorer tissue seal after the procedure with FNAs.[69] Although there is a transient reduction in semen quality while antisperm antibodies are present,[71] this has not been shown to be permanent following biopsy procedures.[70,71,73,74] This same transient drop in semen quality has been shown in other species such as man,[75,76] llamas,[77] and farm animals.[78] Other potential consequences to testicular biopsy are coagulation necrosis, hematoma formation, tubular degeneration, interstitial fibrosis, and inflammation[71,72]; however, the severity of these sequelae is less so with the use of the Trucut needle.[72]

Animals with severe oligozoospermia or teratozoospermia may benefit from testicular biopsy to ascertain a definitive cause of the oligozoospermia or teratozoospermia. This has been recommended in humans,[79] when other less invasive tests have yielded no answers. There are no published reports on fertility effects after testicular biopsy, only on the semen quality after biopsy.[70,71,73,74] This may be due to the fact that the humans[75,76,79] or animals undergoing the procedure were already infertile and/or were part of a scientific study in which the animals were castrated at the end of the study and had histopathology performed on the testicles.[71,72,77,78]

Possible results from testicular biopsy include but are not limited to Sertoli cell only syndrome, orchitis, immune-mediated orchitis, inflammation, and tubular degeneration. The difficult part of testicular biopsies is there is a lack of research studies indicating possible successful treatments, so in many cases anecdotal treatments may be applied.[6,80] Recent studies suggest that the most common cause of nonobstructive azoospermia in dogs may be chronic immune-mediated orchitis.[6] This begs the question as to whether the histological changes seen with azoospermia are the primary condition or a manifestation of another disease process whether it be infertility from environmental chemicals[60,62] or low-grade bacterial disease[80] wherein the primary disease has since past.

Traditionally, testicular biopsies have been avoided due to perceived risks of the procedure making the problem worse, or due to the belief "what can be done anyhow?" However, with evidence that biopsies do not seem to affect future fertility of the animal, the potential gains in knowledge obtained to help understand why there is a declining fertility in dogs and other species, well outweighs the risks in the author's opinion. Core biopsies are preferred over FNAs to allow the analysis of the histological structure of the testis. FNAs are limited in value to the presence or absence of infection or inflammation, and evidence of spermatogenesis occurring. The questions pertaining to reducing fertility and azoospermia suggest that performing testicular biopsies in dogs with declining fertility rather than waiting until azoospermia is evident may in fact indicate a disease process that could then be treated and prevent the sequelae of chronic immune-mediated orchitis; more research is needed in this area and the analysis of more testicles with declining sperm quality/fertility. Additionally, infertility appears to be an inherited issue, with many relatives in familial lines becoming affected,[6,81,82] so the more data that are obtained earlier in the infertility process, the more we can potentially understand the heritability of some of these fertility issues in dogs as inheritance is not yet proven.[82]

SUPPLEMENTS TO IMPROVE FERTILITY
Zinc

Semen zinc levels have been shown to change with sperm quality in dogs and man.[22] As the quality of the ejaculate reduces so too does the level of zinc, suggesting that zinc is required for good quality sperm to be produced.[22] Zinc is thought to help prevent chromatin decondensation and has positive effects on sperm motility and antioxidant activity of semen.[83,84] Zinc may be supplemented at 3 mg/kg daily to enhance spermatozoa quality and motility.[84]

Carnitine

Carnitine has effects as an antioxidant to remove acetyl-CoA from mitochondria and prevent lipid peroxidation of polyunsaturated fatty acids in cell membranes. Carnitine levels in the semen of infertile men are lower than fertile men,[85] suggesting addition of carnitine to diets of infertile males may improve sperm quality and number when supplemented at 50 mg/kg per day.[1]

Fish Oil

Fish derived n-3 polyunsaturated fatty acids are not synthesized by mammals and must be provided in the diet. Contrasting effects have been shown, with supplementation shown to improve sperm counts, motility, and fertility,[86–88] and others showing no difference in reducing susceptibility of the sperm membrane to lipid peroxidation, and no effect on sperm motility and fertility.[89] It is recommended to supplement with fish oil of composition: 25% docosahexaenoic acid and 10% eicosapentaenoic acid[84] at 54 mg/kg once daily.[88]

Vitamin E

Vitamin E is an antioxidant, which protects the testis from oxidative damage and stabilizes sperm membranes to improve sperm quality. This has been shown in other species[90–93] but the effect would be expected to occur in dogs as well. Vitamin E may be supplemented at 5 mg/kg once daily.[84]

Folic Acid

Folic acid (vitamin B9) is essential for the synthesis of proteins and DNA and is not stored in the body, so must be delivered in food. Its use is more theoretical, with publications being limited to use in bitches to reduce the incidence of cleft palate puppies in bitches fed grain-deficient diets.[94] Although commonly recommended, there is no published evidence of folic acid supplementation with sperm quality; however, it is not expected to be problematic to supplement dogs to improve semen quality.

Semen Analysis and When to Expect Improvement

The process of spermatogenesis can be imagined to be like a long car production line. During the production process, there are lots of steps along the way and the use of lots of building blocks to end up with the final product, the car, or in this case the sperm. The spermatozoa, which are ejaculated from the epididymis are like a snapshot in time of the sperm production process, and anything that may affect the production process at any time may manifest in defective products being produced. Some sperm abnormalities are produced by primary defects of the testicles and epididymis; others are the result of inadequate testicular function, or are the manifestation of some sort of insult including iatrogenic insults.

Spermatogenesis in the dog consists of 4.5 cycles (each cycle is 13.6 days[95]) resulting in a 62-day process plus 2 weeks epididymal transit time. This means to go from a single cell to a single ejaculated fertile sperm, the process will take 76 days, or approximately 11 weeks. Through a series of mitotic divisions of spermatogonia more spermatogonia are produced to replace themselves and others produced go on to produce spermatozoa. The first spermatogonia (A1), divide to produce A2 spermatogonia that divide to produce A3 spermatogonia, which divide to produce A4 spermatogonia that divide to produce I spermatogonia that divide to produce B spermatogonia. B spermatogonia, through another mitotic division, give rise to primary spermatocytes that undergo the first meiotic division to produce haploid secondary spermatocytes. Through a second meiotic division, secondary spermatocytes give rise to spermatids. Spermatids are haploid and go through a series of changes to form spermatocytes. The time taken to form spermatids from A1 spermatogonia takes 3.5 cycles, or 48 days in the dog. Defects in the sperm head can result from any disruption in these first 48 days. Through the next 14 days of the sperm cycle, which beings as the Golgi phase (which is responsible for the beginning of the acrosome formation) through to the end of the spermatogenic cycle (after the maturation phase) of the spermatid to produce the spermatozoans that are finally released from the Sertoli cells into the lumen of the seminiferous tubule. Defects in the tail will usually be from issues with the formation of the tail, so the last 12 days of the spermatogenic cycle and the next 14 days of epididymal transit time.

As the spermatozoa migrate through the epididymis, the cytoplasmic droplet, which forms as a package of waste material from the original spermatogonia that are no longer required by the developed spermatozoa, under the head of the sperm, migrates from a proximal position on the midpiece to a distal position on the midpiece and allow the spermatozoa to attain motility. Distal droplets are removed during the ejaculation process and are often seen detached from the spermatozoa during a semen motility examination. Defects in migration of the cytoplasmic droplet may be due to the inappropriate release of immature sperm, or a problem with epididymal motility or low-testosterone levels, all of which are required for migration of the cytoplasmic droplet and attainment of motility by the spermatozoa. Spermatozoa containing distal cytoplasmic droplets do not seem to affect the fertility of fresh semen in dogs; however, they seem to affect the post-thaw motility of frozen semen samples suggesting they will affect the fertility of frozen semen samples containing a high proportion of distal cytoplasmic droplet sperm (observed, unpublished data by author, S Mason, 2006-2023). In contrast, semen samples containing a high proportion of proximal cytoplasmic spermatozoa will be expected to have reduced fertility due to the ability of these proximal droplet spermatozoa to compete with normal sperm and also to fertilize oocytes and prevent cleavage of these fertilized oocytes.[96] A discussion of other abnormalities and effects of the abnormalities is discussed in a previous article in this periodical.[1]

As should be clear, any event at any point in time will potentially affect the quality of the spermatozoa released by the male. **Table 2** indicates the time to reassess semen wherein a reduction in the defect would expect to be seen if there was a single insult to the process of spermatogenesis.

Table 2
Morphological defects of spermatozoa and anticipated time to resolution

Defect	Time to Analyze to Expect Improvement
Head and midpiece primary defects	14–76 d depending on stage of insult
Tail defects	14–28 d depending on stage of insult
Proximal droplets	14 d
Distal droplets	7 d
Detached heads	1–4 d

Detached heads are an interesting defect, which are usually a result of epididymal dysfunction. Because there is a continuous production of spermatozoa, there should be a continuous efflux of "old" spermatozoa from the epididymis and passed in the urine. In some animals, the male suffers from epididymal dysfunction wherein the spermatozoa are not removed from the epididymis and remain there too long and eventually they start to degenerate, and the head neck junction becomes weak, and the heads detach from the tails.[10] In these animals, if the semen sample is collected daily and the sperm analyzed, then it would be expected after 2 to 4 days that the old sperm are removed and what are then ejaculated are "nonstagnant" appropriately mature sperm, that is, the proportion of sperm with detached heads will reduce and in turn improve the fertility of the male in question.

Although morphological assessment of sperm is imperative in any infertility investigation, the classification of the types of abnormalities used by different authors can be confusing. Many authors classify sperm defects as primary or secondary abnormalities. Primary abnormalities are defects created by abnormal production from the testicles, whereas secondary abnormalities are defects caused by epididymal dysfunction or processing and handling after ejaculation. The author finds this nomenclature confusing, as for some defects like proximal droplet sperm, they could be due to a defect of the sperm formation (primary) or a defect of the epididymis (secondary). The author prefers the use of the terms compensable and noncompensable defects, wherein compensable defects are those wherein if enough normal sperm are added the defect would be overcome and fertilization of oocytes would be expected, an example of this would be coiled tail sperm or detached head sperm, where adding more normal sperm would overcome the deformed spermatozoa. Noncompensable defects are those wherein adding more normal sperm would not overcome the defective sperm. An example of noncompensable spermatozoa would be proximal droplet sperm as they interfere with, and prevent the function of the normal sperm in the ejaculate when there is a high proportion of proximal droplet sperm.[97]

If the observed sperm defects are not improved in the appropriate period as above, then it is assumed the defects were not due to a one-off assault and more involved fertility assessments as described earlier should be undertaken.

SUMMARY

Assessment of semen in a male infertility investigation is just a small proportion of the workup that can be undertaken. Assessment of semen to confirm a problem regarding azoospermia, oligozoospermia, or teratozoospermia is imperative to ascertain if there is a semen issue or not. If the spermiogram is normal, then in most cases this will rule out the male as a cause of infertility. To investigate male infertility issues then the less invasive tests should be conducted before the more invasive tests. It is recommended to analyze the diet of the dog, perform quantitative AP analysis if suggested, semen culture, reproductive ultrasound, and hCG response testing before the more invasive testing of testicular biopsy, which must be performed under anesthesia. If indicated, it may be worthwhile to perform testicular biopsies early in the course of the disease before azoospermia has ensued.

CLINICS CARE POINTS

- AP levels are high in normal ejaculates of dogs.

- Hormone response testing allows clinicians to assess the dogs response to stimulation with respect to hormone levels.
- Testicular biopsies early in investigation procedures increases the chances of finding something fixable.
- Response to treatment for poor spermiograms is a protracted process of 2-4 months.

DISCLOSURE

The author has no commercial or financial conflicts of interest. No funding was used for this article.

REFERENCES

1. Kolster KA. Evaluation of Canine Sperm and Management of Semen Disorders. Vet Clin Small Anim Pract 2018;48(4):533–45.
2. Lopate C. The Problem Stud Dog. Vet Clin Small Anim Pract 2012;42(3):469–88.
3. Canine fresh and cryopreserved semen evaluation. Anim Reprod Sci 2004;82-83: 209–24.
4. Johnston SD. Performing a Complete Canine Semen Evaluation in a Small Animal Hospital. Vet Clin Small Anim Pract 1991;21(3):545–51.
5. Olson PN. Clinical Approach for Evaluating Dogs with Azoospermia or Aspermia. Vet Clin Small Anim Pract 1991;21(3):591–608.
6. Goericke-Pesch S, Reifarth L, Behrens Mathiesen C, et al. Chronic Immune-Mediated Orchitis Is the Major Cause of Acquired Non-obstructive Azoospermia in Dogs. Original Research. Front Vet Sci 2022;9. https://doi.org/10.3389/fvets.2022.865967.
7. Johnston S, Root Kustritz M, Olson P. In: Kersey R, LeMelledo D, editors. Canine and feline theriogenology. Philadelphia, PA: Saunders; 2001. p. 312–28, 322-323.
8. Linde Forsberg C. Artificial Insemination. Presented at: ESAVS-EVSSAR-ENVN reprouciton in companion, exotic and laboratory animal ; 2005; Nantes.
9. Oettle EE. Sperm morphology and fertility in the dog. J Reprod Fertil 1993;257–60.
10. Barth AD, Oko JR. Abnormal morphology of bovine spermatozoa. IA, USA: Iowa State University Press; 1989.
11. Frenette G, Dubé JY, Tremblay RR. Origin of Alkaline Phosphatase of Canine Seminal Plasma. Arch Androl 1986;16(3):235–41.
12. Kutzler MA, Solter PF, Hoffman WE, et al. Characterization and localization of alkaline phosphatase in canine seminal plasma and gonadal tissues. Theriogenology 2003;60(2):299–306.
13. Gobello C, Castex G, Corrada Y. Serum and seminal markers in the diagnosis of disorders of the genital tract of the dog: a mini-review. Theriogenology 2002; 57(4):1285–91.
14. Schäfer-Somi S, Fröhlich T, Schwendenwein I. Measurement of Alkaline Phosphatase in Canine Seminal Plasma - An Update. Reprod Domest Anim 2013;48(1): e10–2.
15. Stornelli A, Arauz M, Baschard H, et al. Unilateral and Bilateral Vasectomy in the Dog: Alkaline Phosphatase as an Indicator of Tubular Patency. Reprod Domest Anim 2003;38(1):1–4.
16. Hess M. Documented and anecdotal effects of certain pharmaceutical agents used to enhance semen quality in the dog. Theriogenology 2006;66(3):613–7.

17. Beaufays F, Onclin K, Verstegen J. Retrograde ejaculation occurs in the dog, but can be prevented by pre-treatment with phenylpropanolamine: A urodynamic study. Theriogenology 2008;70(7):1057–64.
18. Collins JP. Retrograde ejaculation. Berlin Heidelberg: Springer; 1982. p. 179–89.
19. Hershlag A, Schiff SF, DeCherney AH. CLINICAL REVIEW: Retrograde ejaculation. Hum Reprod 1991;6(2):255–8.
20. Christensen BW. Canine Prostate Disease. Vet Clin Small Anim Pract 2018;48(4): 701–19.
21. Ruel Y, Barthez PY, Mailles A, et al. Ultrasonographic evaluation of the prostate in healthy intact dogs. Vet Radiol Ultrasound 1998;39(3):212–6.
22. Ferré-Dolcet L, Frigotto L, Contiero B, et al. Prostatic fluid composition and semen quality in dogs with benign prostatic hyperplasia undergoing treatment with osaterone acetate. Reprod Domest Anim 2022;57(1):72–9.
23. Tsutsui T, Hori T, Shimizu M, et al. Regression of Prostatic Hypertrophy by Osaterone Acetate in Dogs. J Vet Med Sci 2000;62(10):1115–9.
24. Tsutsui T, Hori T, Shimizu M, et al. Effect of Osaterone Acetate Administration on Prostatic Regression Rate, Peripheral Blood Hormone Levels and Semen Quality in Dogs with Benign Prostatic Hypertrophy. J Vet Med Sci 2001;63(4):453–6.
25. Trigg TE, Wright PJ, Armour AF, et al. Use of a GnRH analogue implant to produce reversible long-term suppression of reproductive function in male and female domestic dogs. J Reprod Fertil Suppl 2000;255–61.
26. Keid LB, Soares RM, Vasconcellos SA, et al. A polymerase chain reaction for the detection of Brucella canis in semen of naturally infected dogs. Theriogenology 2007;67(7):1203–10.
27. Keid LB, Soares RM, Vasconcellos SA, et al. Comparison of agar gel immunodiffusion test, rapid slide agglutination test, microbiological culture and PCR for the diagnosis of canine brucellosis. Res Vet Sci 2009;86(1):22–6.
28. Keid LB, Soares RM, Vieira NR, et al. Diagnosis of Canine Brucellosis: Comparison between Serological and Microbiological Tests and a PCR Based on Primers to 16S-23S rDNA Interspacer. Vet Res Commun 2007;31(8):951–65.
29. Walker WH, Cheng J. FSH and testosterone signaling in Sertoli cells. Reproduction 2005;130(1):15–28.
30. Chłopik A, Wysokińska A. Canine spermatozoa—What do we know about their morphology and physiology? An overview. Reprod Domest Anim 2020;55(2): 113–26.
31. de Kretser DM, Buzzard JJ, Okuma Y, et al. The role of activin, follistatin and inhibin in testicular physiology. Mol Cell Endocrinol 2004;225(1):57–64.
32. Hess RA, Fernandes SAF, Gomes GRO, et al. Estrogen and Its Receptors in Efferent Ductules and Epididymis. J Androl 2011;32(6):600–13.
33. Koivisto M, Eschricht F, Urhausen C, et al. Effects of Short-term Hyper- and Hypoprolactinaemia on Hormones of the Pituitary, Gonad and -Thyroid Axis and on Semen Quality in Male Beagles. Reprod Domest Anim 2009;44:320–5.
34. De Rosa M, Zarrilli S, Di Sarno A, et al. Hyperprolactinemia in Men: Clinical and Biochemical Features and Response to Treatment. Endocrine 2003;20(1–2): 75–82.
35. Mogheiseh A, Vara N, Ayaseh M, et al. Effects of Cabergoline on Thyroid Hormones and Semen Quality of Dog. Top Companion Anim Med 2017;32(1):13–5.
36. Wudy SA, Schuler G, Sánchez-Guijo A, et al. The art of measuring steroids: Principles and practice of current hormonal steroid analysis. J Steroid Biochem Mol Biol 2018;179:88–103.

37. de Gier J, Buijtels JJCWM, Albers-Wolthers CHJ, et al. Effects of gonadotropin-releasing hormone administration on the pituitary-gonadal axis in male and female dogs before and after gonadectomy. Theriogenology 2012;77(5):967–78.

38. Knol BW, Dieleman SJ, Bevers MM, et al. GnRH in the male dog: dose-response relationships with LH and testosterone. Reproduction 1993;98(1):159–61.

39. Meij BP, Mol JA, Hazewinkel HAW, et al. Assessment of a combined anterior pituitary function test in beagle dogs: Rapid sequential intravenous administration of four hypothalamic releasing hormones. Domest Anim Endocrinol 1996;13(2): 161–70.

40. Romagnoli S, Baldan A, Righetti C, et al. Use of the gonadotropin-releasing hormone (GnRH) stimulation test to monitor gonadal function in intact adult male cats. Reprod Domest Anim 2017;52(1):24–7.

41. Spruijt A, Kooistra H, Oei C, et al. The function of the pituitary-testicular axis in dogs prior to and following surgical or chemical castration with the GnRH-agonist deslorelin. Reprod Domest Anim 2022. https://doi.org/10.1111/rda.14266.

42. Günzel-Apel AR, Hille P, Hoppen HO. Spontaneous and GnRH-induced pulsatile LH and testosterone release in pubertal, adult and aging male beagles. Theriogenology 1994;41(3):737–45.

43. Purswell BJ, Wilcke JR. Response to Gonadotropin-relaesing-hormone by the intact male dog - serum testosterone, lutenizing-hormone and follicle-stimulating-hormone. Article. J Reprod Fertil 1993;335–41.

44. Ortega-Pacheco A, Bolio-Gonzalez M, Colin-Flores R, et al. Evaluation of a Burdizzo Castrator for Neutering of Dogs. Reprod Domest Anim 2006;41(3):227–32.

45. Santana M, Batista M, Alamo D, et al. Influence of Sexual Stimulation and the Administration of Human Chorionic Gonadotrophin on Plasma Testosterone Levels in Dogs. Reprod Domest Anim 2012;47(3):e43–6.

46. Kawakami E, Hori T, Tsutsui T. Changes in plasma luteinizing hormone, testosterone and estradiol-17β levels and semen quality after injections of gonadotropin releasing hormone agonist and human chorionic gonadotropin in three dogs with oligozoospermia and two dogs with azoospermia. Anim Reprod Sci 1997;47(1): 157–67.

47. Tremblay Y, Belanger A. Changes in plasma steroid levels after single administration of hCG or LHRH agonist analogue in dog and rat. J Steroid Biochem 1985; 22(3):315–20.

48. Gonzalez G, Guendulain C, Maffrand C, et al. Comparison of the Effect of the Aromatase Inhibitor, Anastrazole, to the Antioestrogen, Tamoxifen Citrate, on Canine Prostate and Semen. Reprod Domest Anim 2009;44:316–9.

49. Kawakami E, Hirano T, Hori T, et al. Improvement in spermatogenic function after subcutaneous implantation of a capsule containing an aromatase inhibitor in four oligozoospermic dogs and one azoospermic dog with high plasma estradiol-17β concentrations. Theriogenology 2004;62(1):165–78.

50. Cerundolo R, Court MH, Hao Q, et al. Identification and concentration of soy phytoestrogens in commercial dog foods. Am J Vet Res 2004;65(5):592–6.

51. Mostrom M, Evans TJ. Chapter 60 - Phytoestrogens. In: Gupta RC, editor. Veterinary toxicology. 3rd edition. MA, USA: Academic Press; 2018. p. 817–33.

52. Bennetts HW, Uuderwood EJ, Shier FL. A specific breeding problem of sheep on subterranean clover pastures in Western Australia. Aust Vet J 1946;22(1):2–12.

53. Shutt D, Braden A. The significance of equol in relation to the oestrogenic responses in sheep ingesting clover with a high formononetin content. Aust J Agric Res 1968;19(4):545–53.

54. Perez-Rivero J-J, Martinez-Maya J-J, Perez-Martinez M, et al. Phytoestrogen treatment induces testis alterations in dogs. Potential use in population control. Vet Res Commun 2009;33(1):87–95.

55. McClain RM, Wolz E, Davidovich A, et al. Subchronic and chronic safety studies with genistein in dogs. Food Chem Toxicol 2005;43(10):1461–82.

56. Darr CR, Moraes LE, Scanlan TN, et al. Sperm Mitochondrial Function is Affected by Stallion Age and Predicts Post-Thaw Motility. J Equine Vet Sci 2017;50:52–61.

57. Fuente-Lara AdI, Hesser A, Christensen B, et al. Effects from aging on semen quality of fresh and cryopreserved semen in Labrador Retrievers. Theriogenology 2019;132:164–71.

58. Pereira A, Borges P, Fontbonne A, et al. The Comet assay for detection of DNA damage in canine sperm. Reprod Domest Anim 2017;52(6):1149–52.

59. Fotuouhi A, Meyers S. Assessment of sperm parameters in North American great danes: a rapidly aging dog breed. Anim Reprod Sci 2020;220:106397.

60. Lea RG, Byers AS, Sumner RN, et al. Environmental chemicals impact dog semen quality in vitro and may be associated with a temporal decline in sperm motility and increased cryptorchidism. Sci Rep 2016;6(1):31281.

61. Grindler NM, Vanderlinden L, Karthikraj R, et al. Exposure to Phthalate, an Endocrine Disrupting Chemical, Alters the First Trimester Placental Methylome and Transcriptome in Women. Sci Rep 2018;8(1). https://doi.org/10.1038/s41598-018-24505-w.

62. Harris I, Lea R, Sumner R. Exposure to environmental contaminants and the impact on reproductive health. Clinical Theriogenology 2022;14(3):138–45.

63. Schug TT, Johnson AF, Birnbaum LS, et al. Minireview: Endocrine Disruptors: Past Lessons and Future Directions. Mol Endocrinol 2016;30(8):833–47.

64. Wang Y, Qian H. Phthalates and Their Impacts on Human Health. Healthcare 2021;9(5):603.

65. Skakkebaek NE, Meyts ER-D, Louis GMB, et al. Male Reproductive Disorders and Fertility Trends: Influences of Environment and Genetic Susceptibility. Physiol Rev 2016;96(1):55–97.

66. Chenoweth P, Lorton S. Animal andrology theroies and applications. MA, USA: CABI; 2014. p. 41–2, chap 3.

67. Maloney SK, Mitchell D. Regulation of ram scrotal temperature during heat exposure, cold exposure, fever and exercise. J Physiol 1996;496(2):421–30.

68. Kumidiaka J, Nagaratnam V, Rwuaan JS. Seasonal and age-related-changes in semen quality and testicular morphology of bulls in a tropical environment. Vet Rec 1981;108(1):13–5.

69. Angrimani DSR, Nichi M, Losano JDA, et al. Fatty acid content in epididymal fluid and spermatozoa during sperm maturation in dogs. J Anim Sci Biotechnol 2017;818. https://doi.org/10.1186/s40104-017-0148-6.

70. Gouletsou P, Galatos A, Leontides L, et al. Impact of Fine- or Large-Needle Aspiration on Canine Testes: Clinical, In Vivo Ultrasonographic and Seminological Assessment. Reprod Domest Anim 2011;46(4):712–9.

71. Attia KA, Zaki AA, Eilts BE, et al. Anti-sperm antibodies and seminal characteristics after testicular biopsy or epididymal aspiration in dogs. Theriogenology 2000; 53(6):1355–63.

72. Lopate C, Threlfall WR, Rosol TJ. Histopathologic and gross effects of testicular biopsy in the dog. Theriogenology 1989;32(4):585–602.

73. Hunt WL, Foote RH. Effect of repeated testicular biopsy on testis function and semen quality in dogs. J Androl 1997;18(6):740–4.

74. James RW, Heywood R, Fowler DJ. Serial percutaneous testicular biopsy in the Beagle dog. J Small Anim Pract 1979;20(4):219–28.
75. Johnson L, Petty CS, Neaves WB. The Relationship of Biopsy Evaluations and Testicular Measurements to Over-All Daily Sperm Production in Human Testes. Fertil Steril 1980;34(1):36–40.
76. Hjort T, Linnet L, Skakkebaek NE. Testicular biopsy: Indications and complications. Eur J Pediatr 1982;138(1):23–5.
77. Heath AM, Pugh DG, Sartin EA, et al. Evaluation of the safety and efficacy of testicular biopsies in llamas. Theriogenology 2002/10/01/2002;58(6):1125–30.
78. Galina CS. EVALUATION OF TESTICULAR BIOPSY IN FARM ANIMALS. Vet Rec 1971;88(24):628–&.
79. Brannen GE, Roth RR. Testicular Abnormalities of the Subfertile Male. J Urol 1979;122(6):757–62.
80. Cassal M. Canine autoimmune orchitis. Clinical Theriogenology 2012;4(3):251–4.
81. Allen WE, Patel JR. Autoimmune orchitis in two related dogs. J Small Anim Pract 1982;23(11):713–8.
82. England GCW, Phillips L, Freeman SL. Heritability of semen characteristics in dogs. Theriogenology 2010;74(7):1136–40.
83. Björndahl L, Kvist U. Human sperm chromatin stabilization: a proposed model including zinc bridges. Mol Hum Reprod 2009;16(1):23–9.
84. Alonge S, Melandri M, Leoci R, et al. The Effect of Dietary Supplementation of Vitamin E, Selenium, Zinc, Folic Acid, and N-3 Polyunsaturated Fatty Acids on Sperm Motility and Membrane Properties in Dogs. Animals 2019;9(2):34.
85. Matalliotakis I, Koumantaki Y, Evageliou A, et al. L-carnitine levels in the seminal plasma of fertile and infertile men: correlation with sperm quality. Int J Fertil Women's Med 2000;45(3):236–40.
86. Rooke J, Shao C, Speake B. Effects of feeding tuna oil on the lipid composition of pig spermatozoa and in vitro characteristics of semen. Reproduction 2001; 121(2):315–22.
87. Mitre R, Cheminade C, Allaume P, et al. Oral intake of shark liver oil modifies lipid composition and improves motility and velocity of boar sperm. Theriogenology 2004;62(8):1557–66.
88. Risso A, Pellegrino FJ, Relling AE, et al. Effect of Long-Term Fish Oil Supplementation on Semen Quality and Serum Testosterone Concentrations in Male Dogs. Article. Int J Fertil Steril 2016;10(2):223–31.
89. Yeste M, Barrera X, Coll D, et al. The effects on boar sperm quality of dietary supplementation with omega-3 polyunsaturated fatty acids differ among porcine breeds. Theriogenology 2011;76(1):184–96.
90. Hong Z, Hailing L, Hui M, et al. Effect of Vitamin E supplement in diet on antioxidant ability of testis in Boer goat. Anim Reprod Sci 2010;117(1):90–4.
91. Yue D, Yan L, Luo H, et al. Effect of Vitamin E supplementation on semen quality and the testicular cell membranal and mitochondrial antioxidant abilities in Aohan fine-wool sheep. Anim Reprod Sci 2010;118(2):217–22.
92. Yousef MI, Abdallah GA, Kamel KI. Effect of ascorbic acid and Vitamin E supplementation on semen quality and biochemical parameters of male rabbits. Anim Reprod Sci 2003;76(1):99–111.
93. Aydilek N, Aksakal M, Karakilcik AZ. Effects of testosterone and vitamin E on the antioxidant system in rabbit testis. Andrologia 2004;36(5):277–81.
94. Elwood JM, Colquhoun TA. Observations on the prevention of cleft palate in dogs by folic acid and potential relevance to humans. N Z Vet J 1997;45(6):254–6.

95. Ibach B, Weissbach L, Hilscher B. Stages of the Cycle of the Seminiferous Epithelium in the Dog. Andrologia 2009;8(4):297–307.
96. Peña A, Barrio M, Becerra J, et al. Infertility in a Dog due to Proximal Cytoplasmic Droplets in the Ejaculate: Investigation of the Significance for Sperm Functionality In Vitro. Reprod Domest Anim 2007;42(5):471–8.
97. Thundathil J, Palasz AT, Barth AD, et al. The use of in vitro fertilization techniques to investigate the fertilizing ability of bovine sperm with proximal cytoplasmic droplets. Anim Reprod Sci 2001;65(3):181–92.

Nutrition and Theriogenology

A Glimpse Into Nutrition and Nutritional Supplementation During Gestation, Lactation, Weaning and Breeding Dogs and Cats

Hyun-tae Kim, DVM, MS[a],*,
Joseph J. Wakshlag, DVM, PhD, DACVIM (nutrition), DACVSMR[b]

KEYWORDS

- Gestation • Lactation • Growth • Large and giant breed puppy growth
- Spermatogenesis • Nutraceutical

KEY POINTS

- Pregnant and growing animals need to consume a complete and balanced diet formulated for respective life stages or all-life stages based on the American Association of Feed Control Officials nutritional adequacy statement.
- Regular body weight and body condition monitoring of pregnant and growing animals at each veterinary visit is important to determine appropriate energy intake.
- Energy demands during growth are often adequately met; however, mineral balance can be a concern in large and giant breed dogs.
- There is little evidence in the canine literature that supplements for conception and gestation are worthwhile.
- Some evidence points to nutritional supplementation for spermatogenesis; however, much of the literature is in normal stud dogs without dysfunctional spermatogenesis.

NUTRITION FOR THE NORMAL INTACT MALE AND FEMALE BEFORE BREEDING

Both breeding female and male should be in an ideal body condition utilizing a common body condition scoring system (eg, 5 out of 9 on a 9-point scale) and fed a complete and balanced maintenance diet as established by the American Association of Feed Control Officials (AAFCO). Overweight or underweight females may have lower

---

[a] Department of Clinical Sciences and Advanced Medicine, School of Veterinary Medicine, University of Pennsylvania, 3800 Spruce Street, Philadelphia, PA 19104, USA; [b] Department of Clinical Sciences, College of Veterinary Medicine, Cornell University, 930 Campus Road, CPC -3-526, Ithaca, NY 14853, USA
* Corresponding author. 300 Alexander Ct., Apt 3104, Philadelphia, PA 19103.
E-mail address: petfoodis@gmail.com

Vet Clin Small Anim 53 (2023) 1083–1098
https://doi.org/10.1016/j.cvsm.2023.05.003
0195-5616/23/© 2023 Elsevier Inc. All rights reserved.

ovulation and conception rate and poor performance (inadequate milk production, higher neonatal mortality, hypoglycemia-prone puppies, dystocia due to larger fetus) throughout the stages of reproduction (see Sones and Balogh's article, "Body Condition and Fertility in Dogs," in this issue).[1,2] Sometime after breeding (usually during gestation growth about half way into gestation) switching to a diet designed to support the life stages of gestation and lactation or all-life stages is recommended for both female dogs and cats, and the diet should be highly digestible and palatable. Feeding a nutrient and energy-dense food (approximately 4000 kcal/kg dry matter or greater) will help queen's or bitch's nutritional demands to be easily met without volume increases during much of gestation.

The concept of "flushing," defined as increasing food intake by 5% to 15% before estrus until breeding, was once suggested to enhance the reproductive performance in that both dogs and cats accumulating body fat reserves during gestation for subsequent lactation, but this practice used mostly in pigs is not necessary in feline and canine females with optimal body condition.[1] Although it seems logical to store more energy in their body, loss of body condition followed by weeks of lactation can be recovered spontaneously later with provision of proper nutrition and management (ie, separating litters from dams earlier).

In the case of breeding males, no specific nutritional requirement is documented, but they should be in optimal physical condition without any clinical disease to ensure breeding performance. Physical examination (plus body and muscle condition scoring) can be performed to assess nutritional status of breeding animals. Intact males in heavy service may experience weight loss or hyporexia, but this can be resolved with increased ration or caloric density of the food. Selection and screening of breeding males is covered elsewhere (see Bart J.G. Broeckx's article, "Incorporating Genetic Testing into a Breeding Program," in this issue).

FEEDING THE GRAVID FEMALE

Energy requirements of cats and dogs during gestation increase in a different manner. Depending on respective fetal growth patterns and weight gain of dams; a queen's body weight increases linearly during gestation, whereas a bitch's body weight does not increase until the last half to third of gestation. The weight gain and energy requirements are correlated, and during gestation, caloric intakes should be gradually increased on an individual basis. For optimal fetal growth and development, approximately 25% to 50% increase in daily intake over maintenance requirement is desired during the last half of pregnancy to the time of whelping for dogs. In case of pregnant dogs with ideal body condition, the increment can be initiated around the fifth week of gestation (10%–15% increase each week from the fifth week). Food intake of queens is gradually increased from the second week of gestation, and 40% to 50% increase in body weight is often recognized at the point of parturition.[3] In part this increase in cats will increase adiposity which is desired considering queens will usually not increase caloric intake as robustly as dogs during lactation that can precipitate weight loss during the lactation phase as they cannot keep up with caloric demands particularly with larger litters.

Overfeeding the dams should be avoided to maintain optimal body condition (to slightly overconditioned in cats) until whelping, as excessive energy intake leads to obesity of dams that may result in heavier fetuses and dystocia (see Sones and Balogh's article, "Body Condition and Fertility in Dogs," in this issue). In cases of females with large litters or giant breed dogs, volume limitation may compromise their food intake by abdominal fill; therefore, the dogs should be fed free choice or small multiple meals throughout the day, particularly if ultrasound shows larger numbers in the litter (greater than 8).[1]

A diet with a nutritional guarantee on the packaging to support the gestation and lactation or all-life stages is necessary and these diets are usually higher than 4000 kcal/kg dry matter for dogs and 4500 kcal/kg dry matter for cats. As fetuses get larger, protein requirements exceed maintenance especially during late gestation, and the formula should provide high-quality protein (ie, animal-based protein) to avoid protein malnutrition (often > 29% dry matter for dogs and 32% dry matter for cats).[4] With cats, optimal levels of taurine and arachidonic acid should be provided in the formula to maintain normal reproduction and prevent fetal loss. Most importantly is that commercial dog foods have an appropriate calcium to phosphorus balance (typically 2:1–1:1); therefore, adding calcium to the diet in the form of eggshell or other calcium carbonate substrates may negatively affect this ratio leading to a predisposition toward periparturient hypocalcemia that should be avoided.

FEEDING DURING LACTATION

Immediately after whelping, the dam's food intake increases dramatically and continues to increase for the first 3 weeks of lactation as it is the period where the growth rate of litters is the greatest. Maintenance energy and nutrient requirements of lactating cats and dogs are directly correlated with milk production and depend on litter size. Based on the current National Research Council guideline, maintenance energy requirements for lactating dogs and cats are approximately 145 kcal/kg $BW^{0.75}$ and 100 kcal/kg $BW^{0.67}$, respectively, and the estimations can be used as a starting point for feeding which must then be adjusted for the number of puppies or kittens in the litter.[5] Energy requirement of lactating dams can simply be estimated as 25% increase of nutrient intake above maintenance for each puppy or kitten in the litter. This is applicable to a maximum of 8 offspring (ie, 300% of maintenance energy requirement) and beyond 8 offspring it can sometimes be difficult for a lactating female to sustain themselves through food consumption without weight loss at the point of weaning. To achieve the adequate energy intake, a diet designed to support the life stages of gestation and lactation should be fed free choice or small multiple meals, and this will help lactating females meet their energy requirement and produce adequate milk, as feeding larger meals less frequently can lead to soft stools or diarrhea. To produce large quantities of milk, the dam's water requirement drastically increases as the moisture content of milk is over 75%.[6] Water requirements (mL) of lactating females are close to energy requirements in kcal, and sufficient clean water should be available (eg, a lactating 30 kg Labrador will require approximately 1800 kcals and with 6 puppies needs 4500 kcals which roughly translates to needing 4500 mL of water each day for milk production).

During lactation, body condition of lactating females should be maintained by providing adequate nutrition throughout the stage. In cats, peak milk production is reached at week 3 and energy requirement peaks around at week 7.[7] At the end of lactation, quantity and nutrient content of the queen's milk no longer can support optimal growth of offspring; therefore, weaning of the kittens should be started as early as week 2 to 4. In the case of dogs, peak lactation occurs in the fourth week, and transitioning to weaning can be started earlier based on breed difference (ie, size) and bitch's body condition.[6,8] Reducing the amount of food available to dam and/or switching back to an adult maintenance diet at around 6 to 7 weeks will decrease milk production and aid in the weaning process. After successfully weaning the litters, females can be fed the same amount of calories as pre-breeding intake.

Hand rearing of litters may be needed in some cases (eg, large litters and/or agalactia, toxic milk syndrome, illness or death of dam, eclampsia). Commercial milk replacers (Esbilac and Kitten milk replacer [KMR]) for puppies and kittens can be fed to meet their both protein and energy requirements, as the formulas approximate the nutrient compositions of bitch's and queen's milk. Milk replacers vary in their nutrient profile and bioavailability and may affect growth and health of growing neonates (eg, development of cataract due to insufficient level of essential amino acid arginine).[9] Use of cow's or goat's milk as an alternative is not recommended because of its nature of lower caloric density, and slightly higher lactose content leading to diarrhea in the neonates due to the volume needed to meet caloric demands compared to bitch's milk (**Table 1**).[10] Energy requirement during the first 4 weeks of life is around 15 to 20 kcal/100 g body weight, which may be greater than 25 kcal/100 g body weight in kittens in the first 4 weeks, and the amount of puppy and kitten formulas fed is increased accordingly as they grow, in general.

FEEDING GUIDELINES FOR WEANING PUPPIES/KITTENS

When puppies and kittens reach 4 weeks of age, the quantity and nutrient content of dam's milk are no longer suitable for optimal development.[5,6] Gestation/lactation or all-life stages formulas given to dams can be soaked in water and made into a "gruel" (particularly if using a commercial kibble ration) and offered to the puppies or kittens as early as around 3 to 4 weeks of age, depending on dam's body condition and the number of offspring in the litter. Placing the food on the paws and face of puppies and kittens will usually promote solid food intake. A canned formula that meets the energy and nutrient requirement for growth or all-life stages can be gradually introduced and weaned at 5 to 6 weeks of age for puppies and 6 to 7 weeks of age for kittens and should also be mixed into a "gruel" to optimize intake. The nutritional adequacy statement of the chosen diet should be checked to ensure that it supports growth or all-life stages, and at the point of weaning, home prepared human or raw formulas should not be fed due to their nutritional imbalance or inadequacy, particularly raw foods due to potential pathogen exposures to young offspring with poor immune system status.

FEEDING THE GROWING PUPPY/KITTEN

Although the National Research Council provides a specific lengthy equation for the energy needs of puppies based on adult body weight and current body weight throughout the growing process, it is cumbersome and difficult to use for most practitioners.[11] A simple postweaning energy requirement assumption can be made for most puppies and kittens which is 3 times resting energy requirement (RER) based on current body weight which is rapidly changing. For example, a 6 kg, 10 week old Labrador would be RER $= 70 \ (6)^{0.75} = 268$ kcal. This would then be tripled to

Table 1 Average milk protein, fat, and lactose concentrations found in dog, goat, and cow milk per 100 mL as per analysis by author and USDA Nutrient Database			
		Per 100 mL	
Species	Protein (g)	Fat (g)	Lactose (g)
Dog	7.9	10.5	3.8
Goat	3.5	4.1	4.3
Cow	3.3	3.2	4.8

approximately 805 kcal a day. When 50% of adult body weight is achieved, the energy intake is reduced to 2.5 times RER, and it is 1.8 to 2 times RER at 80% of adult body weight until the puppy reaches desired adult body weight (**Fig. 1**).[12] Though simple to calculate it should be noted that for most breeds (except some giant breed dogs) that the calories consumed between 4 to 5 months of age are likely to be the peak of calorie consumption and that to maintain an ideal body condition increasing caloric consumption is often not necessary beyond this point in development. The recommendation is a starting point for estimation of energy requirement for maintenance based, and frequent monitoring of body weight and condition and caloric adjustments should be involved for optimal growth. A complete and balanced diet designed for growth or all-life stages must be fed to prevent nutritional deficiencies in the face of high nutrient demand. Avoiding excessive energy intake during the growth period is also crucial to prevent obesity and skeletal developmental disorders especially in large and giant breeds. Feeding kittens is slightly different and less well studied; however, recommendation is to feed them at approximately 3 times their RER until they are approximately 50% of their predicted adult body weight and to then feed them at 2 x their RER until they are at adult status which is around 6 to 7 months of age and to then feed between 1.2 to 1.5 x RER into adulthood (see **Fig. 1**).

PROTEIN REQUIREMENTS

Protein requirements of growing dogs are highest in 4 to 14 weeks (56.3 g/1000 kcal) and decreased gradually at 14 weeks and older (43.8 g/1000 kcal).[13] Dry commercial foods formulated for puppy growth should provide high-quality protein content of at least 25% dry matter or greater. Adult maintenance diets may provide adequate levels of protein for growing dogs, but energy density (3500–4500 kcal/kg recommended for growth) of the foods and other essential nutrients such as calcium and phosphorus may not be balanced for appropriate growth. Provision of higher protein levels in growing dogs was thought to accelerate growth and contribute to development of skeletal deformities in large and giant breed puppies.[14] Faster growth rate was observed in Great Dane puppies fed higher protein (32% dry matter) compared to 15% dry matter and 23% dry matter, but the difference in protein intake across the groups did not have a deleterious effect on skeletal development.[15]

After weaning, growing kittens have a protein requirement of 56.3 g/1000 kcal throughout their growth, and this reflects their need for particular essential amino acids and nitrogen metabolism. The amount of sulfur-containing amino acids (ie, taurine, methionine) needed is greater in kittens than puppies or other growing animals, and to meet the amino acid requirement, at least 19% of a diet must originate

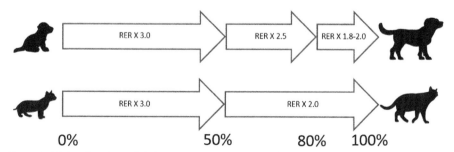

Fig. 1. Initial estimation of daily energy requirements of growing dogs and cats for maintenance and growth.

from animal protein sources for growing kittens; hence, animal-based protein sources are generally used.[16] Arginine is another essential amino acid that is needed in greater quantity in growing kittens, especially when a diet is high in protein content (56% dry matter), to support growth and normal functioning of urea cycle.[17] Optimal protein levels in kitten growth diets are 30% to 36% metabolizable energy calories or 35% to 50% dry matter, in general.[18]

FISH OIL AND DOCOSAHEXAENOIC ACID

Long-chain omega-3 polyunsaturated fatty acids, especially docosahexaenoic acid (DHA, 22:6 n-3), are essential in neural and retinal tissue development in puppies and kittens. This is based on the presence of DHA in the tissues, and dogs and cats have limited ability to convert alpha-linolenic acid (18:3 n-3) to DHA as they mature.[19,20] As prenatal and postnatal DHA supplementation is considered crucial for enhancing neural development and performance, many pet foods formulated for growth and reproduction contain about 0.5% omega-3 fatty acids with omega-6 and omega-3 ratio of 5:1 to 10:1.[21,22] Omega-3 content in the diets can be increased by incorporating omega-3 sources such as marine oils (fish, crustacean, and algal oils high in n-3 fatty acids).[23] Supplementing reproducing female's nutrition with omega-3 during gestation and lactation would have the similar effects for developing fetuses and neonates, as dam's milk becomes enriched with omega-3 fatty acids.[24] When a complete and balanced diet designed for growth or gestation/lactation contains fore-mentioned amount of omega-3 fatty acids and proper omega-6 and omega-3 ratios, additional supplementation of omega-3 is not necessary, yet it should be recognized that this enrichment of DHA should also be in the lactating dam's diet as well as the offspring for optimal development.

OBESITY AND BODY CONDITION SCORE

Diets formulated for growth are higher in fat as energy density of a food is largely determined by fat content. Despite increased nutrient needs during growth, excessive energy intake can result in obesity at an early age. In large or giant breed puppies, the excess food intake involves overconsumption of nutrients such as calcium and can lead to developmental orthopedic problems, since intake of all required nutrients in commercial formulas is increased as energy intake increases.[14] On the other hand, excessive growth rate in kittens does not involve such skeletal or developmental disorders, but obesity can become an issue leading to increased risk for critical feline diseases such as diabetes mellitus and idiopathic hepatic lipidosis.[25] Therefore, regular body condition monitoring of growing puppy and kitten at each veterinary visit is important for determining appropriate energy intake to optimize proper growth of individuals.[26,27] Depending on body condition score, reduction of food intake or portion-controlled feeding is recommended. Switching to a food with a lower energy density (<3500 kcal/kg) seems logical preventing further excessive weight gain in growing animals as long as nutrient intake is still sufficient for growth, particularly in the obesity prone animal.

CALCIUM AND PHOSPHORUS: LARGE BREED CONSIDERATIONS

Growing large and giant breed puppies have special needs with respect to calcium and phosphorus. Contrary to the belief that additional calcium would be helpful for the puppies' skeletal health, use of supplemental amounts of the minerals is of no value and can be deleterious. During their growth from weaning to 6 months of age, passive absorption of calcium in the small intestine is upregulated, and the calcium absorption is directly proportional to calcium concentrations in their diets. Excessive dietary calcium (>4.5 g/1000 kcal) leading to hypercalcitoninism, which reduces osteoclast activity and interferes with normal bone remodeling, is likely to negatively affect skeletal development (eg, articular cartilage development) and cause the beginnings of clinical signs (shifting lameness, pain on musculoskeletal examination) of osteochondrosis.[28] Several pet food manufacturers have responded to this by formulating large breed puppy formulas with lower amounts of Ca and P per 1000 kcal of diet, and the diets are formulated to contain calcium levels no more than 1.1% (dry matter) and calcium and phosphorus ratio between 1:1 and 1.5:1, with a dietary range of calcium per 1000 kcals of 2.0 to 4.5 g[15,29,30] For large and giant breeds puppies it is very important to examine the nutritional guarantee regarding life-stage feeding to ensure that the product is appropriate for growth of large and giant breed dogs which will be on all appropriate commercial dog foods per AAFCO regulations. Phosphorus intake in skeletal development is not considered as critically important as the calcium intake, but low phosphorus intake in growing dogs led to impaired growth and development of musculoskeletal abnormalities (muscle weakness).[31] Therefore, supply and balance of both essential bone forming minerals are crucial for skeletal health of growing puppies. In mature dogs, passive calcium absorption is downregulated and begins to rely on vitamin D metabolism to regulate calcium absorption and retention which does not seen to occur in puppies; therefore, adult dogs are able to tightly regulate the calcium homeostasis mechanisms even with higher calcium intake.[32] Small and medium canine breeds also possess the same passive calcium absorption pattern during their growth, but probably because of genetic differences in calcium metabolism and slower growth rates, the breeds' skeletal development is unlikely to be impacted by excessive dietary calcium.[33,34]

NUTRITION AND NUTRACEUTICALS: OVULATION AND CONCEPTION

As previously stated, the fact that commercial dog foods approved by AAFCO are replete in vitamins and minerals and are typically approved for all-life stages or gestation and lactation the addition of nutrients is not essential for ovulation or conception. The complete and balanced nature of dog and cat foods are a significant disconnect between human ovulation, conception, and gestation studies where there are sometimes modest benefits supplementing vitamins and minerals due to the incomplete nature of the common western diet.[35,36] There is a paucity of research in companion animals to suggest that vitamin or mineral supplementation can improve fertility of female dogs or cats. In human medicine a majority of nutraceutical (eg, nonessential nutrients and herbals) research involves libido rather than improving conception with considerable research around endocrine disruptors from estrogenic compounds found in soy product.[37,38] In the current dog food market there are less expensive products that still use soy as an ingredient; however, because of client perception it is not utilized in premium products very often and even at levels utilized in less expensive foods, it is unlikely that the ability for dogs to conceive and carry conceptuses to whelping is concerning due to endocrine disruptors in foods. Water contamination particularly when using well water has the potential to be issues that are not within the scope of this review. A recent publication examining dog food formulation suggests that a diet containing additional flaxseed meal (which is known to contain phytoestrogens), fermentable fibers, calcium, and phosphorus may have some utility in improving litter size; however, there were different breeds represented and often larger dogs have increased litter numbers making the data somewhat suspect.[39] Ironically, as an author (JW), it is commonly reported by breeders that flaxseed may have some anti-conceptus properties that are not founded in the scientific literature, and considering the test diet from the study above had additional flaxseed meal or other ingredients with phytoestrogens as a major addition to the diet negates this theory to some extent, particularly with new evidence in rodent models suggesting that flaxseed phytoestrogens may be beneficial in polycystic ovaries.[39,40] These dietary concerns related to cumulative phytoestrogen exposure in humans are still heavily questioned in the emerging vegetarian trends with no firm conclusions and our pet foods are typically meat rich rather than vegetable and legume heavy and the fact that dam reproductive lifespan is much shorter than human makes this less of a concern.[41]

There is some literature in the human arena suggesting that there are nutraceuticals with equivocal improvements in oocyte quality for women undergoing in vitro fertilization; however, this was not associated with live births. In humans undergoing in vitro fertilization oocyte quality was enhanced modestly by using a supplement that included folic acid, selenium, vitamin E, catechins, glycyrrhizin, diosgenin, damiana, and omega-3-fatty acids; however, in humans the dietary history often reveals modest nutrient deficiency which is not commonly observed in dogs.[35,36,40] In human medicine folic acid is supplemented in many foods and prenatal vitamins to diminish midline defects in fetuses; however, complete and balanced pet foods make this issue irrelevant to canine and feline theriogenology. In addition, the use of herbal nutraceuticals like the ones utilized above are generally considered safe, yet there is little information on the safety of such herbal nutraceuticals in dogs and cats, which should be a first step in understanding toxicity and pharmacology of the active ingredients which can be vastly different between species. Rodent studies, which are a better example of a multiparous species and more relevant to the dog and cat, often use intraperitoneal injection of high concentrations of herbal extracts that bypasses the gastrointestinal system and may not be relevant to oral application of these herbal remedies further distancing some rodent studies from the reality of oral supplementation in dogs and cats. Furthermore, the herbal remedies in meta-analyses often show equivocal improvements in ovulation or litter size and the studies are not rigorously performed suggesting bias in interpretation.[40] In dogs and cats, the study of ovulation and live births is difficult since they are multiparous and there are many confounding factors such as oocyte maturation and release, typical breed differences in live births, and poorly validated research tools to follow ovulation and conception.

Regardless, of these trepidations one herbal remedy worth mentioning is the use of *Foeniculum vulgare seeds (aka* Fennel Seed) that has some evidence in improving lactation and has been used for centuries.[42] It is thought that fennel seed supplementation provides possible estrogenic effects and inhibition of dopamine that is a negative regulator of prolactin release from the specific polyphenolics dianethole and photoanethole, inducing galactogenic effects.[42] The proestrogen effects may also have utility as fennel seed at 2% and 4% of the diet has improved litter size in rats, further proving that this may be a globally beneficial nutraceutical for conception and lactation within limits[43]; however, there are no dog or cat studies to prove that this would be an effective supplement for breeding females.

NUTRITION AND NUTRACEUTICALS FOR SPERMATOGENESIS

Spermatogenesis and dysfunctional sperm production are often related to heritable issues in dogs. When feeding a complete and balanced diet in the normal stud dog, there is no real need to provide supplemental nutrition or nutraceuticals; however, if a veterinary theriogenologist finds issues with sperm production or motility issues there may be some interesting nutritional supplements and nutraceutical supplements that can be offered. Of course, unlike ovulation the study of spermatogenesis is much easier considering the ease of enumerating sperm, motility, and functional versus dysfunctional sperm. In the human literature specific supplements have been shown to increase sperm count or even improve motility issues including selenium, omega-3 fatty acids eicosapentaenoic acid (EPA) and DHA, coenzyme Q, and carnitine. These data are relatively low in quality with selenium being the universally studied nutrient that has some benefits in humans, but again most human diets are relatively low in selenium due to the poor diet.[44–47] There are a number of herbal and nutritional supplements that may have some utility in human studies, and a few canine studies mentioned below appear to be safe, and are not phytochemicals typically found in commercial dog foods.

A relatively well-designed study in dogs where both control and treatment groups were assessed for semen volume, sperm number, motility, and dysfunctional sperm was performed using a nutritional supplement over 90 days.[48] The dietary supplement was designed to provide vitamin E (1.5 times dietary intake), zinc (1 times dietary intake), folic acid (30 times dietary intake), and selenium (2.5 times dietary intake) at higher intake concentrations than the standardized diet between control and treatment groups. Results showed a decrease in semen volume and an increase in total sperm counts by approximately 2-fold, respectively. Though deemed positive, in these fertile dogs it would be difficult to extrapolate the effects on overall fertility in subfertile dogs, and the lower semen volume may be detrimental to fertilization since the accessory sex gland contributions to semen quality cannot truly be assessed. Though the use of such nutrients cannot be definitively recommended, supplements of the nature at these modest increases are likely safe and may be worthwhile (**Table 2**).

Maca root

Lepidium meyenii is a plant native to the Peruvian Andes region, also known as Latin Ginseng (which may be the reason that Asian Ginseng is thought to be a fertility enhancer), that has been studied extensively for improvements on male fertility.[49] The root and its extract have a range of phytochemicals that are thought to have the medicinal properties beyond just fertility enhancement, and the macerate cooked root can be ingested as a powder or the filtrate can be consumed as a beverage. There is limited data in rodents to suggest the exact dose or phytochemicals involved in increased spermatogenesis, with dosing ranging from 10 mg/kg to 1 g/kg per day with positive results.[50] A study in young bulls using a dose of 233 mg/kg improved semen quality in one study showing interspecies benefits.[49] It should be noted that

Table 2 Potential nutrients and nutraceutical agents to potentially aid in spermatogenesis in dogs	
Supplement	**Dosing (mg or IU/kg)**
ʟ-Carnitine	20–30
Vitamin E (alpha tocopherol – 1 IU = 1 mg)	10
Selenium	0.02–0.05
Folic acid	0.1–0.2
Peruvian Maca root	10–100
Fish oil (25% EPA/DHA formulation)	60–100
Pinus taeda	50
Ashwaghanda root	100

there is no data in dogs and cats and those considering this extract should likely start at lower dosing regimens such as 10 mg/kg and working up from there. A note of caution is that in studies there were discrepancies in results depending on the preparations whether powders or tinctures and modest differences between subspecies plant differences (red, yellow, or black root extracts) and it appears that Peruvian grown extracts may be superior to those grown in Asia.[49]

Ashwagandha

The root of *Withania somnifera*, otherwise known as Ashwagandha root, has been purported to have many different medicinal properties, similar to Maca root.[51] This is a native plant to India and has been termed "Indian Ginseng" by some. Unlike Maca root whose exact actions on spermatogenesis and the exact polyphenols involved remain elusive, Ashwagandha root has 3 major polyphenols that are thought to exert a majority of the pharmacological properties of this plant. A number of rodent studies suggest that doses of 100 to 300 mg/kg of Ashwagandha root extract show 50% plus increases in sperm motility and enhanced sperm counts over 30 to 90 days.[51] Further human clinical assessments in subfertile men suggest that 3 to 5 g a day of Ashwagandha root extract improves sperm counts and motility with 14% improvement in conception rates.[51] There is currently no data on the safety and efficacy of such supplements or the quality of supplements available; hence, utilizing the lowest doses effective in rodent studies above may be the most prudent way forward realizing that this would require approximately 3 g a day for the average Labrador Retriever and more concentrated products are likely to be more cost-effective.

Pinus Taeda

A recent study in dogs was performed over 90 days of supplementation with 50 mg/kg of a hydrolyzed lignin extracted as byproduct waste from the "loblolly pine," which is abundant in the southeastern and southwestern United States.[52] The hydrolysis of these lignans liberates a plethora of polyphenols that may have medicinal properties. This study examined the antioxidant properties in serum samples that was prominent and may have protective properties for spermatogenesis. The mean sperm counts and semen volume were doubled within 90 days of supplementation; however, a significance over 90 days was not found because of the large variation in these parameters across dogs, and motility and viability appear to be no different between the control and treated dogs.[52] Again, these were samples from normally fertile dogs and not from dogs with low or abnormal sperm motility populations giving pause to whether they would be effective, yet this supplement appears to be safe for longer term use allowing for confidence that supplementation is not harmful.

Carnitine

Carnitine is a quaternary amino acid derivative that is important in mitochondrial energy utilization that is essential to normal sperm function. Carnitine is not an essential amino acid and is commonly synthesized in the liver due to its importance in fatty acid metabolism in all organ systems and deficiency is not commonly observed without distinct heritable defects.[53] There is evidence in the human arena that supplementation with carnitine or acylcarnitine has some utility in improving sperm function that cannot be ignored. This provides some nidus for potential supplementation in dogs and possibly cats with dietary carnitine. In human theriogenology tentative recommendation of 2 to 3 g per day are often recommended for spermatogenesis; however, there have been no studies in dogs or cats. A size-based algorithm of approximately 20 to 30 mg/kg body weight can be made as carnitine supplementation does not appear harmful unless super supplementing with very high amounts which leads to some carnitine reaching the colon that can be metabolized to tri-methylamine dioxide which has been associated with increased risk of chronic disease; hence, moderation is advised.[54]

Eicosapentaenoic Acid and Docosahexaenoic Acid

The long-chain omega-3 fatty acids EPA and DHA are highly important in puppy development and proper nutritional supplementation in the form of marine oils is often found in well-formulated gestational and puppy growth products. There appears to be a relationship between sperm counts and quality of sperm and the presence of EPA and DHA intake in humans, and the human diet is often quite devoid of these marine fatty acids.[47] There is trepidation in making global recommendations regarding fish oil additions to provide a better profile as all dog and cat feeds are different regarding their EPA and DHA levels. Based on the author's opinion, there is little detriment in supplementing marine oils (fish, krill, algae) to dogs, as there are health benefits to these oils regardless of the current diet that is being consumed. Typical recommendations are to supply approximately 25 to 65 mg/kg of EPA/DHA and based on dietary energy requirements if a dog or cat food is formulated with approximately 1% fish oil this recommendation is typically reached.[55] A typical Labrador consuming 300 g of a typical 400 kcal per cup of dog food will get approximately 1 g of EPA/DHA (assuming the fish oil used in the product is around 25%–30% EPA/DHA) per day which translates to around 30 mg/kg on average. If 1 teaspoon per 20 kg body weight of a high-quality marine oil is supplemented, the intake of EPA and DHA would increase by approximately 1200 mg. In a typical well-conditioned 30 kg Labrador (1.5 teaspoons in a 30 kg Lab), the total EPA/DHA intake would be approximately 1800 mg that translates to 60 mg/kg of additional EPA/DHA in the diet. This is a common recommendation for a variety of ailments and may also be beneficial in the male dog with fertility issues.

Nontraditional dietary approaches

The rise in feeding nontraditional diets (raw and cooked home prepared) is growing and may be as high as 20% in the dog owning population.[56] Exactly how these numbers transpire among breeding populations is unknown. There are 2 major concerns around these practices that include the incomplete nature of the diet and the potential for zoonotic pathogen exposure. Survey literature suggests that when providing home prepared diets whether cooked or raw to dogs, approximately 60% or greater will have one or more nutrient deficiencies which have the potential to be catastrophic for the parturient female and potentially for reproductive efficiency.[57] The benefits of home prepared diets are that they are often highly digestible and lead to better fecal quality particularly in the whelping and lactating female where energy demands are high.[58,59] One issue surrounding lactation is that many of the home prepared diets are relatively high in protein and fat and lower in carbohydrate which is antithetical to appropriate milk production and diet need to be relatively high in protein so the mammary tissue can synthesize lactose which is a primary nutrient for the growing puppy and addition of minimally 25% of calories as a carbohydrate source is recommended for appropriate milk production.[60] Similarly, at least 26% protein as dry matter in a typical 4000 kcal/kg diet is necessary in the lactating dam, with cats likely requiring more.[13] To this end for breeders who are using home prepared diet plans it is ideal to get both a veterinary theriogenologist and a veterinary nutritionist involved to ensure the dietary plan can support reproduction and lactation.

The more tenuous debate around home prepared diets is the utilization of raw meats in the diet plan. We always recommend cooking meats to reduce the likelihood of pathogen exposure to the reproducing dog or cat, and carbohydrates require cooking for optimal digestibility. A recent case report of abortion related to microbial exposure (ie, salmonella) set the tone for discouraging raw feeding to gravid breeding females.[61] The exposure to pathogenic microbial or protozoal contaminants (eg, salmonella, enteropathogenic *Escherichia coli*, toxoplasmosis, *Listeria*, and *Neospora*) has been associated with illness and/or death in some case reports where dogs, particularly puppies or gravid females, have been exposed to raw feeding practices or pre-weaning periods for puppies.[62–67] It is recommended to not employ these practices in gravid dogs and cats and puppies/kittens in particular. If owners are adamant about these feeding practices, they provide these sorts of diets only when dogs and cats are mature (over 6 months of age) and not actively reproducing.

SUMMARY

The complexity of life-stage nutrition surrounding feeding the gravid and lactating female centers around optimizing intake for proper development and ensuring proper caloric intake during the time of high demand. From there, proper weanling growth and bone formation and developmental issues center around ensuring proper muscling with adequate protein and caloric intake, as well as calcium and phosphorus nutrition whose window in very small between excess and deficiency, particularly in the larger and giant breed dogs. It is essential to choose commercial diets whose nutritional guarantee states that these feeds are adequate for large and giant breed dogs ensuring a proper diet for growth minimally for the first 6 months and potentially even longer in giant breed dogs. Feeding breeding males and females is a more simple requisition unless there are issues with spermatogenesis, ovulation, or conception where using safe supplements in an incremental fashion can be tried in an effort to improve conception if necessary; however, there are few studies in subfertile and fertile dogs to support these efforts. As feeding practices have become more diverse over the years, the first and foremost effort should be doing things in a safe and reliable manner to foster success, ensuring that puppies and kittens and their parents remain healthy for years to come.

CLINICS CARE POINTS

- Lactation: Energy demands during lactation will increase approximately 200% to 300% from energy requirements to maintain an average female dog and weight loss may still occur with large litters.
- Lactation and weaning: Often feeding a puppy or kitten food with higher energy density is recommended for the lactating female and for the weaning puppies or kittens.
- Pregnancy: Energy demands for cats begin to increase from the day of conception, whereas dogs do not require energy intake increases (30%–50%) until about 30 days into pregnancy.
- Breeding females: Optimal body condition is ideal for breeding and nutritional supplementation is not necessary if well-balanced nutritionally complete foods are being used.
- Puppy weaning: It is ideal to use puppy foods that are well balanced energy dense and have a calcium to phosphorus ratio of 1:1 to 2:1 and have a calcium content in the window of 2.0 to 4.5 g/1000 kcal.
- Infertility: Nutritional or herbal supplements to improve fertility in males and females is an inexact science and often starting with lower dosing working toward higher dosing is recommended with veterinary-guided health screens to ensure proper organ function when using herbals is warranted.

DISCLOSURE

The authors have nothing to disclose.

REFERENCES

1. Debraekeleer J, Gross K, Zicker S. Feeding reproducing dogs. Small Anim Clin Nutr 2010;281–94.
2. Lawler DF, Monti KL. Morbidity and mortality in neonatal kittens. Am J Vet Res 1984;45(7):1455–9.
3. Loveridge G. Bodyweight changes and energy intake of cats during gestation and lactation. Anim Technol 1986;37:7–15.
4. Wichert B, Schade L, Gebert S, et al. Energy and protein needs of cats for maintenance, gestation and lactation. J Feline Med Surg 2009;11(10):808–15.
5. National Research Council. Nutrient requirements of dogs and cats. Washington, DC: National Academies Press; 2006. p. 37–8, chap 3. Energy.
6. Oftedal OT. Lactation in the dog: milk composition and intake by puppies. J Nutr 1984;114(5):803–12.
7. Munday HS, Earle KE, Anderson P. Changes in the body composition of the domestic shorthaired cat during growth and development. J Nutr 1994; 124(suppl_12):2622S–3S.
8. Scantlebury M, Butterwick R, Speakman JR. Energetics of lactation in domestic dog (Canis familiaris) breeds of two sizes. Comp Biochem Physiol Mol Integr Physiol 2000;125(2):197–210.
9. Heinze CR, Freeman LM, Martin CR, et al. Comparison of the nutrient composition of commercial dog milk replacers with that of dog milk. J Am Vet Med Assoc 2014;244(12):1413–22.
10. BAINES FM. Milk substitutes and the hand rearing of orphan puppies and kittens. J Small Anim Pract 1981;22(9):555–78.
11. National Research Council. Nutrient requirements of dogs and cats. Washington, DC: National Academies Press; 2006. p. 354–70, chap 15. Nutrient Requirements and Dietary Nutrient Concentrations.
12. Debraekeleer J, Gross K, Zicker S. Feeding growing puppies: postweaning to adulthood. Small animal clinical nutrition. 5th edition. Topeka, Kansas: Mark Morris Institute; 2010. p. 311–9.
13. National Research Council. Nutrient requirements of dogs and cats. Washington, DC: National Academies Press; 2006. p. 111–44, chap 6. Protein and Amino Acids.
14. Hedhammar A, Wu F, Nunez E, et al. Overnutrition and skeletal disease. An experimental study in growing Great Dane dogs. Cornell Vet 1974;64:53–7 (2): Suppl 5.
15. Nap RC, Hazewinkel HA, Voorhout G, et al. Growth and skeletal development in Great Dane pups fed different levels of protein intake. J Nutr 1991;121(suppl_11): S107–13.
16. MacDonald M, Rogers Q, Morris J. Nutrition of the domestic cat, a mammalian carnivore. Annu Rev Nutr 1984;4(1):521–62.
17. Rogers QR, Taylor TP, Morris JG. Optimizing dietary amino acid patterns at various levels of crude protein for cats. J Nutr 1998;128(12):2577S–80S.
18. Gross K, Becvarova I, Debraekeleer J. Feeding growing kittens: postweaning to adulthood. Small Anim Clin Nutr 2010;5:21–8.
19. Dunbar BL, Bauer JE. Conversion of essential fatty acids by Delta 6-desaturase in dog liver microsomes. J Nutr 2002;132(6 Suppl 2):1701S–3S.

20. Bauer JE, Dunbar BL, Bigley KE. Dietary Flaxseed in Dogs Results in Differential Transport and Metabolism of (n-3) Polyunsaturated Fatty Acids. J Nutr 1998; 128(12):2641S–4S.
21. Zicker SC, Jewell DE, Yamka RM, et al. Evaluation of cognitive learning, memory, psychomotor, immunologic, and retinal functions in healthy puppies fed foods fortified with docosahexaenoic acid-rich fish oil from 8 to 52 weeks of age. J Am Vet Med Assoc 2012;241(5):583–94.
22. Holman RT, Johnson SB, Ogburn PL. Deficiency of essential fatty acids and membrane fluidity during pregnancy and lactation. Proc Natl Acad Sci U S A 1991;88(11):4835–9.
23. Heinemann KM, Bauer JE. Docosahexaenoic acid and neurologic development in animals. J Am Vet Med Assoc 2006;228(5):700–5, 655.
24. Heinemann KM, Waldron MK, Bigley KE, et al. Long-chain (n-3) polyunsaturated fatty acids are more efficient than alpha-linolenic acid in improving electroretinogram responses of puppies exposed during gestation, lactation, and weaning. J Nutr 2005;135(8):1960–6.
25. Lund EM, Armstrong P, Kirk CA, et al. Prevalence and risk factors for obesity in adult cats from private US veterinary practices. Intern J Appl Res Vet Med 2005;3(2):88–96.
26. Laflamme D. Development and validation of a body condition score system for dogs, Canine Pract, 22, 1997, 10-15.
27. Laflamme D. Development and validation of a body condition score system for cats: a clinical tool. Feline Pract 1997;25:13–8.
28. Kealy R, Olsson S, Monti K, et al. Effects of limited food consumption on the incidence of hip dysplasia in growing dogs. J Am Vet Med Assoc 1992;201(6): 857–63.
29. Schoenmakers I, Hazewinkel H, Voorhout G, et al. Effect of diets with different calcium and phosphorus contents on the skeletal development and blood chemistry of growing Great Danes. Vet Rec 2000;147(23):652–60.
30. Goedegebuure S, Hazewinkel H. Morphological findings in young dogs chronically fed a diet containing excess calcium. Veterinary Pathology 1986;23(5): 594–605.
31. Kiefer-Hecker B, Kienzle E, Dobenecker B. Effects of low phosphorus supply on the availability of calcium and phosphorus, and musculoskeletal development of growing dogs of two different breeds. J Anim Physiol Anim Nutr 2018;102(3): 789–98.
32. Stockman J, Watson P, Gilham M, et al. Adult dogs are capable of regulating calcium balance, with no adverse effects on health, when fed a high-calcium diet. Br J Nutr 2017;117(9):1235–43.
33. Nap RC, Hazewinkel HA, van den Brom WE. 45Ca kinetics in growing miniature poodles challenged by four different dietary levels of calcium. J Nutr 1993; 123(11):1826–33.
34. Dobenecker B. Apparent calcium absorption in growing dogs of two different sizes. J Nutr 2004;134(8 Suppl):2151S–3S.
35. Buhling KJ, Grajecki D. The effect of micronutrient supplements on female fertility. Curr Opin Obstet Gynecol 2013;25(3):173–80.
36. Grieger JA, Grzeskowiak LE, Wilson RL, et al. Maternal selenium, copper and zinc concentrations in early pregnancy, and the association with fertility. Nutrients 2019;11(7):1609.
37. Rizzo G, Feraco A, Storz MA, et al. The role of soy and soy isoflavones on women's fertility and related outcomes: an update. J Nutr Sci 2022;11.

38. Cerundolo R, Michel KE, Shrestha B, et al. Effects of dietary soy isoflavones on health, steroidogenesis, and thyroid gland function in dogs. Am J Vet Res 2009;70(3):353–60.
39. Orlandi R, Vallesi E, Calabrò S, et al. Effects of two commercial diets on several reproductive parameters in bitches: Note one—From estrous cycle to parturition. Animals 2020;11(1):23.
40. Arentz S, Abbott JA, Smith CA, et al. Herbal medicine for the management of polycystic ovary syndrome (PCOS) and associated oligo/amenorrhoea and hyperandrogenism; a review of the laboratory evidence for effects with corroborative clinical findings. BMC Complement Altern Med 2014;14(1):1–19.
41. Mehraban M, Jelodar G, Rahmanifar F. A combination of spearmint and flaxseed extract improved endocrine and histomorphology of ovary in experimental PCOS. J Ovarian Res 2020;13:1–8.
42. Abbas A, Ikram R, Hasan F, et al. Fennel fortified diet: New perspective with regard to fertility and sex hormones. Pak J Pharm Sci 2020;33(6):2595–600.
43. Badgujar SB, Patel VV, Bandivdekar AH. Foeniculum vulgare Mill: a review of its botany, phytochemistry, pharmacology, contemporary application, and toxicology. BioMed Res Int 2014;2014:842674.
44. Ross C, Morriss A, Khairy M, et al. A systematic review of the effect of oral antioxidants on male infertility. Reprod Biomed Online 2010;20(6):711–23.
45. Mora-Esteves C, Shin D. Nutrient supplementation: improving male fertility fourfold. New York, NY: Thieme Medical Publishers; 2013. p. 293–300.
46. Buhling K, Schumacher A, Zu Eulenburg C, et al. Influence of oral vitamin and mineral supplementation on male infertility: a meta-analysis and systematic review. Reprod Biomed Online 2019;39(2):269–79.
47. Safarinejad MR, Hosseini SY, Dadkhah F, et al. Relationship of omega-3 and omega-6 fatty acids with semen characteristics, and anti-oxidant status of seminal plasma: a comparison between fertile and infertile men. Clinical nutrition 2010;29(1):100–5.
48. Alonge S, Melandri M, Leoci R, et al. The effect of dietary supplementation of vitamin E, selenium, zinc, folic acid, and N-3 polyunsaturated fatty acids on sperm motility and membrane properties in dogs. Animals 2019;9(2):34.
49. Beharry S, Heinrich M. Is the hype around the reproductive health claims of maca (Lepidium meyenii Walp.) justified? J Ethnopharmacol 2018;211:126–70.
50. Qureshi M, Muhammad S, Siddiqui FA, et al. Phytochemical and biological assessments on Lipidium meyenii (maca) and Epimidium sagittatum (horny goat weed). Pak J Pharm Sci 2017;30(1):29–36.
51. Sengupta P, Agarwal A, Pogrebetskaya M, et al. Role of Withania somnifera (Ashwagandha) in the management of male infertility. Reprod Biomed Online 2018; 36(3):311–26.
52. Aiudi GG, Cicirelli V, Maggiolino A, et al. Effect of Pinus taeda Hydrolyzed Lignin on Biochemical Profile, Oxidative Status, and Semen Quality of Healthy Dogs. Front Vet Sci 2022;9:866112.
53. Agarwal A, Said TM. Carnitines and male infertility. Reprod Biomed Online 2004; 8(4):376–84.
54. Gatarek P, Kaluzna-Czaplinska J. Trimethylamine N-oxide (TMAO) in human health. EXCLI journal 2021;20:301.
55. Bauer JE. Therapeutic use of fish oils in companion animals. J Am Vet Med Assoc 2011;239(11):1441–51.
56. Dodd S, Cave N, Abood S, et al. An observational study of pet feeding practices and how these have changed between 2008 and 2018. Vet Rec 2020;186(19):643.

57. Dillitzer N, Becker N, Kienzle E. Intake of minerals, trace elements and vitamins in bone and raw food rations in adult dogs. Br J Nutr 2011;106(S1):S53–6.

58. Algya KM, Cross T-WL, Leuck KN, et al. Apparent total-tract macronutrient digestibility, serum chemistry, urinalysis, and fecal characteristics, metabolites and microbiota of adult dogs fed extruded, mildly cooked, and raw diets. J Anim Sci 2018;96(9):3670–83.

59. Do S, Phungviwatnikul T, de Godoy MR, et al. Nutrient digestibility and fecal characteristics, microbiota, and metabolites in dogs fed human-grade foods. J Anim Sci 2021;99(2):skab028.

60. National Research Council. Nutrient requirements of dogs and cats. Washington, DC: National Academies Press; 2006. p. 49–80, chap 4. Carbohydrates and Fiber.

61. Allen-Durrance A, Mazzaccari KM, Woliver CL. Bacteremia and Late-Term Abortion Secondary to Salmonellosis in a Dog. J Am Anim Hosp Assoc 2022;58(5):262–4.

62. Taques IIGG, Barbosa TR, de Cássia Martini A, et al. Molecular assessment of the transplacental transmission of Toxoplasma gondii, Neospora caninum, Brucella canis and Ehrlichia canis in dogs. Comp Immunol Microbiol Infect Dis 2016;49:47–50.

63. Morley PS, Strohmeyer RA, Tankson JD, et al. Evaluation of the association between feeding raw meat and Salmonella enterica infections at a Greyhound breeding facility. J Am Vet Med Assoc 2006;228(10):1524–32.

64. Arsenault AC, Carr SV, Fraser RS, et al. Protothe003osis and Toxoplasma gondii coinfection in a dog from Nova Scotia, Canada. Can Vet J 2022;63(11):1114–8.

65. Basso W, Venturini M, Bacigalupe D, et al. Confirmed clinical Neospora caninum infection in a boxer puppy from Argentina. Vet Parasitol 2005;131(3–4):299–303.

66. da Costa Reis RP, Crisman R, Roser M, et al. Neonatal neosporosis in a 2-week-old Bernese mountain dog infected with multiple Neospora caninum strains based on MS10 microsatellite analysis. Vet Parasitol 2016;221:134–8.

67. Davies R, Lawes J, Wales A. Raw diets for dogs and cats: a review, with particular reference to microbiological hazards. J Small Anim Pract 2019;60(6):329–39.

Canine Pregnancy, Eutocia, and Dystocia

Autumn Davidson, DVM, MS, DACVIM (Internal Medicine)[a],*,
Janis Cain, DVM, DACVIM (Internal Medicine)[b]

KEYWORDS

- Pregnancy • Periparturient • Eutocia • Dystocia • Newborn

KEY POINTS

- Health of a successful pregnancy depends on proper husbandry, nutrition, and veterinary care. Veterinary preventative oversight requires knowledge of normal versus abnormal conditions in the brood bitch during breeding, gestation, and whelping, as well as appropriate interventions when indicated (obstetrics).
- State of the art equipment as is used in human obstetrics is now available to veterinarians, enabling uterine monitoring (tocodynamometry) and fetal stress/wellbeing evaluation (doppler); these can be used in the clinic or in the client's home.
- Client education about normal labor enables early recognition of dystocia and improves outcome by promoting early veterinary intervention.

 Video content accompanies this article at http://www.vetsmall.theclinics.com.

INTRODUCTION

Working with breeder clients to successfully produce a healthy litter of puppies entails attention to detail from the moment a breeding is planned to the moment the puppies set out in the world (or remain in the kennel) for their destinies. So many things can go wrong. So many of these problems can be avoided or minimized through wise veterinary input. There are many excellent Veterinary Clinics of North America (VCNA) editions concerning reproduction and pediatrics already, and the authors are looking forward to this issue with anticipation. This article begins the journey with the prebreeding examination.

THE PREBREEDING PERIOD

Breeding soundness examinations in the prospective dam should include evaluation of her physical condition, appropriate infectious disease screening (canine brucellosis

[a] School of Veterinary Medicine, University of California, Davis, 1 Garrod Drive, Davis, CA 95616, USA; [b] Canine Reproduction Center at Ironhorse Vet Care, 7660 Amador Valley Boulevard, Suite E, Dublin, CA 94568, USA
* Corresponding author.
E-mail address: apdavidson@ucdavis.edu

Vet Clin Small Anim 53 (2023) 1099–1121
https://doi.org/10.1016/j.cvsm.2023.05.004
0195-5616/23/© 2023 Elsevier Inc. All rights reserved.

before each breeding [Chapter 8]), herpes serology (to guide quarantine management), vaccination status (doi:10.1016/j.cvsm.2013.11.006), available genetic screening appropriate for the breed (Chapter 3), current diet and all medications/supplements (including folic acid where indicated and essential fatty acids), and the diet planned for pregnancy (Chapter 10). Prebreeding vaginal cultures of the normal bitch are not indicated.[1] The physical examination should pay specific attention to the external genitalia and mammary glands. Bitches should be evaluated for vestibule-vaginal malformations, which could interfere with copulation or whelping. Abnormalities in the development of the Müllerian duct or with the normal fusion between the Müllerian duct and the urogenital sinus during embryogenesis can result in atresia of the tubular genitalia or the formation of septa. Septa can be circumferential (hymen-like) or dorsoventral bands; both are usually located just cranial to the urethral papilla. Dorsoventral bands, if narrow, can usually be easily resected with palpation or vaginoscopy before breeding and whelping, even during proestrus (**Fig. 1**). A short general anesthetic is sometimes indicated if the band is thick. Circumferential (annular) strictures are more difficult to resolve surgically because they require an episiotomy and commonly reform and restricture. Artificial insemination and elective cesarean delivery are usually advised instead. Rarely anomalous uterine structures (agenesis, duplication) accompany vaginal septa and preclude breeding.[2] The heritability of most of these anomalies is not known.[3] Bitches should be evaluated for mammary gland normalcy and nipple duct patency. Nonpatent or inverted nipples can predispose bitches to galactostasis and mastitis (**Fig. 2**). Based on the type of mating intended, plans should then be made for appropriate veterinary ovulation timing and breeding assistance. Ovulation timing (Chapter 12) improves conception rates and litter size and permits accurate calculation of gestational age, permitting elective cesarean delivery safely (Chapter 12).

Clinical Care Point: Abnormalities found in the prebreeding examination can avoid critical problems with breeding and whelping.

PREGNANCY DIAGNOSIS

Pregnancy is most commonly confirmed and best evaluated with abdominal ultrasonography, conclusively at 25 to 30 days postbreeding. Ultrasonography can be attempted as early as 17 to 20 days after the luteinizing hormone (LH) surge if concerns exist about early gestational loss of embryos.[4] Testing serum relaxin levels of

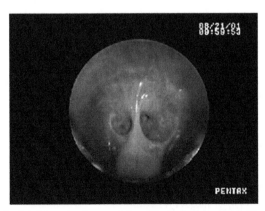

Fig. 1. Septate vaginal stricture in the cranial vestibule, just caudal to the vestibular-vaginal junction. This stricture may not obstruct breeding but would cause an obstructive dystocia.

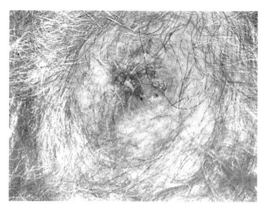

Fig. 2. Inverted, occluded, and exudative, inflamed nipple.

placental origin lacks information about fetal health and litter size. Radiography requires fetal skeletal ossification. Conception, implantation, normal litter size, and fetal health are all evaluated ultrasonographically. Unusually small litters or fetal anomalies should trigger conversation about obstetrics (Chapter 12).

PHARMACOLOGY

Following fertilization and before fixation and implantation, the canine blastocysts become evenly spaced throughout the uterine horns via efficient transuterine migration. Implantation actually occurs 18 to 20 days after the preovulatory LH surge, about diestrus days 8 to 10.[5] During the first month of pregnancy organogenesis occurs and the impact of potentially teratogenic drugs is most critical. At therapeutic levels, most drugs in the maternal bloodstream can cross the placenta to reach fetal circulation. Even before implantation, drugs in maternal circulation reach the blastocysts. Any drug that later reaches the fetal circulation must be metabolized and excreted by the immature fetal kidney and/or through subfunctional hepatic metabolism.[6] Clinicians should evaluate the package insert on any drug before prescribing its use in pregnant or lactating bitches. Cautions for use in pregnant or lactating individuals will be outlined as "safe, untested/unknown, or problematic." Extrapolation across species may not be reliable (ie, tested in laboratory mice). Dose reduction of many drugs is advised, but guidelines are lacking.

PROBLEMS DURING PREGNANCY
Acute Abdomen

The differential diagnoses for a sexually intact bitch with acute onset of signs of abdominal pain include pyometra, uterine rupture, and uterine torsion. Acute peritonitis secondary to deposition of semen into the abdominal cavity should also be considered in the estrual bitch with acute signs of abdominal pain and a history of possible exposure to an intact male dog, or with a recent history of artificial insemination. Semen is forced into the uterus during the copulatory lock because of the large amount of prostatic fluid in the final fraction of the canine ejaculate. Normally the semen should not enter the peritoneal cavity of bitches after mating, but in the case of mates mismatched in size or a diseased uterus, semen could be forced into the peritoneal cavity through a tear in the uterus or vagina or through the oviducts. Intraperitoneal deposition of semen results in peritonitis because prostatic fluid contains significant foreign antigens. Severe suppurative peritonitis and the systemic inflammatory response syndrome are likely sequelae.[7] Ultrasonography can support the diagnosis. Stabilization followed by exploratory laparotomy and extensive lavage of the abdomen are indicated. Inspection of the vagina (endoscopically) and uterus (grossly) for perforation should be carefully performed. This syndrome has high morbidity and mortality for the bitch.

Hyporexia

Bitches can experience a transient loss of appetite and sometimes have periodic vomiting during the second and third weeks of gestation.[8] This condition usually resolves spontaneously, but sometimes marked anorexia hinders adequate nutrition during gestation. Antiemetic therapy can be helpful with metoclopramide (0.10–0.20 mg/kg by mouth or subcutaneously [SC] every 12 hours). Alternative antiemetic drugs may not be safe or recommended for pregnancy; clinicians must evaluate the risk versus benefit. In uncommon cases, force feeding should be considered. Hyperemesis gravidarum in women is believed to occur secondary to an acute elevation of human chorionic gonadotropin; no pregnancy gonadotropin has been identified in the bitch.[9]

Preterm Labor

Mid- to late-term gestational loss attributed to premature labor (PTL) occurs in the bitch. Both myometrial irritability accompanied by cervical changes (softening) and hypoluteoidism have been implicated in the pathophysiology of idiopathic preterm birth in veterinary medicine. Uterine activity and cervical changes leading to the loss of pregnancy via resorption or abortion before term have no metabolic, infectious, congenital, traumatic, or toxic cause identified. Progesterone levels can be normal for pregnancy (5–90 ng/mL) when increased myometrial contractility is first detected. Premature deliveries occur when progesterone levels are less than 2.0 ng/mL. Premature labor is often a retrospective diagnosis achieved after thorough evaluation of the dam and stillborn fetuses has been performed. This evaluation should include metabolic screening of the dam for systemic disease and infectious disease (brucellosis), histopathology and microbiologic evaluation of expelled fetuses and placentae, and review of kennel husbandry, including nutrition, medications, supplements, and environmental factors. All results are normal or negative. Dams experiencing premature myometrial activity in one pregnancy might or might not exhibit it during subsequent pregnancies, but the syndrome can be a chronic cause of failure to successfully reproduce. In human medicine, preterm birth complicates 10% to 12% of human pregnancies, but it accounts for 80% of fetal morbidity and mortality. The early (<40 days' gestation) use of tocodynamometry in bitches with historical or suspected PTL can detect myometrial irritability before the development of luteal insufficiency and facilitate therapy using the tocolytics. Tocolytic therapy inhibits myometrial contractility and is indicated in the management of PTL when no contributory pathologic condition is identified. Elaboration of prostaglandins from the endometrium and placenta associated with premature myometrial activity can result secondarily in luteolysis. The authors' preference is the drug terbutaline, a betamimetic, which avoids the potential complications of progesterone supplementation during pregnancy (masculinization of female fetuses, primary failure of lactation)[10] (**Fig. 3**). Tocolytic therapy can prevent the eventual development of critically low (<2 ng/mL) progesterone levels preterm.[11] The main contraindication to tocolytic therapy in veterinary medicine is undetected uterine, fetal, or placental pathologic condition, making forced maintenance of the pregnancy problematic for the dam. Terbutaline at 0.03 mg/kg by mouth every 8 hours has been used to suppress uterine contractility in bitches, and the dose is ideally titrated to effect using tocodynamometry; monitoring for maternal tachycardia is

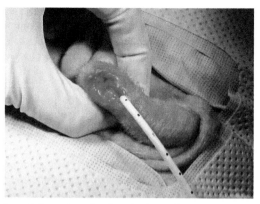

Fig. 3. Masculinization of the vulva of a female dog subjected to progesterone therapy en utero.

advised (www.veterinaryperinatalspeciatlies.com). Diltiazem at 0.5 mg/kg by mouth every 8 hours can be used if response to terbutaline is inadequate. Therapy is discontinued 24 to 48 hours before term to allow labor to proceed. In the authors' experience, poor-quality labor requiring cesarean delivery is common posttocolytic therapy. An elective cesarean delivery should be discussed with clients (Chapter 12).

Clinical Care Point: Preterm labor resulting in the loss of a pregnancy before diagnosis can be mistaken as failure to conceive.

METABOLIC DISORDERS
Gestational Diabetes

Gestational diabetes occurs infrequently in the bitch and is attributed to elevated progesterone levels, mediated by increased levels of growth hormone, during the long luteal phase. Polydipsia, polyuria, and polyphagia with weight loss occur. Higher-fiber diets can promote euglycemia in the bitch, but nutritional adequacy for gestation must be observed. Mild exercise can help. Insulin is not likely indicated or helpful. Oversized fetuses can result from an increased production of insulin in response to maternal hyperglycemia and may cause dystocia due to fetal-maternal mismatch.[12]

Pregnancy Ketosis/Toxemia

Pregnancy toxemia in the bitch is due to altered carbohydrate metabolism in late gestation, resulting in ketonuria without glycosuria or hyperglycemia. Hypoglycemia can occur uncommonly. The most common cause is poor nutrition or anorexia during the last half of gestation. Hepatic lipidosis can occur. An improved plane of nutrition can resolve the condition in most cases, but termination of the pregnancy with management of metabolic disorders may be indicated in severe cases.[13]

Pregnancy Thrombosis

Hypercoagulability has been recognized in pregnant dogs. Pregnancy is a recognized hypercoagulable state that becomes problematic in women with genetic prothrombosis; women are managed aggressively.[14] Affected bitches have an increased tendency for thrombosis, as evidenced by an elevated D-dimer level, with variable clinical appearances. One report documented thrombosis after cesarean delivery.[15] Ultrasonography can be used to document thrombosis, which occurs commonly in the caudal vena cava, resulting in venous congestion in the pelvic limbs (**Fig. 4**). Antithrombotic therapy with low-molecular-weight heparin is well documented in women but undocumented in the bitch. Anticoagulants can result in congenital defects (aspirin-induced cleft palates) or loss of pregnancy due to placental or fetal hemorrhage. Warfarin is contraindicated in pregnancy because it crosses the placenta. Termination of the pregnancy may be indicated enabling antithrombotic therapy if not curative. The condition is believed to be inherited in women; affected bitches should be removed from the breeding pool.

Pregnancy Edema

Marked edema of the distal pelvic limbs, caudal mammary glands, and perineum has been observed, usually in large-breed bitches with large litter size.[16] These bitches are not hypoalbuminemic. Venous thrombosis should be ruled out with Doppler ultrasonography. Mild walking or swimming is helpful. Diuretics are contraindicated in pregnancy. Furosemide can cause a decrease in placental intervillous blood flow, and spironolactone is a pregnancy category D (positive evidence of fetal risk) drug in humans. Mild sodium restriction can help. Severe edema of the perineum can cause dystocia (**Fig. 5**); this differs from maternal hydrops allantois and amnion, in which large volumes of fluid collect within the respective cavities, putting the pregnancy and bitch at risk, and an indication for cesarean delivery.[17]

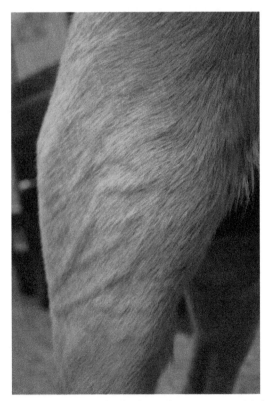

Fig. 4. Venous distension of the upper thigh of a midterm pregnant bitch with thromboembolic disease.

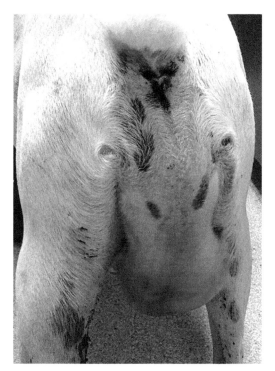

Fig. 5. Severe vulvar edema secondary to lymphatic compression due to a large litter, late gestation.

Vaginal Hyperplasia

Vaginal hyperplasia can recur/occur at term and be mistaken for pregnancy edema. Mild elevation of estradiol at the end of gestation in the bitch can induce reformation of vaginal hyperplasia, seen more commonly during estrus, and cause compromise of the birth canal (**Fig. 6**). Elective cesarean delivery is then indicated. Vaginal hyperplasia can be confirmed by digital examination of the vagina, finding a mass originating cranial to the urethral papilla. A temporary surgical manipulation permitting vaginal delivery has recently been described.[18] The condition is likely to recur with subsequent elevation of estrogen levels.

Eclampsia

Puerperal tetany or eclampsia (Chapter 10) occurs most commonly during the first 4 weeks postpartum, but clinicians should be aware it can occur in the last few weeks of gestation.[19] Eclampsia results from faulty prenatal nutrition, commonly with calcium supplementation, which causes parathyroid atrophy, making the normal response to high calcium demands of lactation blunted. Eclampsia can result from large litters' nursing despite a correct diet postpartum. Calcium supplementation can be considered postpartum. Clients should be educated about early signs of hypocalcemia (facial pruritus, panting, nausea, and stiff gait progressing to tetany). The diagnosis is presumptive based on these classic signs and confirmed by total serum calcium levels less than 7 mg/dL or preferably iCa less than 1.18 mmol/L. Immediate treatment is a slow intravenous (IV) administration of 10% calcium gluconate 0.5 to 1.5 mL/kg, to effect, while monitoring for cardiac arrhythmias. The effective dose

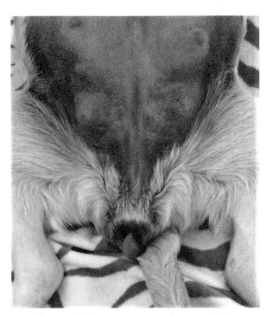

Fig. 6. Recurring vaginal hyperplasia at term gestation, producing a vestibulovulvar mass impacting the birth canal.

of 10% calcium gluconate diluted 50% with normal saline is then repeated SC every 6 to 8 hours until the bitch is eucalcemic, stable, and eating such that oral supplementation (elemental calcium at 25–50 mg/kg/d) can be initiated. Postpartum, weaning or partial weaning should be initiated if the pups are old enough to start eating on their own.

WHELPING
Eutocia and Dystocia

Bitches typically enter stage I labor within 24 hours of a decline in serum progesterone levels to less than 2.0 ng/mL, which occurs in conjunction with elevated levels of circulating prostaglandins and is commonly (~60% detection, https://www.veterinaryperinatalspecialties.com/) associated with a transient drop in body temperature, usually to less than 99°F (37.2°C). Monitoring serial progesterone level for impending labor is problematic because in-house equipment enabling rapid results are inherently less accurate between 2.0 and 5.0 ng/mL, making previous validation of in-house equipment with commercial laboratory results important. Rapid declines in the progesterone level can occur over a period of a few hours after the bitch is sent home. Commercial laboratories offering quantitative progesterone by chemiluminescence typically have a 12- to 24-hour turnaround time, which is not rapid enough to enable decisions about an immediate indication for elective obstetric intervention. If progesterone level is less than 2 ng/mL, with any assay system, labor is imminent. The timing of elective cesarean deliveries (Chapter 12) is best accomplished with previous ovulation timing.

Stage I labor in the bitch normally lasts from 12 to 24 hours, during which time the uterus has myometrial contractions of increasing frequency and strength, associated with cervical dilation. No abdominal effort (visible external contractions) is evident during stage I labor. Bitches can exhibit changes in disposition and behavior during stage

I labor, becoming reclusive, restless, and nesting intermittently, often refusing to eat and sometimes vomiting. Panting and trembling can occur. Vaginal discharge is clear and watery, sometimes voluminous.

Stage II labor in the bitch begins when external abdominal efforts can be seen, accompanying myometrial contractions, to culminate in the delivery of a newborn. Presentation of the fetus at the cervix triggers the Ferguson reflex, promoting the release of endogenous oxytocin from the hypothalamus. Normal stage II labor should result in delivery within an hour; however, great variation exists. The entire delivery can take from 1 to more than 24 hours, but normal labor is associated with shorter total delivery time (4–5 h) and shorter intervals (30–60 minutes) between births. Vaginal discharge can be clear, serous to hemorrhagic, or green (uteroverdin). Bitches continue to nest between deliveries and may nurse and groom newborns intermittently. Anorexia, panting, and trembling are common. Stage III labor is defined as delivery of the placenta. Bitches normally vacillate between stages II and III of labor until the litter delivery is complete. During normal labor, all fetuses and placentae are delivered vaginally, although not delivered together in every instance.

Dystocia is difficulty with a normal vaginal delivery of a newborn from the uterus and must be diagnosed in a timely fashion for medical or surgical intervention to improve outcome.[20] Dystocia results from maternal factors (uterine inertia, pelvic canal anomalies, intrapartum compromise), fetal factors (oversize, malposition, malposture, anatomic anomalies), or a combination of both. For effective management, prompt recognition of dystocia and correct identification of etiologic factors are essential to making the best therapeutic decisions. Uterine inertia is the most common cause of dystocia. Primary uterine inertia results in the failure of delivery of any neonates at term and is thought to be multifactorial, including metabolic defects at the cellular level. Intrinsic failure to establish a functional, progressive level of myometrial contractility occurs. A genetic component could be present. Secondary uterine inertia results in cessation of labor once initiated and consequential failure to deliver the entire litter. Secondary inertia can be due to metabolic or anatomic (obstructive) causes and might have a genetic component when no contributory cause can be identified. Birth canal abnormalities such as vaginal strictures, stenosis from previous pelvic trauma or particular breed conformation, and intravaginal or intrauterine masses can cause obstructive dystocia. In most cases, canal abnormalities should be detected in the prebreeding examination and resolved or avoided by elective cesarean delivery. Causes of intrapartum compromise rendering the dam unable to complete delivery include metabolic abnormalities such as hypocalcemia and hypoglycemia, systemic inflammatory reaction, sepsis, and hypotension (due to hemorrhage or shock).

Fetal factors contributing to dystocia most commonly involve mismatch of fetal and maternal size, fetal anomalies, and fetal malposition and/or malposture. Prolonged gestation with a small litter size (fetal stress/cortisol initiates labor) can cause dystocia due to an oversized fetus. Fetal anomalies such as twinning (shared in placenta), hydrocephalus, and anasarca similarly can cause dystocia because of fetal-maternal birth canal mismatch. Fetal malposition (ventrum of fetus proximal to the dam's dorsum) and fetal malposture (flexed neck and scapulohumeral joints most commonly) promote dystocia because the fetus cannot transverse the birth canal smoothly.

An efficient diagnosis of dystocia depends on taking an accurate history and performing a thorough physical examination in a timely manner. The clinician must quickly obtain a careful reproductive history, detailing breeding dates, any ovulation timing performed, historical and recent labor, as well as a general medical history. The physical examination should address the general status of the dam and include a digital and/or vaginoscopic pelvic examination for patency and content of the birth canal, evaluation of the litter and individual fetal sizes, and assessment of fetal viability (Doppler or real-time ultrasonography, ideally) and uterine activity (tocodynamometry most useful). A radiograph can confirm fetal count.

An accepted approach to veterinary obstetric monitoring involves the use of external monitoring devices using tocodynomometry (Tocodynamometer, Healthdyne Inc, Marietta, GA, USA) and a handheld Doppler (Sonicaid, Oxford Instruments, England) to detect and record uterine activity and fetal heart rates (https://doi.org/10.1016/j.cvsm.2012.01.010) (**Fig. 7**). These devices can be used either in the home setting or at the veterinary clinic; a veterinarian must be involved with use of the service. Their use requires that the hair coat be lightly clipped caudal to the ribcage, over the gravid area of the lateral flanks, to allow proper contact of the uterine sensor and fetal Doppler. The uterine sensor detects changes in intrauterine and intra-amniotic pressures. The sensor is strapped over the lightly clipped area of the bitch's caudo-lateral abdomen using an elasticized strap. The sensor's recorder can be worn in a small backpack or set aside the bitch. Bitches are at rest in the whelping/queening box or in a crate or clinic cage during the monitoring sessions (**Fig. 8**). The monitoring equipment is well tolerated (Video 1). After each recording session, data are transferred from the recorder digitally to the vendor for interpretation. Fetal Doppler monitoring is performed bilaterally with a handheld unit with bitches in lateral recumbency, using acoustic coupling gel (**Fig. 9**). Directing the Doppler perpendicularly over a fetus results in a characteristic amplification of the fetal heart sounds, distinct from maternal arterial or cardiac sounds, which enables determination of fetal heart rates.

Interpretation of the contractile pattern produced by the uterine monitor requires training and experience. Data are digitally transferred to obstetric personnel (24/7) capable of interpretation, who subsequently consult with the attending veterinary clinician and client. Recordings are made on a twice-daily, hour-long basis when home monitoring is performed, then intermittently on bitches or queens at home as indicated during active labor, or on site in the veterinary clinic for shorter periods (minimally 20 minutes) when patients are being evaluated for suspected dystocia. The canine uterus has characteristic patterns of contractility, varying in frequency and strength before and during the different stages of labor (**Fig. 10**).

Serial tocodynamometry in the bitch permits evaluation of the progression of labor. During late term, the uterus may contract once or twice an hour before actual stage I labor is initiated. During stage I and II labor, uterine contractions vary in frequency from 0 to 12 per hour, and in strength from 15 to 40 mm Hg, with spikes up to 60 mm Hg. Contractions during active labor can last 2 to 5 minutes in duration. Recognizable patterns exist during prelabor and active (stages I–III) labor (**Fig. 11**). Abnormalities in uterine contractility can be detected during monitoring. Dysfunctional labor patterns are often associated with

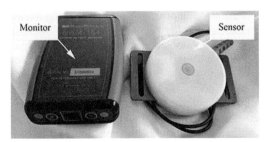

Fig. 7. Tocodynamometry sensor (right) and recorder/transmitter. (Courtesy Veterinary Perinatal Services, inc.)

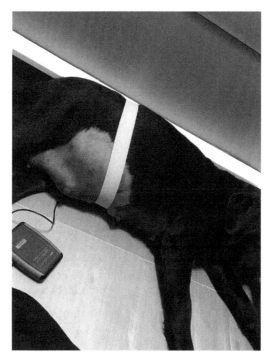

Fig. 8. Tocodynamometer session, stage I labor; Labrador retriever at rest in whelping box. (*Courtesy* of Lisa Colombani, Clarion Reproductive Services, Three Rivers, CA)

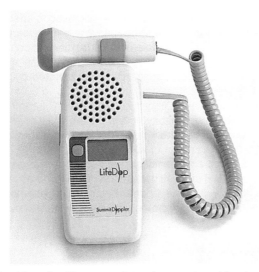

Fig. 9. Handheld fetal Doppler. (*Courtesy of* Veterinary Perinatal Services, Inc., Wheat Ridge, CO, USA)

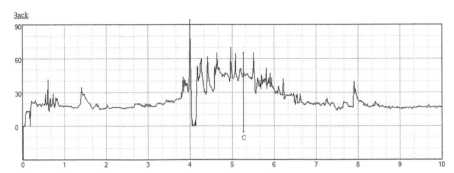

Fig. 10. Tocodynamometry session, contraction just before delivery of a neonate. x-Axis, uterine contraction strength; y-axis, time in minutes.

fetal distress (bradycardia). In addition, the completion of deliveries of fetuses and placentas (or lack thereof) can be evaluated via tocodynamometry.

Clinical Care Point: Familiarity with novel obstetric instruments such as tocodynamometers and fetal Dopplers can greatly facilitate obstetrics and should be described to breeders at the prebreeding examination and consultation.

Medical management of dystocia and indications for emergency surgical management of dystocia (cesarean delivery)

Medical therapy for dystocia, based on administration of calcium gluconate and oxytocin, can be guided and tailored by maternal and fetal monitoring. Calcium increases the strength of uterine contractions, and oxytocin increases their frequency. Calcium gluconate 10% solution with 0.465 mEq Ca^{++}/mL is given SC (the authors caution against giving calcium IV for labor management) at 1 mL/5.5 kg body weight as indicated by the strength of uterine contractions (best measured with tocodynamometry), but generally no more frequently than every 4 to 6 hours. Oxytocin, 10 USP units/mL (American Pharmaceutical Partners), is most effective at minidoses, starting with 0.25 units SC or intramuscularly per bitch regardless of weight, to a maximum dose of 5 U. The dose can be gradually increased to effect (delivery) or until fetal distress is detected; generally, no more than 2 U is necessary. Higher doses of oxytocin or IV boluses can cause tetanic, ineffective uterine contractions that can further compromise fetal oxygen supply by placental compression, or cause uterine rupture. The frequency of oxytocin administration is dictated by the labor pattern, and it is usually not given more frequently than every 30 to 60 minutes. Calcium is given before oxytocin in most cases, improving contraction strength before increasing contraction frequency. The action of oxytocin improves when given 10 to 15 minutes after giving calcium. Most bitches are actually eucalcemic, suggesting the benefit of calcium administration is at a cellular or subcellular level.

Absolute indications for an emergency cesarean delivery include failure to respond to medical management, fetal distress despite adequate to increased uterine contractility suggesting obstructive dystocia, aberrant contractile patterns noted by tocodynamometry, or stillbirths resulting from vaginal delivery of previously viable fetuses (Chapter 12).

NEWBORN RESUSCITATION

Newborn resuscitation entails assisting a pup during the transition from intrauterine to extrauterine life, primarily involving establishing a patent airway ("A"), to enable

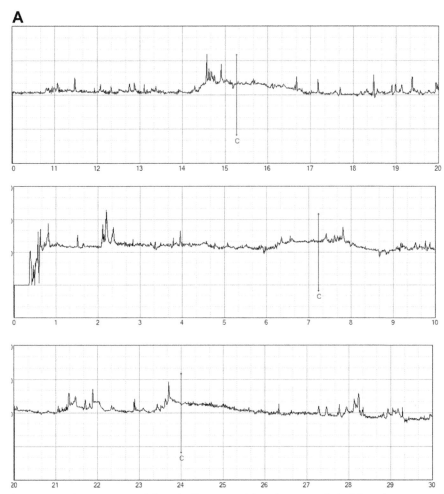

Fig. 11. Tocodynamometry. (*A*) Early first-stage labor in a French bulldog that was well timed, elective cesarean scheduled 2 days after this session was recorded. Bitch was asymptomatic for labor; no temperature change. Cesarean was performed, and all 5 puppies did well and were full term, two with minor meconium expelled. Contractions (*B*) are in a pattern of almost exactly every 10 minutes. Contractions (*B*) are in a pattern of almost exactly every 10 minutes. (*B*) Good pushing. (*C*) Cavalier King Charles spaniel: good contraction pattern (top). Same bitch, onset of inertia (bottom). (*D*) Inertia after both oxytocin and calcium (cane corso) (top). After 5 mL CaGl (middle). ½ Unit of oxytocin (bottom). (*E*) Large breed inertia (top); small breed, good quality Stage II (bottom). Center of contraction marked with the red "C." (*F*) Contraction pattern with fetal/pelvic engagement. With the presence of close coupled contractions, a delivery should be within 1 hour of time, and a good majority of the time when this type of contraction pattern is noted presenting fetal part may be palpated on vaginal examination. The bitch was sleeping during this session, so once again subjective symptoms are not adequate markers of labor progression. (Permission for image Veterinary Perinatal Services, Inc.)

B

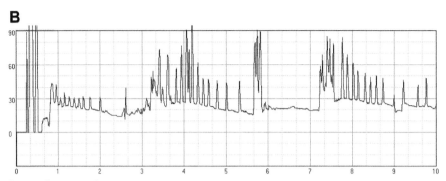

Fig. 11. (continued).

C

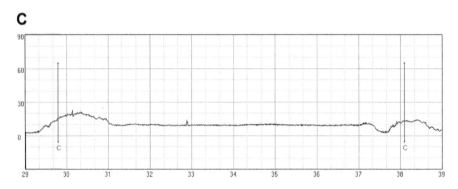

Same bitch, onset of inertia

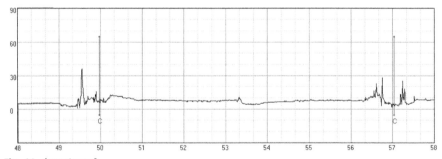

Fig. 11. (continued).

breathing for ventilation ("B") and circulation for cardiac oxygenation ("C"). Actual cardiopulmonary arrest in the newborn can result from asphyxiation following hypoxia and resultant bradycardia. Newborn resuscitation follows a natural whelp if the dam fails to do so, and promptly after removal from the uterus during cesarean delivery. Intervention for resuscitation of newborns following vaginal delivery should take place if the dam fails to stimulate respiration, vocalization, and movement within 1 minute of birth. Examples of a newborn resuscitation kit are found in **Box 1**.

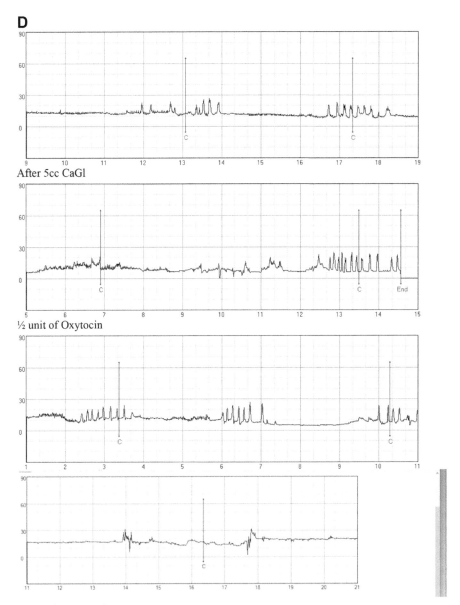

Fig. 11. (*continued*).

After removing amniotic membranes from the neonatal muzzle, the airways should be cleared promptly by gentle oropharyngeal suction with a preemie bulb syringe or DeLee mucous trap while the head is lowered (**Fig. 12**). Neonates should not be swung to clear airways because of the potential for cerebral hemorrhage from concussion (**Fig. 13**).[21] Compression of the diaphragm ("accordion fashion") can traumatize the liver. After checking for a heartbeat and evaluating the heart rate (normal > 180–200 bpm) by digital palpation or auscultation, drying and stimulating the neonate to promote respiration should be performed with appropriate thermal support.

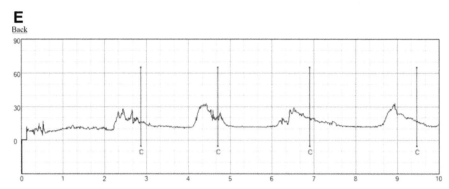

Fig. 11. (*continued*).

Spontaneous breathing and vocalization at birth are positively associated with survival through 7 days of age. Oxygen support can include constant flow-by O_2 delivery by face mask using room air or 40% to 60% O_2. If this is ineffective after 1 minute, and the airway is clear, positive pressure ventilation with a snugly fitting mask to gently expand the lungs (releasing surfactant) is advised (**Fig. 14**). Endotracheal catheterization is challenging and potentially traumatic in the newborn. Anecdotal success with Jen Chung acupuncture point stimulation has been claimed when Jen Chung GV26 acupuncture or a 27-gauge needle is inserted into the nasal philtrum and rotated when the cartilage is contacted (**Fig. 15**).[22] An improvement in heart rate should follow ventilatory support, because myocardial hypoxemia is the most common cause of neonatal bradycardia. Atropine is currently not advised in newborn resuscitation. The mechanism of bradycardia is hypoxemia-induced myocardial depression rather than vagal mediation, and anticholinergic-induced tachycardia can actually exacerbate myocardial oxygen deficits. The use of doxapram as a respiratory stimulant does not improve hypoxemia associated with hypoventilation and is not recommended. If no heartbeat is detected, direct transthoracic cardiac compressions are advised as the first step; epinephrine diluted 1:9 is the drug of choice for cardiac arrest/standstill (0.0002 mg/g administered best by the IV or intraosseous [IO] route). Venous access in the newborn is challenging; the single umbilical vein is one possibility if not thrombosed. The proximal humerus, proximal femur, and proximomedial tibia offer easy intraosseous sites for drug administration (**Fig. 16**).

Chilled newborns can fail to respond to resuscitation. Loss of body temperature occurs rapidly when a newborn is damp. During resuscitation, placing a chilled newborn's trunk and limbs into a warm water bath (95° F–99° F) while ventilating can improve response (**Fig. 17**). Working under a heat lamp or within a (3M™ Bair Hugger™, United States) warming device is helpful. After resuscitation, newborns should be placed in a warm box with warm bedding until they can be safely placed with their dam. Veterinary newborn incubators with an optional oxygen source and puppy cameras exist; caution against overheating is essential.

Newborns lack glucose reserves and have minimal capacity for gluconeogenesis. Providing energy during prolonged resuscitation efforts becomes critical. Clinical hypoglycemia involves blood glucose levels less than 30 to 40 mg/dL and is best treated with IV or IO dextrose at a dose of 0.1 to 0.2 mL of a 2.5% to 5.0% (25–50 mg/mL) dextrose solution. Single administration of parenteral glucose is adequate if the pup can then be fed or nurses. Because of the potential for phlebitis if administered IV,

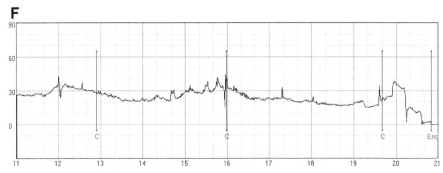

Fig. 11. (*continued*).

50% dextrose solution should only be applied to mucous membranes; however, circulation must be adequate for absorption from the mucosa. Newborns repeatedly administered dextrose should be monitored for hyperglycemia because of immature metabolic regulatory mechanisms. If a newborn is too weak to nurse or suckle, a mixture of a warmed, balanced crystalloid (1/2 strength saline) and 2.5% dextrose may be administered SC at a dose of 1 mL/30 g body weight until the pup can be fed or nurses; however, SC administration of glucose can result in abscessation. Five percent dextrose in lactated Ringer or Normosol solution is hypertonic and contraindicated with dehydration. A balanced and warmed nutrient-electrolyte solution or preferably colostrum from the dam can be administered by stomach tube every 15 to 30 minutes until the newborn is capable of suckling. If colostrum replacement therapy is instituted for newborns where concern about nursing of colostrum exists, oral supplementation should ideally occur within 8 hours of birth, 15 hours at the most. Otherwise parenteral administration is advised.[23]

Clinics Care Point: Trained veterinary technicians and assistants can provide invaluable assistance with neonatal resuscitation once trained and provided with appropriate equipment and technique. Breeders can be included with similar orientation.

The umbilicus of newborns should be treated with 2% tincture of iodine immediately after birth or resuscitation to reduce contamination and prevent ascent of bacteria into the peritoneal cavity (omphalitis, peritonitis); the alcohol-based tincture of iodine promotes faster desiccation of the umbilicus than water-based Betadine (**Fig. 18**). Omphalitis resulting from umbilical contamination in the postpartum period places the neonate at risk for bacterial septicemia. Tetanus has been noted. The umbilicus should be closed and dry 24 hours postpartum; erythema or purulent drainage indicates antibiotics should be instituted because of the potential for peritonitis (**Fig. 19**). Excessive umbilical attention by the dam can result in exposure of the SC tissues with risk of peritonitis. Urine leakage (confirm with a dipstick) from the umbilicus suggests a urachal defect may be present; ultrasonography is indicated.

Several useful modifications of the human APGAR scoring system have been proposed for veterinary medicine (see Sophie A. Grundy article, "Canine Neonatal Health," by Grundy in this issue) (**Box 2**).[24–26] After resuscitation or within the first 24 hours of a natural delivery, a complete physical examination with vital signs should be performed, preferably at home. The oral cavity, hair coat, limbs, digits, umbilicus, and urogenital structures should be visually inspected. Severe congenital defects can result in morbidity and mortality; breeders may elect euthanasia if the prognosis is poor or the cost of therapy prohibitive. In the normal newborn, the mucous

---

Box 1
Neonatal resuscitation kit

- Syringes tuberculin (tb) and acupuncture or less than 25-gauge needles
- Preemie pediatric bulb syringes
- DeLee aspirators
- Small face masks, piglet resuscitators, puppy ventilators (https://www.heritageanimalhealth.shop/products/aspirator-resuscitator-kit-puppy-one-puff)
- Towels (prewarm in drier)
- Heat sources (Baer, warm water blanket, infrared lamp)
- Puppy box (styrofoam, insulated, or incubator style) with thermal support
- Multiple clean mosquito forceps and small scissors
- 3-0 monofilament suture cut in 5″ lengths
- Tincture of iodine 2%
- Bowls for warm water baths
- Thermometers
- Pediatric/neonatal stethoscope ± Doppler
- Neonatal (kitchen) gram scale
- Oxygen sources
- Neonatal drugs on hand: naloxone, epinephrine freshly diluted 1:9, 50% dextrose diluted to 2.5% to 5%

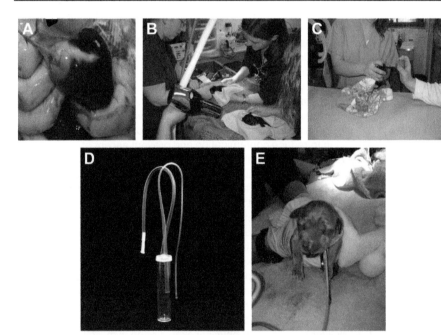

Fig. 12. (*A*) Removal of newborn amniotic membrane. (*B*) Drying and warming newborn Labrador retrievers. (*C*) Aspirating oropharyngeal fluid with pediatric bulb syringe. Best to lower the newborn head. (*D*) DeLee aspirator. White tip is placed in operator's mouth for suction, and clear tip in newborn's oropharyngeal space to aspirate fluid. (*E*) Newborn held with head below thorax for optimal oropharyngeal drainage and aspiration of airway with DeLee aspirator.

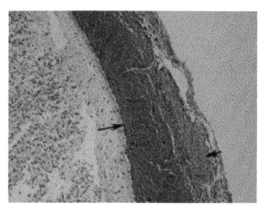

Fig. 13. Histopathology, subdural hematoma, 1-day-old golden retriever postswinging to clear airway. Hematoxylin and eosin stain; 100X. *Arrows* indicate an area of meningeal and intraparenchymal hemorrhage.

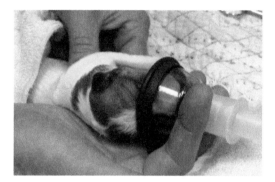

Fig. 14. Positive pressure ventilation with snug face mask; palpation of heart rate.

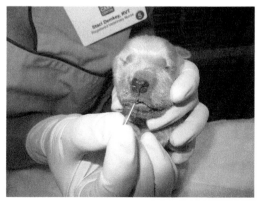

Fig. 15. Acupressure point (nasal philtrum) for breathing using an acupuncture needle, rotating briefly.

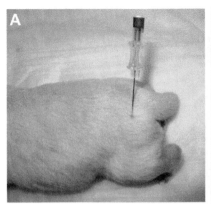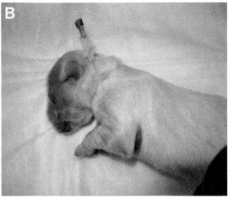

Fig. 16. (A) Intraosseous catheterization, trochanteric fossa, intended for short-term IV administration in newborn during resuscitation. (B) Intraosseous catheterization, proximal humerus, intended for short-term IV administration in newborn during resuscitation.

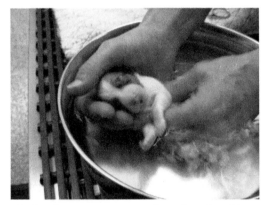

Fig. 17. Warm water bath submersion to reverse hypothermia, with cardiac palpation during newborn resuscitation.

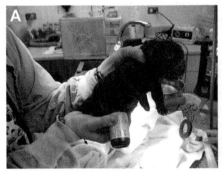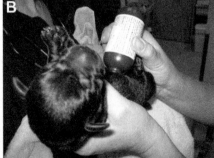

Fig. 18. (A) Method to dunk umbilicus in 2% tincture of iodine. the bottle is pressed gently into the newborn abdomen. (B) The newborn is turned briefly onto dorsum to saturate the umbilicus and then righted.

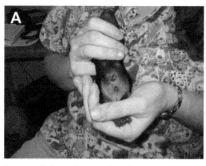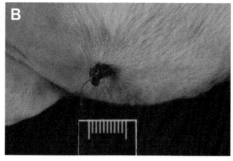

Fig. 19. (A) Umbilicus has been clamped, ligated, trimmed, and dunked in 2% tincture of iodine. (B) Normal umbilicus, 24 hours after umbilical care.

membranes should be pink and moist, a suckle reflex present, the coat full and clean, and the urethra and anus patent. The thorax should be auscultated; vesicular breath sounds and a lack of murmur are normal; and subtle murmurs, if present, should resolve within 14 to 21 days. The abdomen should be pliant and not painful. A normal newborn will squirm and vocalize when examined and nurse and sleep quietly when returned to the dam. Normal newborns will attempt to right themselves and orient by rooting toward their dam. Newborns are highly susceptible to environmental stress, infection, and malnutrition. Proper husbandry is critical and should include daily examination of each for vigor and recording of weight, as well as careful evaluation of the postpartum bitch.

Box 2
Veterinary small animal APVAR key

A is Appearance/color of mucus membranes (mm) 2 = pink, 1 = pale/bluish, 0 = cyanotic

P is Pulse/heart rate 2 = normal ~200 bpm, 1 = bradycardia less than ~160 bpm, 0 = none

V is Vocal/crying: 2 = immediate, 1 = minimal, 0 = none

A is Activity: 2 = moving vigorously, 1 = weakly, 0 = limp

R is Respiration: 2 = normal, 1 = intermittent/agonal, 0 = none

Additional notes
  A: normal physical examination
  B: meconium significant
  C: physical anomaly

Vital neonate score 8 to 10

Fair neonate score 6 to 8

Poor neonate score < 6

APVAR (Appearance, Pulse, Vocalization, Activity, and Respiration) scoring of newborns is a veterinary modification of APGAR (Appearance, Pulse, Grimace, Activity, and Respiration) scoring in humans, and has been proposed for assessment of likelihood of survival during the newborn period. In veterinary medicine, low APVAR scores immediately after birth might not predict eventual mortality, but assessment at 10 to 60 minutes after birth may be useful to indicate need for further recovery/resuscitation intervention.[20]

SUPPLEMENTARY DATA

Supplementary data related to this article can be found online at https://doi.org/10.1016/j.cvsm.2023.05.004.

REFERENCES

1. Groppetti D, Pecile A, Barbero C, et al. Vaginal bacterial flora and cytology in proestrous bitches: Role on fertility. Theriogenology 2012;77(8):1549–56.
2. Palm CA, Segev G, Shipov A, et al. Treatment of a Congenital Imperforate Vestibulovaginal Junction and Secondary Hydrocolpos With Endoscopic Laser Ablation in Two Dogs. Top Companion Anim Med 2021;45:100576.
3. Colaço B, Pires MA, Payan-Carreira R. Congenital aplasia of the uterine-vaginal segment in dogs. A birds-eye view of veterinary medicine. Croácia: InTech; 2012. p. 165–78.
4. Yeager AE, Concannon PW. Association between the preovulatory luteinizing hormone surge and the early ultrasonographic detection of pregnancy and fetal heartbeats in beagle dogs. Theriogenology 1990;34(4):655–65.
5. Concannon P, Tsutsui T, Shille V. Embryo development, hormonal requirements and maternal responses during canine pregnancy. J Reprod Fertil Suppl 2001; 57:169–79.
6. Wiebe VJ, Howard JP. Pharmacologic Advances in Canine and Feline Reproduction. Top Companion Anim Med 2009;24(2):71–99.
7. Slater LA, Davidson AP, Dahlinger J. Theriogenology question of the month: Semen Peritonitis. J Am Vet Med Assoc 2004;225:1535.
8. Kustritz MV. Pregnancy diagnosis and abnormalities of pregnancy in the dog. Theriogenology 2005;64(3):755–65.
9. Dypvik J, Pereira AL, Tanbo TG, et al. Maternal human chorionic gonadotrophin concentrations in very early pregnancy and risk of hyperemesis gravidarum: A retrospective cohort study of 4372 pregnancies after in vitro fertilization. Eur J Obstet Gynecol Reprod Biol 2018;221:12–6.
10. Curtis EM, Grant RP. Masculinization of Female Pups by Progestogens. J Am Vet Med Assoc 1964;144(4):395–8.
11. Davidson AP. Tocodynamometry Detects Preterm Labor in the Bitch Before Luteolysis. Top Companion Anim Med 2015;30(1):2–4.
12. Kruger EF. Pregnancy diabetes. In: Greco DS, Davidson AP, editors. Blackwell's five minute veterinary consultant clinical companion: small animal endocrinology and reproduction. MA, USA: Wiley Blackwell; 2017. p. 423–5.
13. Kruger EF. Pregnancy Ketosis. In: Greco DS, Davidson AP, editors. Blackwell's five minute veterinary consultant clinical companion: small animal endocrinology and reproduction. MA, USA: Wiley Blackwell; 2017. p. 433–5.
14. James AH. Pregnancy and thrombotic risk. Crit Care Med 2010;38:S57–63.
15. Lago-Alvarez Y, Rose H, Campanale D, et al. Thromboembolic disorder in a dog after cesarean surgery. Clinical Theriogenology 2022;14(2):106–9.
16. Davidson AP, Cain J, Goodman M. Pregnancy edema in the bitch. In: Greco DS, Davidson AP, editors. Blackwell's five minute veterinary consultant clinical companion: small animal endocrinology and reproduction. MA, USA: Wiley Blackwell; 2017. p. 427–32.
17. Feliciano MA, Cardilli DJ, Crivelaro RM, et al. Hydrallantois in a female dog: a case report. Arq Bras Med Vet Zootec 2013;65:1091–5.
18. Bucci R, Fusi J, Robbe D, et al. Management of Vaginal Hyperplasia in Bitches by Bühner Suture. Animals 2022;12(24):3505.

19. Davidson AP. Reproductive causes of hypocalcemia. Top Companion Anim Med 2012;27(4):165–6.
20. Runcan EE, da Silva MA. Whelping and dystocia: Maximizing success of medical management. Top Companion Anim Med 2018;33(1):12–6.
21. Grundy SA, Liu SM, Davidson AP. Intracranial trauma in a dog due to being "swung" at birth. Top Companion Anim Med 2009;24(2):100–3.
22. Cavanagh A. Neonatal resuscitation. OK, USA: Veterinary Team Brief; 2017.
23. Rossi L, Lumbreras AEV, Vagni S, et al. Nutritional and Functional Properties of Colostrum in Puppies and Kittens. Animals (Basel) 2021;11(11):3260.
24. Groppetti D, Pecile A, Del Carro AP, et al. Evaluation of newborn canine viability by means of umbilical vein lactate measurement, apgar score and uterine toco-dynamometry. Theriogenology 2010;74(7):1187–96.
25. Plavec T, Knific T, Slapsak A, et al. Canine Neonatal Assessment by Vitality Score, Amniotic Fluid, Urine, and Umbilical Cord Blood Analysis of Glucose, Lactate, and Cortisol: Possible Influence of Parturition Type? Animals 2022;12:1247.
26. Wilborn RR. Small animal neonatal health. Veterinary Clinics: Small Animal Practice 2018;48(4):683–99.

Canine Cesarean Section
Emergency and Elective

Janice Cain, DVM, DACVIM (Internal Medicine)[a],*,
Autumn Davidson, DVM, MS, DACVIM (Internal Medicine)[b]

KEYWORDS

• Cesarean section • Anesthesia • Preparturient • Newborn

KEY POINTS

• A properly performed Cesarean section (CS) with current techniques for anesthesia will result in improved newborn survival.
• If a dystocia situation with evidence of fetal distress (fetal heart rates <180 bpm), moving to an emergency CS without delay will improve chance for successful outcomes.
• A planned, elective CS is a reasonable alternative to emergency surgery in many cases.

Cesarean section (CS) is performed primarily to improve newborn survival. There are situations in which CS is indicated to preserve maternal health or future fertility but in most cases, the choice of CS is all about saving pups! Canine CS is well covered in the literature, comparing anesthesia techniques and methods for improved newborn recovery. In this edition, pertinent literature is reviewed, with an added focus on refined techniques from the authors' experience of more than 1300 successful CS cases over several decades. Although management of the emergency CS (Em-CS) is important for all small animal veterinarians, the authors additionally encourage an acceptance of the elective CS as a planned event.

EMERGENCY CESAREAN SECTION

The decision for Em-CS is based on a variety of factors (See article "Canine Pregnancy, Eutocia, and Dystocia" by Davidson and Cain in this issue) and occurs in approximately 60% of dystocia cases.[1,2] After assessment of the dam for complications of dystocia (eg, dehydration, hypoglycemia, hypocalcemia, and hemorrhage), it is important to assess fetal heart rates (HR) via ultrasonography (US), or fetal Doppler. Fetal distress (persistently low fetal HR of <180bpm) indicates that medical management to continue vaginal delivery could further compromise fetus(es). Proceeding to Em-CS should be done as soon as the decision is made to go forward with surgery. Continued delay could

[a] Canine Reproduction Center at Ironhorse Vet Care, 7660 Amador Valley Boulevard, Suite E, Dublin, CA 94568, USA; [b] School of Veterinary Medicine, University of California, Davis, 1 Garrod Dr, Davis, CA 95616, USA
* Corresponding author.
E-mail address: janicecain@comcast.net

Vet Clin Small Anim 53 (2023) 1123–1146
https://doi.org/10.1016/j.cvsm.2023.04.007
0195-5616/23/© 2023 Elsevier Inc. All rights reserved.

compromise both the dam and any remaining fetuses. In one report, Em-CS for a dystocia patient after vaginal delivery of at least one pup had a higher fetal mortality rate compared with an Em-CS that was started before any vaginal births.[3]

When Not to do an Emergency CS

If anesthesia/surgery would be harmful to the dam, medical support is indicated, not surgery. It would be unusual for an owner to choose to compromise their bitch; her survival is paramount. Moreover, the veterinarian and owner should together consider the status of vaginal delivery in a dystocia situation. If most fetuses have been successfully delivered, then a choice can be discussed whether to do an Em-CS to deliver the remaining pup(s) or stop intervention (See article "Canine Pregnancy, Eutocia, and Dystocia" by Davidson and Cain in this issue). If a large litter and exhausted dam, it is not required to go forward with Em-CS to deliver remaining fetus(es), so long as the bitch is not in distress due to fetal obstruction or uterine trauma. Similarly, if all fetuses are nonviable (no heartbeats), and the bitch is not in distress, then Em-CS is not indicated. Often owners and veterinarians are under the impression that Em-CS is required, or the dam will have medical complications (toxicity, sepsis) but that is not true in most cases. A remaining viable fetus can survive dystocia and be delivered numerous hours later, after treatment is stopped but can also die and pass eventually. If the owner accepts this outcome, then Em-CS is not needed. The authors emphasize that US is needed to provide correct assessment of viability of remaining fetuses. Deceased fetuses will usually pass vaginally after 2 to 14 days. In the rare instance that a deceased fetus or decayed fetal material remains (confirmed via US), hysterotomy for removal can be considered on a nonemergency basis several weeks later.

ELECTIVE CESAREAN SECTION

The elective Cesarean section (El-CS) has gained acceptance among veterinarians with an interest in canine reproduction. Improvement of anesthesia and newborn recovery techniques results in successful outcomes. Ovulation timing to determine the expected due date has improved the ability to plan and perform the El-CS successfully. The planned El-CS is a practical procedure for veterinarians outside of emergency facilities and a reasonable alternative to natural whelping for some dogs and owners.

The primary indication for El-CS is improved newborn survival. Natural vaginal birth is a stressful event and can result in death of some pups. In one study, all pups from El-CS survived, whereas newborn death rate ranged from 3% to 20% in litters born from both natural whelping or Em-CS.[4] Investigators have reported higher average lactate concentrations in cord blood of newborn pups (indicating hypoxic stress) born by vaginal delivery or Em-CS as compared with El-CS.[5,6] Other reports confirm the benefit of elective over Em-CS: obstructive dystocia increased newborn mortality more than 8-fold[7] and others documented a higher newborn mortality rate in Em-CS compared with El-CS.[3,8–10] It can be difficult to always predict when whelping will result in dystocia but a discussion between the veterinarian and owner regarding the whelping plan or arrangements for an El-CS should be considered at time of pregnancy diagnosis.

Additional Considerations for an Elective CS

- Uncertain availability of a reliable, experienced emergency team if an Em-CS is needed.
- Indication based on breed: brachycephalic, "bully" breeds, Molosser type and other giant breeds, Scottish and Norwich Terriers can have whelping difficulty or historically poor newborn survival.

- Indication based on anatomy: for example, postpelvic trauma or unrepairable vaginal septum.
- History of need for CS due to previous primary or secondary uterine inertia.
- Litter size: avoidance of dystocia due to either single pup or very large litter.
- Age of first parturition: advanced age increases risk of dystocia.[3]
- If tocolytic drugs used to treat preterm labor, an impaired contraction pattern can occur when whelping (See article "Canine Pregnancy, Eutocia, and Dystocia" by Davidson and Cain in this issue).
- Maintenance of the bond, trust, and confidence between owner and their veterinarian, rather than referral to an emergency facility with staff unfamiliar to the owner.
- Owner preference: (1) owner questions their ability to handle or make decisions in stressful situations and (2) owner's negative experience with an earlier emergency event.
- Owner concerns about cost difference between an Em-CS versus planned El-CS.

Negative Aspects to Elective CS

- Any anesthesia/surgery carries some inherent patient risk.
- Pain for the dam.
- Some will debate the ethics of the El-CS: (1) possible unnecessary surgery; (2) breeding any dog for which a CS is wanted/needed rather than natural whelping; and (3) *encouraging* breeders to select breeds or dams that *require* CS.
- Potential complications of wound healing, risk of infection, adhesions.
- Possible delay in mothering behavior by the dam after anesthesia/surgery.
- Possible decrease in milk production/milk letdown.
- More work for the owner to care for pups and strictly observe dam/pups for several days after surgery.
- Cost to owner as opposed to uneventful natural whelping.

PLANNING THE ELECTIVE C-SECTION
Selecting the Surgery Date

Determining the expected due date is the key to successfully planning and performing a preparturient El-CS. This is best achieved by precise ovulation timing: techniques to determine the date of ovulation. The interval between ovulation and whelping is relatively consistent as 63 $\pm$ 1 days (or 64–66 days from preovulatory luteinizing hormone [LH] peak).[11,12] There can be a 1 to 2-day variation for large litters (whelp early) and 1 to 2 pup litters (whelp late) but the accuracy of this due date prediction is quite remarkable. The authors also recognize some breed-specific variations for gestational length could be possible, including Cavalier King Charles Spaniels expected due date earlier at 62 $\pm$ 2 and Greyhounds later at 68 $\pm$ 1.5 (both measurements are days from LH peak).[12,13] As well, it might be prudent to consider familial history, when available.

A planned El-CS can be safely performed, with excellent neonatal survival, 1 to 2 days before the median expected due date. At this time, labor is not usually evident (preparturient) but the dam should have adequate colostrum and fetuses will be mature (organ and surfactant development). The choice when to plan the El-CS will depend on.

- Breed of dog and earlier history of whelping.
- Litter size: US to assess pregnancy at 23 to 28 days postbreeding is helpful to further confirm the expected due date and to determine relative litter size.

- Comfort level of the owner to seek emergency veterinary care should the dam go into labor before the planned surgical day.

METHODS FOR OVULATION TIMING
Progesterone testing

Serum progesterone concentration determination is the primary tool of ovulation timing due to ease, convenience, and economy. Progesterone starts to increase with the preovulatory luteinization of follicles at approximately the time of the preovulatory LH peak.[11,14] Ovulation occurs approximately 2 days after the LH peak, and then ova require approximately another 2 days to mature.[14,15] The peak fertile window is 4 to 6 days after the LH peak. The authors prefer the reliability of reference laboratory testing using a chemiluminescence assay (the values that follow reflect this type of assay result ranges). Note: many in-clinic assays are also available, with different result ranges and variable reliability (See article "Progesterone Analysis in Canine Breeding Management" by Conley and Gonzales of this issue).

- Interpretation of the progesterone profile:[11,14]
  - Basal value of less than 1.5 ng/mL
  - Association with LH peak: 1.6 to 2.5 ng/mL
  - Association with ovulation: 3.8 to 6 ng/mL
  - Level at time of breeding: 6 to 20 ng/mL
  - Bitches with very low basal values (eg, <0.5 ng/mL) tend to have lower progesterone levels that indicate the LH peak (eg, 1.6–1.8 ng/mL), whereas those with a higher basal level (eg, 1.4–1.5 ng/mL) tend to have a relatively higher progesterone level at time of LH peak (eg, 2.5 ng/mL).
- The authors prefer to start testing on day 5 to 7 after appearance of vaginal bleeding or based on progression of vaginal epithelial cell cornification. The goal is for the first test to be in the basal range. Testing is then repeated every other day until a pattern consistent with ovulation occurs. Note: It is advisable to evaluate the curve over time and not look for a specific target level to indicate ovulation. The range to determine the LH peak is narrow, whereas progesterone level at breeding can vary significantly. The goal is to determine the LH peak (first increase of progesterone) and confirm this finding by additional progesterone testing (continued increase > 5–7 ng/mL). Rarely, progesterone can start to increase but then declines to basal levels, pause, and then increases several days later.

LH Testing

This can be done in association with progesterone testing. In-clinic test kits are available and affordable (Witness LH Rapid Test, Zoetis, USA). Nonhemolyzed serum samples are obtained daily (starting when progesterone testing begins) and frozen. Key samples are then thawed and analyzed to confirm the LH peak (as estimated by progesterone testing). It is possible that the LH peak can be less than 24 hours and missed, even with daily testing, hence the need to couple LH and progesterone testing (and not use as a sole testing method).

Other indicators of ovulation

- US and vaginoscopy can be additional tools to determine ovulation but are nonspecific and more difficult to interpret for precise determination of ovulation.
- Daily vaginal cytology to determine the onset of diestrus can be used to determine the due date (57 ± 4 days from onset of diestrus),[16] and although not as

accurate as hormonal testing when done alone, can be done by owners at home to augment hormonal testing.

When Ovulation Timing was not Conducted or not Possible

Owners often request a planned El-CS for a pregnancy in which no ovulation timing was conducted or was not done in a precise manner. This presents a dilemma for the veterinarian who tries to proactively help the owner but also needs to ensure a proper surgery date is selected to assure newborn viability. Although not as reliable as precise ovulation timing, some additional methods can be used to further assess fetal maturity. It is important to note, however, that this may eliminate the "planned" part of the El-CS and thus necessitate referral to an emergency facility for surgery.

Tocodynamometry

- Uterine contractions consistent with onset of early stage I labor (See article "Canine Pregnancy, Eutocia, and Dystocia" by Davidson and Cain in this issue).

"Reverse" Progesterone Testing

- The term "reverse" is used to indicate progesterone testing at the end of diestrus. This method is based on the decline of progesterone to values of 2.0 ng/mL or less at the time, or just before natural parturition.[14]
- Test daily near the anticipated due date and do surgery when progesterone is 2.0 ng/mL or less.
- Drawbacks of "reverse" progesterone testing include unreliability because progesterone levels can drop precipitously: The authors have experienced planned C-sections canceled due to a progesterone level of 3 to 6 ng/mL but the bitch goes into active labor that night.
- Moreover, the authors have observed progesterone values of 2 to 4 ng/mL at both the onset of spontaneous labor and at the time of successful El-CS; thus, using progesterone testing to assess term maturity can be unreliable.

Ultrasonography and Radiology

These and other parameters are used to assist gestational aging and/or assessment of term development. Factors can vary based on breed and accuracy is inconsistent.[17–22]

- Early in pregnancy: inner chorionic cavity (vesicle) diameter
- Measurement of diameter of fetal skull (biparietal diameter)
- Mature appearance and peristalsis of fetal small intestinal tract (at/near term)
- Mature appearance and architecture of fetal kidney (at/near term)
- Fetal HR oscillations in early stage I of labor.
- Radiographic appearance of dental buds (near term; **Fig. 1**)
- Calcification of extremities (near term)

Maternal Vaginal Discharge

Clear or mucoid discharge is normal during pregnancy and an increase in clear fluid discharge can occur as pregnancy progresses (See article "Canine Pregnancy, Eutocia and Dystocia" by Davidson and Cain of this issue). Dogs do not usually "break the water sac" as do humans, so increased clear discharge is difficult to interpret, and can be seen for several days to weeks before onset of labor. Appearance of uteroverdin in vaginal discharge (black-green colored discharge) indicates placental separation. This is not proof that fetuses are term because this can occur with preterm

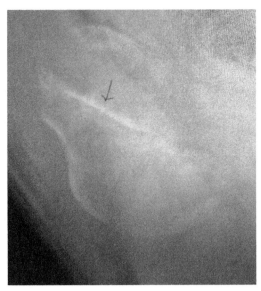

Fig. 1. Radiograph of fetal skull in utero. Arrow indicates line of dentition formation. This is an indication of term/near term fetal development.

delivery or abortion and is concerning for fetal viability if bitch is not in productive labor.

ANESTHETIC CONSIDERATIONS FOR CESAREAN SECTION

The anesthesia goal for CS is similar for all canine surgical patients: delivery of the correct agents in a manner to ensure alleviation of pain and consciousness while affording minimal physiologic risk to the patient. Added factors for CS are the well-being of the fetuses, soon to be newborns, and a rapid, functional recovery of the dam to encourage appropriate mothering behavior.

The metabolic changes that occur during pregnancy that can affect anesthesia have been reviewed[23–25] (See **Table 1**, Physiologic Factors of Pregnancy).

DRUG SELECTION

Assume all anesthetic agents cross the placenta, unless specifically known otherwise, and may induce depression of cardiovascular and neurologic function in newborns.[23,24] Factors that can increase placental drug transfer include high lipid solubility, low molecular weight, and low protein binding.[23,26] Choose drugs that can be reversed when possible.

PREANESTHESIA MEDICATIONS

Many published CS protocols avoid the use of sedatives or analgesics before delivery of all pups. This may be due to study design to evaluate how a specific protocol will affect newborns without interference of other factors. It is recognized, however, that preanesthetic administration of a sedative/analgesic can alleviate stress to the dam and reduce the total dose of anesthetic agents needed; both can improve newborn recovery. In a debilitated patient presenting for an Em-CS, premedication with a sedative might be contraindicated.

Table 1
Some physiologic changes of pregnancy and potential impact for anesthesia and surgery

Physiologic System	Potential Impact
Hematological: Increase in reb blood cell (RBC) mass but a greater increase in plasma volume. Result is anemia of pregnancy	If hematocrit is normal, concern for dehydration
Cardiovascular: Decrease in vascular resistance, resulting in slight decrease in systolic blood pressure but not of clinical significance in the normal patient. Increase heart rate and stroke volume results in increased cardiac output	If patient is compromised, can see hemodynamic affects. Monitor blood pressure, pretreat with IV fluids to stabilize. If a pressor agent is necessary, consider ephedrine (0.03–0.1 mg/kg IV) to improve maternal arterial pressure while not adversely affecting uterine perfusion[23]
Respiratory: Increased oxygen demand, increased minute ventilation and decreased functional residual capacity. Coupled with increased abdominal pressure at term (especially for a small dog with large litter), can induce respiratory compromise and risk of hypoxia and hemoglobin desaturation	Preoxygenation important, intubate quickly and efficiently, monitor for apnea after induction
Gastrointestinal: Progesterone, elevated during pregnancy, causes decease tone of LES, delayed gastric emptying, and decreased gastrointestinal (GI) motility	Increased risk of regurgitation and aspiration. Be sure patient has fasted 12 h, when possible. Watch carefully for regurgitation/aspiration. Intubate quickly and extubate with care and attention
Uterine specific: Any change in perfusion pressure will affect uterine blood flow thus important to maintain normal hydration and alleviate stress (increased catecholamines can decrease uterine blood flow)	Move to CS quickly if an emergency situation. Maintain normal blood pressure and hydration for all cases

Sedative/Analgesic Agents

- *Opioids*: Some investigators use morphine (0.1–0.3 mg/kg IV) before induction, due to its relatively low lipid-solubility.[26–28] Fentanyl is highly lipid soluble with high placental transfer and is typically avoided until after all pups are delivered. Hydromorphone (0.05–0.075 mg/kg IV) is intermediate as regards lipid solubility and is used commonly by the authors (see protocol below). Some investigators use methadone (0.2 mg/kg SQ), which has similar action as morphine but might be less sedating.[29] All opioids can cause respiratory depression and the dam must be monitored accordingly. Similarly, if newborns are sluggish or not breathing spontaneously, naloxone can be administered as a reversal agent: 0.002 to 0.02 mg/kg intramuscularly or subcutaneously, or one drop (approximately 0.1 mL) of 1 mg/mL solution sublingual. Buprenorphine, a partial mu receptor agonist, has relatively low placental transfer but effects cannot be completely reversed with 0.4mg/ml solution.
- *Dexmedetomidine*: An alpha-2 adrenergic agonist has been shown to reduce the dose of induction agents without adverse effects to newborn recovery (2 μg/kg IV).[30,31] Evidence to suggest a placental barrier preventing effective transmission to fetuses was found in one study.[30] Reversal can be considered (atipamezole

20–50 µg/pup SQ or sublingual), although Gropetti[30] reported this was not needed as has been the authors' experience. Reversal in bitch if desired at recovery: (atipamezole 10–20 µg/kg SQ or IM) but then any analgesic benefit is removed.

- *Phenothiazines and benzodiazepines* are not recommended due to prolonged sedation in newborns.[32,33]

Anticholinergics

Increased vagal tone due to intubation and handling of the gravid uterus can induce bradycardia. The use of atropine to counteract maternal bradycardia is questionable due to placental transfer that can increase the HR of fetuses. Low fetal HR is primarily due to hypoxemia and an indicator of stress. Artificial increase in fetal HR, without correction of the underlying cause of bradycardia, could be contraindicated. The use of glycopyrrolate (0.005–0.01 mg/kg IV) is a more common choice, and preferred by the authors, to maintain normal HR in the dam while not affecting fetal HR; its large polar structure and low lipid solubility prevents significant placental transfer.[23,34] Additionally, anticholinergics can increase gastric stasis, so one approach is to use only if necessary to treat maternal bradycardia.[34]

Commonly Used Induction Agents

- *Ketamine and barbiturates* cause significant neonatal neurologic depression and are not recommended.[24,32,35,36] Induction by inhalant is also not recommended because rapid induction and control of airway is needed.
- *Propofol:* Largely accepted as an excellent induction agent for stable patients, allowing rapid induction and ease of intubation (2–6 mg/kg IV titrated to effect). It is rapidly cleared from maternal circulation by redistribution and hepatic metabolism. Propofol is also rapidly cleared from fetal/neonatal circulation by redistribution and resorption of drug back from fetuses to dam can occur.[23,24] The drug does not accumulate with repeated doses. Recovery is typically smooth, with rapid return to consciousness and minimal residual effects. Depression of cardiovascular function is possible[37,38] but is unlikely to be clinically significant in a young, stable patient at recommended doses. Postinduction apnea can occur with rapid infusion.[38] Some authors instituted a waiting period of 15 to 20 minutes after induction to allow propofol redistribution before delivery of the first pup.[30,39] Others, including the authors, have found this delay is not necessary and might be detrimental to newborn viability, especially if fetuses are compromised.[40]
- *Alfaxalone:* A neuroactive steroid, alfaxalone is successfully used to induce anesthesia for CS (1.6–3 mg/kg).[40–42] It has a half-life of approximately 25 minutes, is less likely to cause cardiovascular depression than other injectable agents (at normal therapeutic dosing) and does not accumulate after repeated dosing. Hepatic clearance is by both cytochrome P450 and conjugation.[24] Newborns exhibit quick recovery.[40–42] Some investigators found improved immediate newborn viability scores when using alfaxalone compared with propofol induction but equal eventual newborn survival.[41,42] Two pups in the alfaxalone group of one study had Apgar scores of zero and did not survive.[41] Alfaxalone can be associated with a reactive or longer recovery.[43,44] Signs such as paddling, rigidity, myoclonus, and vocalization have been reported. Although this is not normally a concern for most postanesthesia patients, it might be more concerning for post-CS because the goal is to initiate nursing as soon as possible postop, often with owner assistance. These signs might be ameliorated with preanesthetic sedation.

Local/Regional Anesthesia

- *Epidural:* Excellent analgesia can be provided by a properly administered epidural; technique described elsewhere.[28,45,46] Dogs will require concomitant general anesthesia but at possibly reduced doses, providing good newborn recovery.[28,35] The greatest disadvantage is the need for expertise to perform the epidural properly and efficiently: there is questionable benefit to an epidural if the time needed for the procedure significantly increases total anesthesia time because this can negatively affect newborn recovery. Other potential disadvantages of epidural anesthesia include residual motor defects at recovery (might prolong recovery time) and potential for an increased maternal hypotension.[47,48] Various protocols have been reported using bupivacaine or lidocaine mixed with saline and possibly an opioid.[28,35,47]
- *Local block:* Infiltrative injection into area of incision can aid analgesia and decrease induction and maintenance doses of anesthetics. Attentive injection technique is required to neither inadvertently inject IV nor disrupt mammary vasculature. Lidocaine (1–2 mg/kg)[29,30,43] is often used and at low doses placental transfer is negligible but total duration of effect is limited.[49] Bupivacaine can also be added to improve postoperative analgesia but its slower onset of action makes use of this as a sole agent less helpful to reduce anesthesia doses.

ANESTHETIC MAINTENANCE
Inhalants

Isoflurane or sevoflurane are the commonly used inhalational anesthesia agents. Both are minimally metabolized and removed from the host by ventilation. That can be a problem for newborns that are not spontaneously breathing at birth. Moon reported that the "use of inhaled anesthetics decreased the odds that the litter would have all puppies breathing or any of the puppies moving at birth."[36] Inhalants depress fetal blood pressure and minute ventilation.[23] The degree of newborn depression is directly correlated to the depth of anesthesia of the dam, however.[24] Minimal use of inhalants is preferable, whenever possible, or at least to reduce vaporizer settings to maintain a light plane of anesthesia. Moreover, the minimum alveolar concentration of inhalants is reduced by 16% to 40% due to the physiology of pregnancy[50]; therefore, the anesthetist must be attentive when using inhalants before the complete delivery of all pups.

Continuous Rate Infusion of Injectable Agents

The concept of a total IV anesthesia protocol has been presented.[51] Both propofol and alfaxalone have been studied to determine if injectables can be used solely to maintain anesthesia to avoid the use of inhalants until all pups are delivered.[28,43] In one report, results with alfaxalone (0.2 mg/kg/min) were similar to isoflurane maintenance.[43] The same investigators found poor results in 2 patients with propofol at a continuous rate infusion (CRI) of 0.4 mg/kg/min but 1 patient had a very prolonged surgery time.[52] The authors routinely use propofol to maintain anesthesia before completion of pup delivery but rather than CRI, titrate in a "to effect" protocol (**Box 1**) with very good results.

OTHER PERIANESTHETIC CONCERNS
Intravascular Fluid Support

Perioperative IV fluid support is indicated. A balanced crystalloid solution, such as lactated ringers solution, is often selected at dose rates of 5 to 10 mL/kg/h.

Box 1
Authors' cesarean section anesthesia and surgery management protocol

1. Dog is admitted to hospital 1.5 h before surgery start time. Complete physical examination is performed. Brief US is done to assess fetal viability for distress and evidence for term development. Evaluate mammary glands for adequate colostrum production.

2. Preanesthesia laboratory evaluation: CBC, chemistry profile including electrolytes.

3. IV catheter is placed in peripheral vein and if possible, abdomen is clipped to remove major hair. If dog is too stressed by this, clipping is done after sedation.

4. Operating room (OR) is prepared, and all neonatal recovery devices are assembled (See article "Canine Pregnancy, Eutocia, and Dystocia" by Davidson and Cain in this issue).

5. Approximately 15 min before induction, preanesthesia medications are administered: hydromorphone (0.05–0.75 mg/kg IV) and cefazolin (22 mg/kg IV). If the patient is fractious or stressed, dexmedetomidine (2 μg/kg IV) is used in place of hydromorphone.

6. Anesthesia, surgery, and neonatal teams are all assembled and ready.

7. Final hair clipping and "dirty scrub" done before moving into OR.

8. Preoxygenation for 3 to 5 min if tolerated.

9. Induction: propofol 2 to 4 mg/kg titrated to effect: intubation and oxygen provided. Apply all standard anesthesia monitoring devices (pulse oximeter, ECG, blood pressure monitor, End-tidal CO_2 monitor).

10. Patient in dorsal recumbency and final surgical prep. Local infiltration of lidocaine 1–2 mg/kg) into area of intended incision.

11. Maintenance of anesthesia with propofol titrated in 0.5 to 1 mg/kg miniboluses to maintain light plane of anesthesia.

12. Surgery is started within 10 min of induction, all pups delivered by 15 min from time of induction (5 min of surgery time).

13. After delivery of the last pup, isoflurane inhalant is started 1% to 1.5% vaporizer setting. Note: important to watch anesthesia depth carefully now because original propofol induction dose has redistributed and effect of inhalant is a bit delayed. The patient can get dangerously too light. An additional minibolus of propofol might be needed.

14. Note in giant breed dogs, isoflurane might be started at 0.5% to 1% vaporizer setting if patient seems to need frequent or larger propofol doses to maintain stable anesthesia.

15. Total surgery time is typically 30 min for small breeds and less than 60 min for giant breeds.

16. Oxytocin administered: 1 to 4 units/dog SQ after delivery of last pup and repeated after 15 min.

Vasopressor Therapy

If low mean arterial blood pressure is detected intraoperatively, treatment with ephedrine is recommended (0.03-0.1 mg/kg IV).[48] This will allow pressor support without decreased uterine/placental blood flow.

Prevention of Reflux, Regurgitation, and Aspiration

Aspiration of highly acidic gastric fluid is a concern for any anesthetic regimen and can be more prevalent in CS as discussed above, especially in brachycephalic breeds. Mendelson syndrome is a severe, often fatal, pneumonitis secondary to aspiration of gastric acid. To prevent this, various drugs have been advised.

- *Metoclopramide* (0.1–0.5 mg/kg IV) is used to increase tone of the lower esophageal sphincter (LES)[30,53–55] and has been shown to decrease nausea in women undergoing CS spinal anesthesia.[56] The benefit to the LES lasts 30 to 60 minutes after a bolus injection.[57] One report of anesthesia for airway surgery in brachyce-phalic dogs found decreased evidence of regurgitation in dogs given metoclo-pramide and famotidine (a histamine-2 receptor antagonist [H2RA] antacid).[55] Metoclopramide will also increase prolactin production (by its dopamine antag-onist effect) and thus can also benefit milk production.

- *Proton-pump Inhibitors:* This class of drugs has been shown to better reduce acid production in dog when compared with the H2RA.[58] In one report, dogs un-dergoing orthopedic surgery were found to have a significant increase in gastric and esophageal pH after esomeprazole was administered twice: 12 to 18 hours and 1 to 1.5 hours before surgery but the protocol did not prevent reflux.[59] A delay for maximal acid reduction might be due to activation of dormant parietal cells, resulting in only a partial effect after a single dose.[58] This might make use of such a compound less effective for single dosing before Em-CS but repeated oral administration could be recommended for home use before presentation for the EI-CS.
- *Maropitant:* A strong antiemetic but no evidence for prevention of reflux. Not approved for pups aged younger than 8 weeks due to the potential for bone marrow hypoplasia, thus not recommended for use in CS cases.
- *Ondansetron:* Serotonin receptor blocker that can reduce nausea and vomiting in women undergoing spinal anesthesia for CS. No reports for this use in dogs.

Promotion of Fetal Maturity

When EI-CS is performed in accordance with accurate ovulation timing, medical inter-vention to promote fetal maturity is not needed. The authors have found that pups born 1 to 2 days before expected due date have high survival and evidence of term development. Some investigators have suggested protocols to promote fetal maturity when considering an EI-CS as follows.

- Aglepristone, a progesterone receptor antagonist (not FDA-approved), has been used to bind to and block progesterone receptors before EI-CS.[30,53,54] The theory used was to simulate the progesterone decline that occurs in the natural preparturient period and to promote fetal maturation and milk produc-tion. Dogs were deemed by a variety of methods to be within 1 to 2 days of the expected due date but with serum progesterone concentrations that re-mained above 2 ng/mL. They were given aglepristone 5 to 15 mg/kg SC 1 day before EI-CS. Limitations of these studies include the lack of negative controls (dogs not given aglepristone). The authors of this article, as well as other investigators, have successfully performed EI-CS on dogs preparturient, with progesterone levels greater than 2 ng/mL, without the use of a progesterone-reducing protocol, when appropriate ovulation timing protocols have been used (see above). More investigation into the use of this product is warranted, perhaps to promote milk production in term pregnancy without adequate colostrum.
- *Corticosteroids* to potentially promote lung maturity and surfactant production. Regazzi and colleagues studied the administration of betamethasone (0.5 mg/kg IM) given day 55 postovulation and its impact on pups subsequently delivered preterm.[60] The treatment resulted in differentiation of pulmonary saccules to sub-saccules but not further development to alveoli. Additionally, preterm pups did not have increased surfactant production. The study also found evidence of improved air-filling of newborn lungs in the preterm treatment group, indicating

fluid clearance by another mechanism, and perhaps due to the betamethasone treatment. They also observed moderate atelectasis in the term-delivered non-treated control group (normal newborns), making the benefit of the betamethasone treatment less obvious. In another report, betamethasone administered day 55 after breeding induced preterm labor.[61] Clearly, more investigation into the use of maternal corticosteroid administration is needed.

Infection Prevention

The use of perioperative IV antibiotics has been an accepted practice in veterinary surgery. The continuation of this application is under discussion in human medicine because there is concern for newborn gut biome establishment.[62,63] At this time, there is insufficient evidence to discontinue administration of an antibiotic preoperative for veterinary CS. To achieve sufficient tissue levels, the preoperative antibiotic should be administered within 1 hour before the start of surgery.[64] Repeated dosing should not be necessary due to short total surgery time. It is not indicated to continue antibiotic therapy as a routine in the postoperative/recovery period.

Additional methods to reduce incisional infection is for the dog to be washed at home with an antibacterial shampoo the day before EI-CS and careful attention given to surgical scrubbing of the incisional site immediately preoperative.

Pain Control Postoperative (for the dam)

- *Nonsteroidal anti-inflammatory drugs (NSAIDs)* are commonly used postoperatively for pain control and are commonly used in human medicine after CS.[65] Early in lactation, NSAIDs can have a high clearance rate.[66] Ferrari and colleagues found very-low concentrations of carprofen in bitch's milk after CS, if the gland was not inflamed (mastitis).[67] NSAIDs can be started parenterally after pups are delivered and can be provided for judicious home pain control for 24 to 48 hours postoperatively. Rarely is pain control required for a longer period after CS; veterinarians and owners are advised to empathetically address postoperative pain control but most bitches seem comfortable without continued pain control after 24 to 48 hours (authors' observation). It is important to note, however, that the use of NSAIDs in dogs after CS has not been thoroughly investigated, and there is concern for idiopathic adverse reactions in some individuals and an unknown potential for detriment to newborns.[23,68] Some protocols report the use of either meloxicam or carprofen postoperatively. Alternatively, grapiprant, a prostaglandin EP4 receptor antagonist and noncyclooxygenase inhibiting product, has shown effect for postop pain control and could be considered.[69] Continued studies into the use of best options for post-CS pain control are clearly needed.
- *Tramadol* as a single agent for postoperative pain control is not recommended because the active metabolite is rapidly metabolized in most dogs.[68] This drug is also a Schedule IV controlled substance in the United States, thus appropriate handling for dispensing is required.

Ecbolic Postdelivery

Oxytocin is naturally secreted in response to newborn suckling and will help continued milk letdown and uterine contractions. Oxytocin can be administered parenterally (1-4 units/dog SQ) to potentially decrease postpartum hemorrhage after all pups are delivered by CS.

Table 2
Select reported anesthesia protocols for canine cesarean section

Induction	Maintenance	Sedative/Analgesic Pre-delivery	Local Incisional Block	Number of Cases	Year Published	Reference
Propofol	Sevoflurane	Methadone	Yes	13	2022	Plavec et al,[29] 2022
Propofol	Isoflurane	Dexmedetomidine	Yes	9	2019	Groppetti et al,[30] 2019
Propofol or alfaxalone	Isoflurane	No	No	10	2019	Melandri et al,[42] 2019
Propofol	Propofol/sevoflurane[a], sevoflurane; or epidural/sevoflurane[b]	Morphine	No	45	2018	Vilar et al,[28] 2018
Propofol	Sevoflurane	Morphine	No	4	2018	Oliva et al,[27] 2018
Propofol	Sevoflurane	Medetomidine	No	292	2017	De Cramer et al,[31] 2017
Alfaxalone	Alfaxalone or isoflurane	No	Yes	22	2016	Ruiz et al,[43] 2016
Propofol or alfaxalone	Isoflurane	No	No	74	2014	Metcalfe et al,[40] 2014
Propofol or alfaxalone	Isoflurane	No	No	22	2013	Doebeli et al,[41] 2013
Propofol	Isoflurane	No	No	37	2009	Levy et al,[54] 2009
Propofol; ketamine with midazolam; thiopentone; epidural	Enflurane	Chlorpromazine	No	24	2004	Luna et al,[35] 2004
Propofol	Isoflurane and nitrous oxide	No	No	141	1997	Funkquist et al,[39] 1996

[a] Propofol titrated until pups delivered, then sevoflurane maintenance.
[b] Sevoflurane started after pups delivered.

SPECIFIC ANESTHESIA PROTOCOLS

There was a significant shift in CS anesthesia protocols from barbiturates, ketamine, or inhalational induction to propofol induction in the late 1990s (**Table 2**).[36,39] During the next decade, propofol induction and isoflurane or sevoflurane for maintenance was common.[27–31,35,40–42,54] The introduction of alfaxalone for induction and in some cases CRI for maintenance, has also been addressed.[40–43] The good news is that all recently reported protocols have similar excellent dam and neonatal survival. Comparison of protocols to formulate recommendations is difficult due to a variety of factors such as doses of agents, use of preanesthetic analgesics/sedatives, use of local anesthesia or epidural, interval of time from induction to surgery, length of surgery, and selection of cases: dystocia or elective. Moreover, for prepartum elective CS, criteria used to select the surgery date differed between studies. Additionally, judgment of successful outcome varied from immediate versus later newborn survival and in the latter group, some reports included puppy death due to other causes (trauma, infection).

The final selection of an anesthesia protocol will also depend on confidence of the anesthetist to use certain drugs and combinations. The authors have found that a major factor to improve successful outcome is not just *what* is used but *how* it is used. Considerable training should be invested in teaching anesthetic technicians to use minimal doses to provide sufficient anesthesia but maintain a light, yet humane, anesthetic plane until all pups are delivered. Organization and efficiency of the total perioperative team will help decrease both time from induction to complete delivery and overall surgery time. The authors have found that this results in excellent newborn and dam recovery. The author's protocol (see **Box 1**) formulated over many years and hundreds of cases has evolved to the use of a narcotic for preanesthetic sedation and analgesia, and a single injection of a perioperative antibiotic for infection prophylaxis. Anticholinergics are not routinely administered but glycopyrrolate is on hand if needed for maternal bradycardia. The authors have favored propofol over alfaxalone because most patients are reunited with their owners early in the recovery process and the quality of recovery after propofol induction is preferable. For anesthesia maintenance, propofol is then titrated in miniboluses to continue the light plane of anesthesia until all pups are delivered. Typically, pups are born quite active and vocal, and only very rarely is reversal with naloxone needed. After delivery, isoflurane is started, and the remainder of anesthesia/surgery is routine.

SURGERY TECHNICAL CONSIDERATIONS

The surgical technique for canine CS has been well described.[70,71] The authors support the recommendation for reduced time from induction to delivery and overall surgery time for best newborn and maternal outcome.[7,9]

Some factors that can aid successful surgery include the following:

- Preparation of surgery packs that include all materials necessary for CS to allow quick set up of the surgical field.
- Dorsal recumbency is recommended; rotation off-center to alleviate caval pressure is not needed for dogs.[72]
- Quick and efficient laparotomy incision: clamp larger subcutaneous mammary vessels to address at closure. Due to abdominal distension of pregnancy, this is usually quite easy.
- Typically, do not exteriorize the entire uterus but rather a segment of one horn depending on size of the litter and dam. This will help to provide temperature support for dam and maintain manageable sterile field. The authors do not favor *en*

bloc removal of uterus (and do not recommend ovariohysterectomy (OVH) at time of CS, see below).

- Location of uterine incision: goal is to deliver all pups through one incision whenever possible. Location will depend on the number of pups and size of dam. In larger dogs with a large litter, the incision can be in the uterine body. The authors have found that incision in a uterine horn, at either side of the uterine bifurcation, allows easy delivery. In some cases, the intercornual septum makes access through one incision to the contralateral horn difficult. Although this septum can be carefully stretched, care is taken not to rip this tissue as excessive hemorrhage can occur.
- If necessary, an additional uterine incision is made (typically in opposite horn if cannot effectively deliver all pups).
- Pups are pushed to hysterotomy incision by both gentle traction of fetus and pressure on serosal surface of uterus (**Fig. 2**). Amniotic sac is immediately removed from pup's muzzle and then pulled back to remove from entire body (**Fig. 3**).
- Clamp umbilicus approximately 1 cm from pup's body wall (**Fig. 4**). Cut umbilicus on maternal size of clamp. Alternatively, the pup can be delivered attached to placenta to allow continued transfusion from placenta to newborn (few moments) and then ligate umbilicus.[73]
- Place pup in a sterile surgery towel and place on a Mayo stand for immediate pick-up by recovery team (**Fig. 5**). This method preserves sterility of surgeon by preventing inadvertent touching of surgeon's gloves by recovery staff.
- Traction is then applied to separate placenta from uterus (**Fig. 6**). The remaining thin layer adherent to endometrium can remain or be removed; note if the latter, hemorrhage can be increased. If the placentas are not easily separated, then better to leave intact and they will usually pass uneventfully over time.

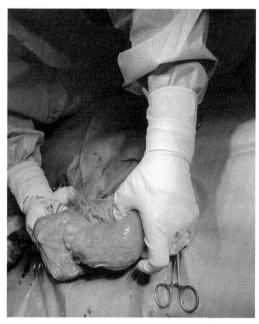

Fig. 2. Using both hands to manipulate the next fetus into the hysterotomy incision. One hand can enter within the uterine lumen to provide gentle traction on the fetus while the other hand pushes the fetus to the hysterotomy incision.

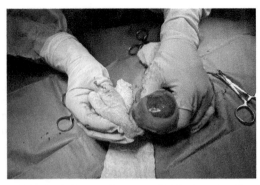

Fig. 3. Surgeon removes amnionic sac from newborns muzzle; the pup might start to breathe at this time.

- On delivery of the last pup, the surgeon palpates both ovarian pedicles and into pelvic canal to assure that truly *all* pups are delivered.
- Removal of all placentas and accumulated blood/clots via hysterotomy incision(s) before closure.
- Closure of uterine incision: 2-layer closure with outer layer in an inverting pattern works well and can be done quite quickly (**Fig. 7**).
- Note: if decomposed, "resorbed" fetuses or placental material is encountered, this can be removed by "wiping" with a surgical sponge and is not a reason to do hysterectomy (**Fig. 8**).
- If the uterus ruptures or tears during surgery, it can be easily repaired and is not a cause for hysterectomy.
- Neonatal recovery is addressed in see article "Canine Pregnancy, Eutocia, and Dystocia" by Davidson and Cain in this issue.

OVARIOHYSTERECTOMY AT TIME OF CESAREAN SECTION

When owners request to have dog desexed, some veterinarians offer OVH as part of the CS surgery (Cesarean Section Spay, CSS). After many years of personal communication to authors from numerous colleagues and attorneys regarding postoperative complications observed after CSS, the authors caution against CSS. The following has been observed.

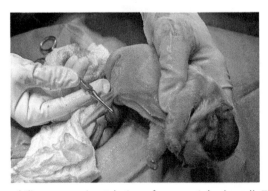

Fig. 4. Clamp the umbilicus approximately 1 cm from pup's body wall. This photo shows a "bulldog" clamp, a nontraumatic clamp that is easy to apply, lightweight and will not interfere with further newborn recovery.

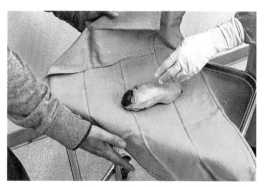

Fig. 5. Surgeon places pup on a sterile towel and then places on a Mayo stand for the recovery technician to then pick-up pup. This method of transfer maintains sterility of surgeon.

- The risk of fatality after a routine CS (without OVH) or routine OVH conducted at another time, in the nonpregnant bitch, is very low.
- The risk of fatality increases with CSS due to hemorrhage from engorged vessels or broad ligament, usually not detected at time of surgery.
- Removal of the enlarged, blood engorged uterus at CSS: depletion of substantial blood volume from which the bitch would otherwise benefit as the uterus involutes.
- Surgery and recovery times can be longer.
- Postoperative pain can be more severe.
- Delay in appropriate mothering behavior can occur.
- The capacity of the uterus to heal is remarkable. Most cannot locate a scar from previous CS at time of a subsequent surgery. Even in cases of uterine rupture, the uterus can be repaired easily, and recovery is typically excellent.
- Hysterectomy is not required due to the presence of decomposed fetal material or placental sites (fetal resorption syndrome). These sites are typically sterile and do not pose a risk of infection to the dam or delayed healing.
- The authors do not have considerable experience with ovariectomy at time of CS. Concern for engorged ovarian vessels remains and can be quite concerning but retention of the uterus is an advantage. More investigation into this practice is

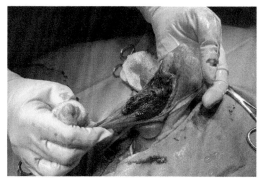

Fig. 6. Use digital manipulation to separate placenta from endometrium, then provide gentle traction to remove placenta.

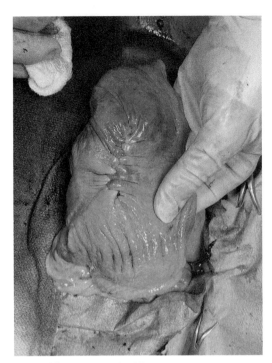

Fig. 7. Completed, inverted hysterotomy incision.

warranted (See article "Decision-making on age of spay-neuter for a specific dog: General principles and cultural complexities" by Hart, Hart, and Thigpen of this issue).

POSTANESTHESIA/SURGERY RECOVERY OF DAM

As with all anesthesia recovery, the dam is carefully observed for optimal timing of extubation. In brachycephalic breeds, or if the dog attempted to regurgitate or vomit after induction, additional care is taken at extubation. English bulldogs were found to have the highest mortality risk in the postoperative period due to respiratory complications.[74] Continued oxygen and IV fluid support in the postoperative period may be necessary and dedicated, continued monitoring in recovery makes a difference! Once the dam has settled, pups can be brought to nurse under direct supervision while the dam is in recovery. Assessment of colostrum production is essential: if deemed inadequate, canine serum/plasma can be administered to the newborn to provide passive immunity (See article "Canine Pregnancy, Dystocia, and Eutocia" by Davidson and Cain of this issue).

DEPARTING FROM HOSPITAL AND ADVICE FOR EARLY NEWBORN PERIOD

Owners are instructed to bring a box or basket with a heat source to safely transport pups home separate from the dam after CS. Once home, nursing must be continued with the advice to encourage/help pups to always nurse under direct supervision, until it is obvious that the dam is alert, recognizes her pups and shows positive mothering behavior. Because the dam might not stimulate (lick) the newborns to eliminate,

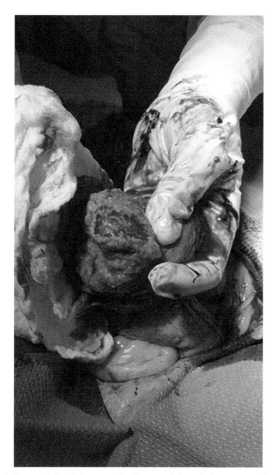

Fig. 8. Example of decayed fetal "resorptive" material and decomposed placenta. This can be removed by wiping with a laparotomy sponge. This tissue is not infected (in nearly all cases) and is not a reason for hysterectomy.

owners are instructed to swab the newborn's genitalia/anal area with a moistened cotton ball to make pups urinate/defecate until the dam takes over this function. Most dams exhibit appropriate mothering behavior within 24 hours post-CS. Owners are advised that continued sanguineous vaginal discharge is expected for the first 24 to 48 hours post-CS and will taper to a trickle (lochia) that can continue (oxidized and brownish) for up to 6 to 8 weeks. If sutures are used in the incision, the owner is instructed to remove them at home in 10 days. Judicious pain control for the dam immediately postop is important (discussed above).

CLINICS CARE POINTS

- In a dystocia situation, if undelivered fetuses are not viable (no fetal HR on US), then there is no need to do an Em-CS, so long as the dam is not in distress due to fetal obstruction or uterine trauma. Deceased fetuses will eventually pass and will not adversely affect the dam.

- An elective CS (El-CS) planned on the basis of ovuation timing, can be offered by primary care veterinarians outside of the emergency clinic setting and usually results in an improved outcome.
- Numerous effective anesthesia protocols are available for CS. Either propofol or alfaxalone are the usual induction agents, followed by repeated IV dosing or low vaporizer settings of an inhalant for maintencence.
- Quick delivery of fetuses can positively affect newborn recovery and survival.
- A well-trained team can effectively manage El-CS and repeated experience will afford great efficiency and high newborn survival.

DISCLOSURE

The authors have no affiliations or conflicts of interest to disclose.

REFERENCES

1. Bergstrom A, Nodtvedt A, Lagerstedt AS, et al. Incidence and breed predilection for dystocia and risk factors for cesarean section in a Swedish population of insured dogs. Vet Surg 2006;35:786–91.
2. Darvelid AW, Linde-Forsberg C. Dystocia in the bitch: A retrospective study of 182 cases. J Small Anim Pract 1994;35:402–7.
3. Schrank M, Contiero B, Mollo A. Incidence and concomitant factors of cesarean sections in the bitch: A questionnaire study. Front Vet Sci 2022. https://doi.org/10.3389/fvets.2022.934273.
4. Jayakumar C, Krishnaswamy A, Sudha G, et al. Planned Cesarean Section and other obstetrical interventions in dogs: A comparative evaluation based on neonatal survival. Indian Journal of Canine Practice 2013;5:136–41.
5. Groppetti D, Pecile A, Del Carro AP, et al. Evaluation of newborn canine viability by means of umbilical vein lactate measurement, apgar score and uterine tocodynamometry. Theriogenology 2010;74:1187–96.
6. Kuttan KV, Joseph M, Simon S, et al. Effect of intrapartum fetal stress associated with obstetrical interventions on viability and survivability of canine neonates. Vet World 2016;9(12):1485–8.
7. Schmidt K, Feng C, Wu T, et al. Influence of maternal, anesthetic, and surgical factors on neonatal survival after emergency cesarean section in 78 dogs: A retrospective study (2002 to 2020). Can Vet J 2021;62:961–8.
8. Alonge A, Melandri M. Effect of delivery management on first-week neonatal outcome: How to improve it in Great Danes. Theriogenology 2019;125:310–6.
9. Proctor-Brown L, Cheong SH, Diel de Amorim M. Impact of decision to delivery time of fetal mortality in canine caesarean section in a referral population. Vet Med Sci 2019;5:336–44.
10. Moon PF, Erb HN, Ludders JW, et al. Perioperative risk factors for puppies delivered by cesarean section in the United States and Canada. J Am Anim Hosp Assoc 2000;36:359–68.
11. Concannon PW, Hansel W, McEntee K. Changes in LH, progesterone and sexual behavior associated with preovulatory luteinization in the bitch. Biol Reprod 1977;17:604–13.
12. Hollinshead F, Hanlon D. Factors affecting the reproductive performance of bitches: A prospective cohort study involving 1203 inseminations with fresh and frozen semen. Theriogenology 2017;101:62–72.

13. Baltutis C, Settle K, Beachler T, et al. Duration of pregnancy is shorter in Cavalier King Charles Spaniels. Clin Theriogenol 2020;12:475–80.

14. Concannon P. Endocrinologic Control of Normal Canine Ovarian Function. Reprod Dom Anim 2009;44(Suppl. 2):3–15.

15. Reynaud K, Fontbonne A, Marseloo N, et al. In vivo meiotic resumption, fertilization and early embryonic development in the bitch. Reproduction 2005;130: 193–201.

16. Holst PA, Phemister RD. Onset of diestrus in the Beagle bitch: definition and significance. Am J Vet Res 1974;35:401–6.

17. Lopate C. Gestational aging and determination of parturition date in the bitch and queen using ultrasonography and radiography. Vet Clin North Am Small Anim Prac 2018;48(4):617–38.

18. Milani C, Artusi E, Drigo M, et al. Ultrasonographic analysis of fetal gastrointestinal motility during the peripartum period in the dog. Anim Reprod Sci 2020;106514. https://doi.org/10.1016/j.anireprosci.2020.106514.

19. Siena G, Milari C. Usefulness of maternal and fetal parameters for the prediction of parturition date in dogs. Animals 2021;11(3):878.

20. Kutzler M, Yeager A, Mohammed H, et al. Accuracy of canine parturition date prediction using fetal measurements obtained by ultrasonography. Theriogenology 2013;60(7):1309–17.

21. Groppetti D, Vegetti F, Bronzo V, et al. Breed-specific fetal biometry and factors affecting the prediction of whelping date in the German shepherd dog. Anim Reprod Sci 2015;152:117–22.

22. Luvoni G, Grioni A. Determination of gestational age in medium and small size bitches using ultrasonographic fetal measurements. J Small Anim Pract 2000; 41:292–4.

23. Aarnes T, Murdock M. Cesarean section and Pregnancy. In: Johnson R, Snyder L, Schroeder C, editors. *Canine and feline anesthesia and Co-existing disease*. Second Edition. Hoboken, NJ: John Wiley & Sons, Inc; 2022. p. 566–84.

24. Raffe M. Anesthetic Considerations During Pregnancy and for the Newborn. In: *Veterinary anesthesia and analgesia the fifth edition of lumb and Jones*. Ames, IA: Wiley Blackwell; 2015. p. 708–19.

25. Allard R, Carlos A, Faltin E. Canine hematologic changes during gestation and lactation. Compan Anim Pract 1989;19:3–6.

26. Kraus B. Anesthesia for cesarean section in the dog. Veterinary Focus 2016;26: 24–31.

27. Oliva V, Queiroz M, Albuquerque V. Vitality evaluation methods for newborn puppies after cesarean section performed under general inhalation anesthesia. Pesq. Vet. Bras. 2018;38(6):1172–7.

28. Vilar JM, Batista M, Pérez R, et al. Comparison of 3 anesthetic protocols for the elective cesarean-section in the dog: Effects on the bitch and the newborn puppies. Anim Reprod Sci 2018;190:53–62.

29. Plavec T, Knific T, Slapsak A, et al. Canine Neonatal Assessment by Vitality Score, Amniotic Fluid, Urine, and Umbilical Cord Blood Analysis of Glucose, Lactate, and Cortisol: Possible Influence of Parturition Type? Animals 2022;12:1247.

30. Groppetti D, Cesare F, Pecile A, et al. Maternal and neonatal wellbeing during elective C-section induced with a combination of propofol and dexmedetomidine: How effective is the placental barrier in dogs? Theriogenology 2019;129:90–8.

31. De Cramer K, Joubert K, Nöthling J. Puppy survival and vigor associated with the use of low dose medetomidine premedication, propofol induction and

maintenance of anesthesia using sevoflurane gas-inhalation for cesarean section in the bitch. Theriogenology 2017;19:10–5.

32. Clarke K, Trim C, Hall L, et al. Anaesthesia for obstetrics. In: Veterinary Anaesthesia. 11th ed. UK: Saunders Elsevier; 2014. p. 587–98.

33. Pascoe PJ, Moon P. Periparturient and neonatal anesthesia. Vet Clin North Am Small Anim Prac 2001;31(2):315–41.

34. Lerche K., Anticholinergics, In: Kurt A., Grimm K., Lamont L., et al., *Veterinary anesthesia and analgesia the fifth edition of lumb and Jones*, 2015, Wiley Blackwell, Ames, IA, 178–182.

35. Luna S, Cassu R, Castro G, et al. Effects of four anaesthetic protocols on the neurological and cardiorespiratory variables of puppies born by caesarean section. Vet Rec 2004;27:387–90.

36. Moon-Massat P, Erb H. Perioperative factors associated with puppy vigor after delivery by cesarean section. J Am Anim Hosp Assoc 2002;38:90–6.

37. Brussel T, Theissen J, Vigfusson G. Hemodynamic and cardiodynamic effects of propofol and etomidate: negative inotropic properties of propofol. Anesth Analg 1989;69(1):35–40.

38. Berry S. Injectable anesthetics. In: Kurt A, Grimm K, Lamont L, et al, editors. Veterinary anesthesia and analgesia the fifth edition of lumb and Jones. Ames, IA: Wiley Blackwell; 2015. p. p277–96.

39. Funkquist P, Nyman G, Löfgren A, et al. Use of propofol-isoflurane as an anesthetic regimen for caesarean section in dogs. J Am Vet Med Assoc 1996;211: 313–7.

40. Metcalfe S, Hulands-Nave A, Bell M, et al. Multicentre, randomised clinical trial evaluating the efficacy and safety of alfaxalone administered to bitches for induction of anaesthesia prior to caesarean section. Aust Vet J 2014;92:333–8.

41. Doebeli A, Michel E, Bettschart R, et al. Apgar score after induction of anesthesia for canine cesarean section with alfaxalone versus propofol. Theriogenology 2013;80:850–4.

42. Melandri M, Alonge S, Peric T. Effects of Alfaxalone or Propofol on Giant-Breed Dog Neonates Viability During Elective Caesarean Sections. Animals 2019;9: 962–73.

43. Ruiz C, Del Carro A, Rosset E, et al. Alfaxalone for total intravenous anaesthesia in bitches undergoing elective caesarean section and its effects on puppies: A randomized clinical trial. Vet Anaesth Analg 2016;43:281–90.

44. Jimenez C, Mathis A, Mora S, et al. Evaluation of the quality of the recovery after administration of propofol or alfaxalone for induction of anaesthesia in dogs anaesthetized for magnetic resonance imaging. Vet Anaesth Analg 2012;39:151–9.

45. Campoy L, Reed M, Peralta S. Canine and Feline Local Anesthetic and Analgesic Techniques. In: Kurt A, Grimm K, Lamont L, et al, editors. *Veterinary anesthesia and analgesia the fifth edition of lumb and Jones*. Ames, IA: Wiley Blackwell; 2015. p. 827–p856.

46. Valverde A. Epidural Analgesia and Anesthesia in Dogs and Cats. Vet Clin North Am Small Anim Prac 2008;38:1205–30.

47. Martin-Flores M, Anderson J, Sakai D. A retrospective analysis of the epidural use of bupivacaine 0.0625–0.125% with opioids in bitches undergoing cesarean section. Can Vet J 2019;60:1349–52.

48. Robertson S. Anesthesia Considerations & Techniques for Caesarian Section. World Small Animal Veterinary Association World Congress Proceedings, 2015. Available at: https://www.vin.com/doc/?id=7259240. Accessed December 15, 22.

49. Garcia E., Local anesthetics, In: Kurt A., Grimm K., Lamont L., et al., *Veterinary anesthesia and analgesia the fifth edition of lumb and Jones*, 2015, Wiley Blackwell; Ames, IA, 332-p354.
50. Palanuik R, Schnider S, Eger E. Pregnancy decreases the requirement for inhaled anesthetic gases. Anesthesiology 1974;42:81–3.
51. Suarez M, Dzikiti B, Stegmann F, et al. Comparison of alfaxalone and propofol administered as total intravenous anaesthesia for ovariohysterectomy in dogs. Vet Anaesth Analg 2012;39:236–44.
52. Ruiz C, Rousset E, Portier K. Poor Apgar score and high mortality in puppies born by caesarean section from bitches anaesthetized with a propofol constant rate infusion. (letter to editor). Vet Anaesth Analg 2017;44:692–3.
53. Roos J, Maenhoudt C, Zilberstein L. Neonatal puppy survival after planned caesarean section in the bitch using aglepristone as a primer: A retrospective study on 74 cases. Reprod Dom Anim 2018;53(Suppl. 3):85–9.
54. Levy X, Fontaine E, Segalini V, et al. Elective caesarean operation in the bitch using aglepristone before the pre-partum decline in peripheral progesterone concentration. Reprod Dom Anim 2009;44:182–4.
55. Costa R, Abelson A, Lindsey J, et al. Postoperative regurgitation and respiratory complications in brachycephalic dogs undergoing airway surgery before and after implementation of a standardized perianesthetic protocol. J Am Vet Med Assoc 2020;256:899–905.
56. Mokini Z, Genocchio V, Forget P, et al. Metoclopramide and Propofol to Prevent Nausea and Vomiting during Cesarean Section under Spinal Anesthesia: A Randomized, Placebo-Controlled, Double-Blind Trial. J Clin Med 2022;11:110.
57. Papich M. Metoclopramide hydrochloride. In: Saunders handbook of veterinary drugs: small and large animal. 4th ed. St Louis: Elsevier Inc; 2016. p. 520–2.
58. Marks S, Kook P, Papich M. ACVIM consensus statement: Support for rational administration of gastrointestinal protectants to dogs and cats. J Vet Intern Med 2018;32:1823–40.
59. Zacuto A, Marks S, Osborn J, et al. The influence of esomeprazole and cisapride on gastroesophageal reflux during anesthesia in dogs. J Vet Intern Med 2012;26:518–25.
60. Regazzi F, Silva L, Lúcio C, et al. Morphometric and functional pulmonary changes of premature neonatal puppies after antenatal corticoid therapy. Theriogenology 2020;153:19–26.
61. Vannucchi C, Regazzi F, Barbosa M. Cortisol Profile and Clinical Evaluation of Canine Neonates Exposed Antenatally to Maternal Corticosteroid Treatment. Reprod Dom Anim 2012;47(Suppl. 6):173–6.
62. Ramasethu J, Kawakita T. Antibiotic stewardship in perinatal and neonatal care. Semin Fetal Neonatal Med 2017;22:278–83.
63. Smaill F, Grivell R. Antibiotic prophylaxis versus no prophylaxis for preventing infection afer cesarean section (Review). Cochrane Database Syst Rev 2014;10. Art. No.: CD007482.
64. Weese JS, Halling K. Perioperative administration of antimicrobials associated with elective surgery for cranial cruciate ligament rupture in dogs: 83 cases (2003–2005). J Am Vet Med Assoc 2006;229:92–5.
65. Al-Waili N. Efficacy and Safety of Repeated Postoperative Administration of Intramuscular Diclofenac Sodium in the Treatment of Post-Cesarean Section Pain: A Double-Blind Study. Arch Med Res 2001;32:148–54.
66. Schneider M, Kuchta A, Dron F, et al. Disposition of cimicoxib in plasma and milk of whelping bitches and in their puppies. BMC Vet Res 2015;11:178.

67. Ferrari D, Lundgren S, Holmberg J. Concentration of carprofen in the milk of lactating bitches after cesarean section and during inflammatory conditions. Theriogenology 2022;181:59–68.

68. Kukanich B. Pain Management in Veterinary Species. In: Mealey KL, editor. Pharmacotherapeutics for veterinary dispensing. John Wiley & Sons; 2019. p. 173–88. https://doi.org/10.1002/9781119404576.ch8.

69. Ross J, Kleine S, Smith C, et al. Evaluation of the perioperative analgesic effects of grapiprant compared with carprofen in dogs undergoing elective ovariohysterectomy. J Am Vet Med Assoc 2023;261:118–25.

70. Traas AM. Surgical management of canine and feline dystocia. Theriogenology 2008;70:337–42.

71. Gilson SD. Cesarean section. In: Slatter D, editor. Textbook of small animal surgery. Philadelphia, PA: Saunders; 2003. p. 1517–20.

72. Probst C, Webb A. Postural influence on systemic blood pressure, gas exchange, and acid/base status in the term pregnant bitch during general anesthesia. Am J Vet Res 1983;44:1963–5.

73. Pereira K, Correia L, Oliveira E, et al. Effects of clamping umbilical cord on the neonatal viability of puppies delivered by cesarean section. J Vet Med Sci 2020;82:247–53.

74. Oda A, Wang W, Hampton A. Perianesthetic mortality in English Bulldogs: a retrospective analysis in 2010-2017. BMC Vet Res 2022;18:198.

Pathology of Perinatal Disorders

Dalen Agnew, DVM, PhD, Diplomate ACVP

KEYWORDS

- Abortion • Canine • Feline • Neonatal death • Pathology • Stillbirth

KEY POINTS

- Perinatal death is a very common, but poorly studied, occurrence in small animal theriogenology.
- A complete postmortem examination, including collection of fetal and placental tissues for histopathology, microbiology, nutritional, and toxicological testing, can identify most causes of neonatal death but may require multiple animals, sometimes from consecutive litters.
- Common causes include viral infections, maternal bacteremia and sepsis, and congenital or developmental abnormalities.
- Further study and comparison to diseases in other species will likely yield a more thorough understanding of perinatal disease.

INTRODUCTION

Death of a single fetus or neonate, let alone an entire litter, can be devastating for a breeder of cats or dogs, regardless of their experience or goals. Significant time and money is typically involved, and the potential secondary effects to the dam's fertility must also be considered. In light of this interest in fertilty, it is surprising that the amount of research or diagnostics invested in perinatal mortality in small animals is scant compared with that in production food animals. In some purebreds, neonatal mortality approaching 25% can be considered "normal," and is an accepted cost of business.[1] Clearly, there is room for considerably more interest and effort in the investigation of perinatal deaths in companion animals.

STANDARDIZED APPROACH TO POSTMORTEM EXAMINATION

More is missed by not looking than by not knowing.
—Thomas McCrae (16 December 1870–30 June 1935), Professor of Medicine
at Jefferson Medical College

Department of Pathobiology and Diagnostic Investigation, Michigan State University College of Veterinary Medicine, 784 Wilson Road D208 VMC, East Lansing, MI 48824, USA
E-mail address: agnewd@msu.edu

Vet Clin Small Anim 53 (2023) 1147–1159
https://doi.org/10.1016/j.cvsm.2023.04.008
0195-5616/23/© 2023 Elsevier Inc. All rights reserved.

The key to identifying the cause of death in any animal, but particularly perinatal deaths, is a thorough postmortem examination, including appropriate sampling for microscopic examination and ancillary testing. Unfortunately, there are few pathognomonic lesions in perinatal deaths, particularly in companion animals where research lags other domestic species, so additional testing is often required and still a cause may not be definitively determined in too many cases. However, the breeder should be reminded that there is virtually no chance of identifying a cause if an examination is not performed.

There are many appropriate approaches to an examination of a fetus, stillborn, or neonate; the key to success is to develop a protocol that allows the prosecutor to examine the entire animal in an organized and repeatable fashion so that nothing is left unexamined.[2] Sample collection should also be done in a standardized fashion—an example of a sample collection checklist is provided in **Table 1**. Note that all samples do not need to be analyzed but should be collected if possible to ensure they are available later if they are needed.

Unfortunately, in perinatal death investigations, there are few pathognomonic lesions, and these diagnostic workups are notoriously unrevealing, grossly and even microscopically. Autolysis is often advanced and lesions subtle. Laboratory testing is critical for a diagnosis and even so, the number of cases that result in no diagnosis can be disappointing to the veterinarian and the client. If multiple aborted fetuses or dead neonates are available, testing more than one can provide a better chance of finding a cause. A complete history, including nutrition, parity, and health history of the dam, is critical.

A minimum sample set would include the following:

1. Fetal membrane (chorioallantois, not amnion), including transfer zone, marginal hematoma, and chorioallantois, fixed and fresh
2. Lung, fixed and fresh
3. Liver, fixed and fresh
4. Kidney, fixed and fresh
5. Brain, fixed and fresh
6. Spleen, fresh
7. Stomach contents, fresh

Table 1
A complete sample set for follow-up testing after a gross examination is critical to success

Sample	Histopathology	Virology	Parasitology	Bacteriology	Nutrition	Toxicology
Placenta	X			X		
Lung	X	X		X		
Liver	X			X	X	X
Kidney	X	X		X		X
Brain	X		X			
Stomach contents	X					
Spleen	X					
Dam serum/ fetal thoracic fluid		X	X	X	X	

Note that the following minimum sample collection protocol does not include samples for karyotyping, which may depend on the laboratory used for testing. In selected cases, additional samples may be needed.

8. Dam serum, acute (at abortion) and convalescent (3–4 weeks later); Alternatively, fetal thoracic fluid can be used for antibody detection, although hemolysis in the sample can substantially impair many assays.
9. Other optional tissues include thyroid (fixed and fresh), tongue (fixed), and skin or eyelid (fixed)
10. If karyotyping is indicated, whole blood collected antemortem from the neonate is the most commonly accepted sample but others such as skin or spleen may be an option depending on the laboratory.

Appropriate fixation requires samples to be less than 4 mm (about 0.25 inch) thick in at least one dimension with a 10:1 ratio of formalin to tissue. To ship samples, the formalin can be drained after 24 to 48 hours and the tissues wrapped in formalin soaked paper towels to minimize weight and leakage during transportation. If shipping in the wintertime, consider adding 10% ethanol to the formalin to prevent freezing.

Fresh unfixed specimens should be refrigerated and not frozen if possible; however, this can depend on how long it takes for the samples to reach the laboratory. If a specimen will not arrive at the laboratory within 2 to 3 days, it may be better to freeze the sample so there is minimal bacterial overgrowth even though this may decrease the ability to grow some pathogens. Regardless, ample ice packs should be used to keep the sample at temperature until its arrival at the laboratory.

Pooling of samples should be done with caution as not all animals in a litter may be affected and pooling can dilute the diagnostic information. It is best to keep the samples unpooled and allow the laboratory to pool later if indicated.

Note that even though samples seem autolyzed, they will still have value, especially for molecular testing. Fetal tissues have a higher percentage of water content making them seem edematous and more friable. Brain is often especially liquefied due to autolysis and incomplete myelination but will congeal when poured into formalin and lesions can be identified histologically. The stress of dystocia or perinatal stress can also leave characteristic but nonspecific lesions including green meconium staining of tissues as well as histologic evidence of meconium and squamous epithelial cells within the pulmonary airways.

Although many practitioners prefer to conduct their own in-house postmortem examination and collect samples as described above to decrease costs and maintain control of the diagnostic process. In many cases, it may be prudent to send the entire neonatal carcass, placenta, and serum from the dam to a diagnostic laboratory experienced in diagnostic investigations.

Placenta can be a very challenging organ to examine, grossly and histologically, but this can be very fruitful in identifying a cause.[3,4] Another challenge is that the bitch or queen will often eat the placenta shortly after delivery—the breeder needs to be aware of this and cautiously collect the placentas when possible. Gloves are important in handling placenta to prevent contamination and to protect the handler from possible zoonotic diseases. Placental compromise can lead to weakness in a neonate, which does not manifest until days after birth, so it is worthwhile for breeders to collect the placentas and store them (refrigerated or frozen) for a few days after birth in case the tissues are needed for diagnostics later.

The placenta in cats and dogs is similar, following the zonary pattern of most carnivores (**Fig. 1**).[2,5] The site of maternofetal attachment forms a girdle around the midsection of the fetus. The attachment is considered endotheliochorial, meaning the chorionic epithelium invades and contacts the endothelium of maternal endometrial blood vessels during placental attachment and development forming a labyrinth, which becomes thicker and more complex as gestation progresses. This region is

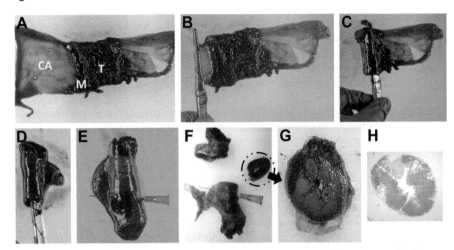

Fig. 1. Canine placental anatomy and procedure for placental sample collection for histopathology. In the carnivore zonary placenta, there are 3 important zones: the transfer zone (T) where the maternal–fetal interface is located, the marginal hematoma (M) where iron storage and transfer occur, and the chorioallantois (CA), which surrounds the allantoic cavity which in turn contains the amnion, amniotic cavity, and fetus. The "Swiss roll" method for placental sample collection involves cutting a 1 to 2 cm wide strip of chorioallantois, marginal hematomas, and transfer zone, incorporating any visible lesions (A). The strip is then gently rolled around a pair of forceps (B–D) and then pierced with a hypodermic needle to hold its position during fixation (E). After fixation in formalin (10:1 ratio of formalin:tissue), a cross-section (F) is cut from the center of the roll (arrow) indicates a larger view (G), laid in a cassette, and processed normally for a histopathology section stained with hematoxylin and eosin (H).

often called the "transfer zone." At the margins of this girdle or "zone," there are regions of iron deposition called the pigmented zone, perizonal hematomas, or marginal hematomas that are much more obvious in dogs than in cats. These are dark green to black regions at the border of the girdle and serve to transfer iron to the fetus. The remaining poles of the placenta are covered by the translucent chorioallantois. Within the chorioallantois and zonary regions is the allantoic cavity and within that cavity is the amnion and amniotic cavity.

One method for collecting a suitable sample of the placenta for histopathology is the "swiss roll" method (see **Fig. 1**). Briefly, a 1-cm wide strip of placenta is cut extending from one pole to the other through the pigmented and transfer zones as well as the translucent chorioallantois (see **Fig. 1**A). This strip is then rolled carefully and pinned in place with a hypodermic needle (see **Fig. 1**B–E). It can then be fixed in formalin and a cross-section cut from the center of the roll for histology, providing a large, oriented sample of placenta for microscopic examination (see **Fig. 1**F–H). Although there may be some value in examination of the amnion, the chorioallantois is usually more diagnostic.

Karyotyping is another important but too infrequently used diagnostic technique to complement gross and microscopic examination. In all unexplained perinatal deaths, particularly with purebred animals, the possibility of chromosomal abnormalities should be considered. There are a few academic and private laboratories currently providing this testing and the particular tissue requirements and preservation protocols will vary by laboratory.

VIRAL CAUSES OF PERINATAL DEATH

Herpesviruses can lead to abortion in most species.[6] In dogs, canine alpha-herpesvirus is a particularly common cause of neonatal weakness and death. In cats, feline herpesvirus-

1 (FHV-1) is a common pathogen but only rarely leads to abortion or stillbirth. It can, however, play a significant role in neonatal death in kittens by causing severe respiratory compromise and systemic generalized infection.

Canine herpesvirus is characterized grossly by subcapsular hemorrhages extending over the entire cortical surface (**Fig. 2**). Similar hemorrhages may be noted on other viscera such as the lung, liver, and spleen as well as on the meninges. Histology shows multifocal hemorrhage and necrosis in the kidney, lung, liver, spleen, and adrenal gland. Intranuclear inclusion bodies are commonly found adjacent to areas of necrosis. Confirmation via polymerase chain reaction (PCR) of fresh or frozen tissue, immunohistochemistry (IHC), or in situ hybridization (ISH) is most common, although virus isolation and serology tests may also be available in some laboratories.

In cats, FHV-1, infection of the kittens may occur at birth or systemically during gestation but determining the pathogenesis can be challenging due to the commonly observed carrier state in many cats.[7] However, identifying virus in diseased lung or other respiratory tissues by PCR, IHC, or ISH is highly suggestive in the absence of other lesions.

Parvoviruses are also common pathogens with notable effects in the perinatal period in companion animals. In dogs, the minute virus of canines (canine parvovirus-1) can lead to abortions and weak neonates.[8] These neonates typically develop enteritis with necrosis and intranuclear inclusion bodies within the enterocytes. Crypt necrosis as seen in canine parvovirus-2 infections has not been described. Interestingly, canine parvoviral DNA has been found in neonatal cerebellar hypoplasia cases but the link has not been well defined.[9]

In cats, cerebellar hypoplasia or abiotrophy is commonly associated with feline panleukopenia virus (feline parvovirus).[10] Early in infection, intranuclear inclusions can be seen in dying cells of the cerebellar external germinal layer but these disappear within 2 weeks when the infected cells die. Purkinje cells are also infected but do not have inclusions, although nuclei show vacuolation and eosinophilia. Visceral organs in the fetus may also be infected but only mild renal hypoplasia is reported.

Canine adenovirus type 1 has also been reported to cause stillbirths, neonatal deaths, and puppies with systemic viremia; however, this may more often be a sequela to disease and compromise of the dam than a fetal infection itself because abortions have been seen with and without CAV-1 in the fetal tissues.[11]

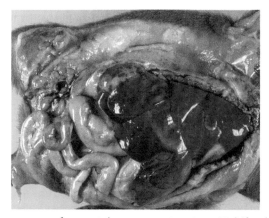

Fig. 2. Whole open carcass of neonatal puppy, postmortem. Multifocal petechial hemorrhages and ecchymoses on the renal capsule as well as less prominent hemorrhages and edema in the lung and liver are characteristic of neonatal infection with canine herpesvirus 1. (*Courtesy of* Dr. Zachary Millman and Courtesy of Dr. Scott Fitzgerald, Michigan State University Veterinary Diagnostic Laboratory.).

Both *feline leukemia virus* and *feline immunodeficiency virus* have been associated with fetal death, weak kittens, decreased litter sizes, and transplacental infection is likely with both viruses. Although the pathogenesis of these viruses' effects on pregnancy is still being worked out, recent study has shown that pregnancies are compromised by placental inflammatory dysregulation when the dam is infected with feline immunodeficiency virus (FIV).[12,13]

Other viruses have been associated with fetal and neonatal death, such as canine distemper virus, feline coronavirus, or feline calicivirus but these may be a result more of the compromise of the dam than direct viral effects on the fetus or neonate. Notably, placental lesions are rare to nonexistent in uncomplicated viral infections.[11,14]

BACTERIAL CAUSES OF PERINATAL DEATH

Bacterial causes of abortion, stillbirth, and neonatal death are numerous but most are secondary to bacteremia in the bitch, damage to and bacterial ascent through the cervix, predisposing conditions, or immune compromise of the bitch rather than pathogens that are strictly venereal.[2,14] The exception in small animal medicine is *brucellosis. Brucella canis*, a zoonotic reproductive pathogen, can spread by venereal and oral means and is an important cause of abortion, weak puppies, and infertility in female dogs and in male dogs (via prostatitis, epididymitis, and orchitis).[15] The organism is shed in affected animals via the urine, semen, milk, vaginal secretions, and infected fetal membranes and taken up in a new host via ingestion or venereally. Once in the body, macrophage traffic the organism to lymph nodes and spleen, from which bacteremia is initiated. The organism seems to hone to the reproductive system and frequently becomes persistent, leading to lifelong infection, often despite treatment. Diagnosis is often made by serology by testing multiple animals in a kennel because individual titers can be quite variable but culture of the organism is definitive.

Although brucellosis-infected bitches can abort after 50 days of gestation or as early as 30 days, term fetuses are commonly born alive and die in the first few hours or days of life.[14,15] These fetuses will have gross and histologic evidence of multisystemic infection, including necrotizing bronchopneumonia, hepatitis, splenitis, lymphadenitis, nephritis, and endocarditis and culture of most organs or body fluids will yield positive cultures. Placentas usually have grossly and histologically apparent necrosis with suppurative inflammation and abundant intracellular bacteria within trophoblastic cells. The bitch will also have serosanguinous (and highly infectious) vaginal discharge for weeks after infection, providing further support for a diagnosis if the fetus or placenta are not available for diagnostics.

Salmonellosis has been occasionally identified in perinatal deaths but is likely secondary to maternal bacteremia.[2,14] *Salmonella enterica* serovar Poona was cultured from one periparturient fetal death and was associated with feeding a raw meat diet to the bitch.

In contrast to *B canis*, the significance of other bacteria cultured from the bitch, fetus, or neonatal puppy should always be carefully investigated. Streptococci, staphylococci, enterococci, mycoplasma, and *Escherichia coli* are all commensal bacteria in the healthy vagina and their significance should be interpreted in the context of histopathology, Gram staining, and whether they are grown abundantly in pure culture (**Fig. 3**).[2] Culturing the same bacterium from both the placenta, which is often contaminated, and the fetal lung, which is not, is also suggestive of a significant bacterial culture. Further examination of the organism for virulence factors such as adherence factors or toxins may be helpful. Host factors such as the competence of the bitch's cervix, immunocompromise, or bacteremia; iatrogenic causes such as grossly contaminated transcervical procedures; or poor

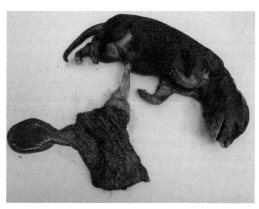

Fig. 3. Canine fetus and placenta, postmortem. This zonary placenta was friable and mottled yellow, tan, red, and green indicating fibrin and areas of necrosis within the transfer zone. The dark red margins of the placenta were the marginal hematomas. A portion of the chorioallantois contained clear, red-tinged fluid. Numerous *Enterococcus* sp were cultured from the placenta and the fetal lung in which there was histological evidence of pneumonia. (*Courtesy of* Dr. Joy Gary and Courtesy of Dr. Jon Patterson, Michigan State University Veterinary Diagnostic Laboratory.).

hygiene during mating may all be factors leading to infection with these opportunistic bacteria.

Very recently, evidence has begun to accumulate that cats and dogs can be infected by *Coxiella burnetii* (Q fever), leading to abortion, stillbirths, and neonatal cases, as well as transmit this zoonotic agent; however, there is little description in the literature of the pathologic condition, although placentitis would be a likely lesion.[16] Further investigations will hopefully shed additional light on this emerging disease.

PROTOZOAL CAUSES OF PERINATAL DEATH

There are several reports of various potential protozoan pathogens such as *Leishmania donovani*, *Cytauxzoon felis*, and the microsporidian *Encephalitozoon caniculi*, which were reported to infect the neonatal dog or cat congenitally or during the immediate perinatal period.[2,17,18] A more recent study questions the possibility of placental transmission of *C felis*, however, so further study is needed.[19] These infections are likely quite rare and present in only a few case reports in the literature.

Although still relatively rare, toxoplasmosis and neosporosis can be vertically transmitted to the bitch or queen, leading to abortion or more commonly neonatal death.[20,21] In most cases, neurologic signs associated with encephalomyelitis is the typical presentation, with organisms and associated necrosis and mixed inflammation observed in the brain as well as skeletal muscle. Although not well documented, infection of the placenta similar to other species would also be expected. PCR on tissue, IHC, or ISH on tissue sections would provide a more definitive diagnosis.

Noninfectious Causes of Perinatal Death

In small animals, noninfectious causes of abortion, stillbirth, and neonatal death are likely more common than infectious causes, at least in North America and Europe. A variety of insults to the dam can lead to placental insufficiency, poor fetal growth, or dystocia, which can damage or weaken the fetus leading to neonatal death shortly after birth. Many of these insults are *metabolic* such as diabetes mellitus, pregnancy toxemia, and hypocalcemia (eclampsia). Other "accidents of pregnancy" such as uterine torsion, dystocia, or maternal trauma can lead to pregnancy loss or the birth of compromised neonates. Besides diabetes mellitus where puppies may be unusually large leading to dystocia, the neonate may have no discernible abnormalities or die from opportunistic bacterial infections, making it critical that a maternal history and physical examination be a part of a neonatal death diagnostic workup.

Maternal malnutrition should also not be discounted as a possible cause of perinatal deaths. Poor caloric intake is the most common type of malnutrition but, historically, taurine deficiency in queens led to significant reproductive losses. An easy diagnostic tool is to collect birthweights on puppies and kittens as a tool for quickly identifying neonates that may be at risk and helping narrow down potential causes for neonatal compromise—recent databases provide excellent breed-specific reference data for birthweights.[22,23]

Intoxications are common in companion animals but infrequently ascribed as the cause of perinatal loss. The most likely source of a potential toxin during this period would be iatrogenic, drugs administered for medical conditions of the dam, particularly if pregnancy was not planned or expected.[24] Hormones such as glucocorticoids can disrupt normal hormonal signaling during pregnancy leading to abortion or premature birth and weak neonates, although a specific mechanism is unknown. Antifungal drugs such as ketoconazole or griseofulvin can lead to teratogenic effects on bones, eyes, and brain, and antineoplastic drugs can similarly have severe teratogenic effects on a variety of organs. Nonsteroidal anti-inflammatory drugs can cause delayed parturition, with subsequent dystocia or weakened neonates.[25]

Hypoluteoidism is likely common in bitches and is commonly defined as deficiency of progesterone (<5 ng/mL) due to insufficient production by the corpora lutea, which ultimately may lead to pregnancy loss. If this happens late in pregnancy, weak neonates or stillbirths will result. Recent research questions the overall importance of hypoluteoidism in companion animal infertility; however, additional research is warranted.[26]

Neonatal isoerythrolysis is a condition seen in kittens but not dogs because cats have 3 distinct blood groups: A, AB, and B.[27] When type A or AB kittens nurse from a type B queen, they will absorb anti-A antibodies from colostrum during the period before gut closure, leading to systemic distribution of the antibodies and destruction of red blood cells. Kittens will present in the first few days of life with red-brown urine, lethargy, failure to thrive, jaundice, and anemia. Disseminated intravascular coagulation and renal failure may follow.

Congenital defects are a common cause of neonatal death. Appreciating the intricate processes in development confirms the large number of points at which this process can go wrong and the wide variety of abnormalities that can develop affecting all systems. Gross examination and description are often sufficient to identify many congenital defects, histologic characterization is necessary for others and may require consultation with diagnosticians with expertise in a particular system. Although many of these abnormalities are nonlethal (in fact, some come to form the basis for breed distinctions), many can also lead to death outside the womb or compromise the animal in such a way that it is susceptible to other causes, such as opportunistic bacteria. Not all are inherited and intense investigation is required to prove causality between a genetic trait and a fatal abnormality; many can be secondary to toxins, infectious agents, or random developmental events. However, it is important to catalog these abnormalities so that trends and associations can be identified. Using the extensive human research and literature in naming and investigating incidents of congenital defects is beneficial.[28] Reporting such events in the veterinary literature or to a research institution may not have immediate value but over time will affect our understanding of disease.

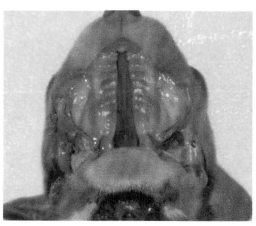

Fig. 4. Canine fetus, head, postmortem. Cleft palate or palatoschisis is a common finding in neonates of all species but in dogs and cats, it is associated with certain breeds, suggesting it is often a heritable trait. Griseofulvin treatment in queens can result in palatoschisis confirming that multiple causes can result in a similar congenital lesion. (*Courtesy of* Dr. David Needle and Dr. Ingeborg Langhor.).

An example of this approach is the growing body of research examining pulmonary dysplasia in puppies. Death following respiratory compromise is commonly reported by breeders who use the nonspecific term "fading puppy syndrome." Recent research suggests that *developmental lung disease* is likely a major factor in these cases, resembling a condition reported in human pediatric patients (K. Williams, unpublished data).[3] Pulmonary dysplasia includes the following: underdeveloped alveoli, pulmonary artery medial hypertrophy, increased numbers of thin-walled venous profiles, and increased capillary profiles. Three-dimensional reconstructions of affected lungs show lesions suggestive of arteriovenous shunts. Continued research, including genetic analyses, is required to better understand this condition in dogs and in humans, with rigorous examination of respiratory disease cases in puppies. Similar comparative, One Health

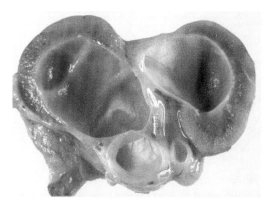

Fig. 5. Canine fetus, kidney, postmortem. Renal dysplasia can take on a variety of characteristics, grossly and histologically. In this case, multiple large medullary cysts and dilation of the pelvis (hydronephrosis) disrupted the normal architecture. Microscopically, lesions of dysplasia, which include abundant mesenchymal stroma, fetal glomeruli, and variably sized collecting ducts lined by pseudostratified columnar epithelium. (*Courtesy of* Dr. Katherine Olstad and Dr. Dodd Sledge.).

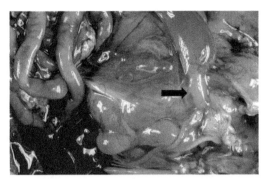

Fig. 6. Canine neonate, open thorax and abdomen, postmortem. Atresia coli (arrow) is the congenital condition in which a section of the colon or large bowel is incomplete (often there is a fibrous remnant still present) or absent. This puppy is the same as illustrated in **Fig. 5** and also had microtia (hypoplastic development of the ear or ears) and palatoschisis. Another puppy in the same litter had cardiac subaortic stenosis demonstrating the frequent occurrence of multiple congenital defects in the same animal or litter. (*Courtesy of* Dr. Katherine Olstad and Dr. Dodd Sledge.).

approaches to other potential developmental diseases would likely yield intriguing results as examinations of perinatal deaths become more common and thorough.

Other common and lethal defects include cleft palate (**Fig. 4**), cardiac defects and vascular transpositions, hydrocephalus, schistosomus reflexus, gastroschisis, ocular lesions, renal dysplasia (including renal cysts and infantile glomeruli) (**Fig. 5**), atresia ani (**Fig. 6**), and anasarca (**Fig. 7**).[29–33] Anasarca is reported but nonspecific finding in abnormal neonates; the fluid accumulation in multiple cavities and the

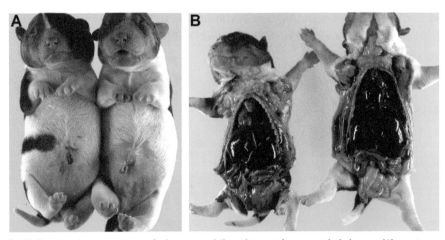

Fig. 7. Two canine neonates, whole carcass (*A*) and open thorax and abdomen (*B*), postmortem. Anasarca is the accumulation of fluid in the subcutaneous space and body cavities, indicating potential congenital abnormalities in the lungs, heart, liver, kidney, or placenta. Besides the preexisting abnormalities leading to anasarca, dystocia can be another complication. One of 2 littermates (left in A; right in B) had severe fluid accumulation in the subcutis, thorax, abdomen, and within the lungs and liver. (*Courtesy of* Dr. Annie Zimmerman, Michigan State University Veterinary Diagnostic Laboratory)

subcutaneous space is suggestive of potential abnormalities in the heart, lungs, liver, or kidney. Notably, congenital defects often come in groups within a single animal because there may be a single insult to multiple developmental processes, or one congenital lesion may cause downstream damage to other organs (eg, pulmonary dysplasia leading to anasarca and/or cardiac abnormalities).

SUMMARY

We currently have a good understanding of the many potential infectious causes of perinatal death in cats and dogs. Vaccination, advanced diagnostics and therapies, and awareness have made these less common. However, many pregnancy and neonatal losses are unexplained and identifying the causes will require increased attention from breeders, veterinarians, diagnosticians, and researchers. This will require increased numbers and more thorough postmortem examinations as well as more research to characterize the many ways that pregnancy and neonatal life can go amiss.

CLINICS CARE POINTS

- The placenta is a key diagnostic sample. Fresh and fixed samples of placenta including chorion, allantois, and amnion should be provided to the diagnostic laboratory and examined.
- Multiple animals (if available) should be submitted for diagnostic testing to ensure that the most important lesions are available to the diagnostician.
- If the gross and microscopic examinations are done by different individuals, shared digital photos will be important when sharing information.
- Always fix specimens in a 10:1 ratio of formalin: tissue and make specimens no thicker than 4 mm (0.25 inches) in at least one dimension.

DISCLOSURE

The author has no conflicts of interest to declare.

REFERENCES

1. Tønnessen R, Borge KS, Nødtvedt A, et al. Canine perinatal mortality: a cohort study of 224 breeds. Theriogenology 2012;77(9):1788–801.
2. Buergelt CD. Disorders of dogs and cats. In: Njaa BL, editor. Kirkbride's diagnosis of abortion and neonatal loss in animals. 4th edition. Ames: Wiley Blackwell; 2012. p. 173–200.
3. Premanandan C, Agnew D. Perinatal mortaility in dogs and cats. Clin Theriogenol 2022;14:70–2.
4. Tesi M, Miragliotta V, Scala L, et al. Gross and histological findings in the canine placenta and amnion at term: What's normal, abnormal or pathological? Reprod Domest Anim 2021;56(5):691–702.
5. Senger PL. Pathways to pregnancy and parturition. 3rd edition. Redmond: Current Conceptions; 2012.
6. Decaro N, Martella V, Buonavoglia C. Canine adenoviruses and herpesvirus. Vet Clin North Am Small Anim Pract 2008;38(4):799–814.

7. Maggs DJ. Update on pathogenesis, diagnosis, and treatment of feline herpesvirus type 1. Clin Tech Small Anim Pract 2005;20(2):94–101.

8. Harrison LR, Styer EL, Pursell AR, et al. Fatal disease in nursing puppies associated with minute virus of canines. J Vet Diagn Invest 1992;4(1):19–22.

9. Schatzberg SJ, Haley NJ, Barr SC, et al. Polymerase chain reaction (PCR) amplification of parvoviral DNA from the brains of dogs and cats with cerebellar hypoplasia. J Vet Intern Med 2003;17(4):538–44.

10. Oliveira IVPM, Freire DAC, Ferreira HIP, et al. Research on viral agents associated with feline reproductive problems reveals a high association with feline panleukopenia virus. Vet Anim Sci 2018;6:75–80.

11. Verstegen J, Dhaliwal G, Verstegen-Onclin K. Canine and feline pregnancy loss due to viral and non-infectious causes: a review. Theriogenology 2008;70(3):304–19.

12. Coats KS, Boudreaux CE, Clay BT, et al. Placental immune pathology in the FIV-infected cat: a role for inflammation in compromised pregnancy? Vet Immunol Immunopathol 2010;134(1–2):39–47.

13. Weaver CC, Burgess SC, Nelson PD, et al. Placental immunopathology and pregnancy failure in the FIV-infected cat. Placenta 2005;26(2–3):138–47.

14. Schlafer DH, Foster RA. Female genital system. In: Maxie MG, Jubb, Kennedy, editors. Palmer's pathology of domestic animals, vol. 3, 6th edition. St Louis (MO): Elsevier; 2016. p. 358–464.

15. Santos RL, Souza TD, Mol JPS, et al. Canine Brucellosis: An Update. Front Vet Sci 2021;8:594291.

16. Ma GC, Norris JM, Mathews KO, et al. New insights on the epidemiology of Coxiella burnetii in pet dogs and cats from New South Wales, Australia. Acta Trop 2020;205:105416.

17. Santaniello A, Cimmino I, Dipineto L, et al. Zoonotic Risk of Encephalitozoon cuniculi in Animal-Assisted Interventions: Laboratory Strategies for the Diagnosis of Infections in Humans and Animals. Int J Environ Res Public Health 2021;18(17):9333.

18. Salant H, Nachum-Biala Y, Feinmesser B, et al. Early onset of clinical leishmaniosis in a litter of pups with evidence of in utero transmission. Parasit Vectors 2021;14(1):326.

19. Wang JL, Li TT, Liu GH, et al. Two Tales of Cytauxzoon felis Infections in Domestic Cats. Clin Microbiol Rev 2017;30(4):861–85.

20. Calero-Bernal R, Gennari SM. Clinical Toxoplasmosis in Dogs and Cats: An Update. Front Vet Sci 2019;6:54.

21. Silva RC, Machado GP. Canine neosporosis: perspectives on pathogenesis and management. Vet Med (Auckl) 2016;7:59–70.

22. Mugnier A, Cane T, Gaillard V, et al. Birth weight in the feline species: Description and factors of variation in a large population of purebred kittens. Theriogenology 2022;190:32–7.

23. Mugnier A, Chastant-Maillard S, Mila H, et al. Low and very low birth weight in puppies: definitions, risk factors and survival in a large-scale population. BMC Vet Res 2020;16(1):354.

24. Wiebe VJ, Howard JP. Pharmacologic advances in canine and feline reproduction. Top Companion Anim Med 2009;24(2):71–99.

25. Landsbergen N, Pellicaan CH, Schaefers-Okkens AC. Gebruik van diergeneesmiddelen tijdens de dracht bij de hond [The use of veterinary drugs during pregnancy of the dog]. Tijdschr Diergeneeskd 2001;126(22):716–22.

26. Hinderer J, Lüdeke J, Riege L, et al. Progesterone Concentrations during Canine Pregnancy. Animals (Basel) 2021;11(12):3369.

27. Bücheler J. Fading kitten syndrome and neonatal isoerythrolysis. Vet Clin North Am Small Anim Pract 1999;29(4):853–70.

28. Gilbert-Barness E, editor. Potter's pathology of the fetus, neonate and Child, vol. 1 and 2, 2nd edition. Philadelphia: Mosby Elsevier; 2007.

29. Cavalera MA, Gernone F, Uva A, et al. Clinical and Histopathological Features of Renal Maldevelopment in Boxer Dogs: A Retrospective Case Series (1999-2018). Animals (Basel) 2021;11(3):810.

30. Estevam MV, Beretta S, Smargiassi NF, et al. Congenital malformations in brachycephalic dogs: A retrospective study. Front Vet Sci 2022;9:981923.

31. Glaze MB. Congenital and hereditary ocular abnormalities in cats. Clin Tech Small Anim Pract 2005;20(2):74–82.

32. Greco DS. Congenital and inherited renal disease of small animals. Vet Clin North Am Small Anim Pract 2001;31(2):393–9.

33. Hyun C, Lavulo L. Congenital heart diseases in small animals: part I. Genetic pathways and potential candidate genes. Vet J 2006;171(2):245–55.

Canine Neonatal Health

Sophie A. Grundy, BVSc (Hons), MANZCVS (Small Animal Medicine), DACVIM
(Small Animal Internal Medicine)

KEYWORDS

- Neonate • Newborn • Canine

KEY POINTS

- The canine neonatal period extends from birth to weaning, but factors outside this time have an impact on neonatal health. Detailed history taking is essential when caring for the neonate.
- Neonates are physiologically unique at birth, and experience rapid growth and organ system maturation during the first few weeks of life. To identify what's abnormal and provide appropriate clinical support, it's important to be familiar with a clinically relevant physiology of the neonate and normal developmental milestones.
- Preventative medicine during the pre-natal period is not always possible as patients are not always presented for care prior to breeding. In these circumstances, owner education regarding the whelping process, and neonatal health monitoring is even more important for positive health outcomes.
- Available clinical monitoring tools for the canine neonate such as birth weight, weight gain, and APGAR scores are objective, and can be utilized by the lay person in a home environment where whelping and neonate care typically takes place. Early identification of at-risk neonates results in prompt intervention.
- Veterinarians working with the canine neonate should be familiar with the prevention, identification, and treatment of disorders associated with the neonatal triad (*hypothermia, hypoglycemia, and dehydration*).

INTRODUCTION

During the past 2 decades there has been a shift from linear thinking to a more global approach in medicine. Models such as the Center for Disease Control's "One Health" and the American Veterinary Medical Association's "Spectrum of Care" speak to the *continuum* rather than the *finite*.[1,2] Neonatal care is no exception to this concept. Neonatal health is not defined by events that occur during the neonatal period; rather, it is a continuum of parent genetics, maternal health, gestation, and the birth process itself, in addition to all other events that occur during the neonatal period. Conceptually, this is important to acknowledge because it means that if we view neonatal care from a *continuum* lens, it begins before conception. Preventative care prior to breeding,

Banfield Pet Hospital, 6081 Florin Road, Sacramento, CA 95823, USA
E-mail address: sophie.grundy@banfield.com

Vet Clin Small Anim 53 (2023) 1161–1193
https://doi.org/10.1016/j.cvsm.2023.05.008
0195-5616/23/© 2023 Elsevier Inc. All rights reserved.

during gestation, and during the whelping period is an essential component of neonatal health. Neonatal health is not limited to the neonatal period. When a canine neonate is presented to a veterinarian the antecedent event may have occurred well before clinical signs developed or were noted. This adds additional layers of history-taking and evaluation that are more complex than for the adult patient.

Lexicon

Within the veterinary literature, there is a lack of clarity regarding the definition of the canine neonatal period. The word perinatal, newborn, and puppy sometimes used as synonyms.[3–5] The word *neonate* is a Latinate noun from: (a) the Latinate root *(g)nasci/(g)natus* "to be born," with the addition of (b) < neo > denoting "new" and (c) <–ate > denoting that the word is a noun:[6]

< neo + **(g)n** + ate → neonate >

The < **(g)n** > is the same base that is present in the words.

(i) *pregnant:* which is formed from the combination of:
(a) < pre > denoting "before," (b) **gn** "born," and (c) < -ant > "adjective"

< pre + **gn** + ant → pregnant >

(ii) *peri(g)natal:* which is formed from the combination of:

(a) < peri > denoting "around," (b) < **(g)n** > "born," (c) < -ate(e) > "noun," and (d) < -al > "pertaining to"

< peri + **(g)n** + at(e) + al > → perinatal >

It is worth mentioning that the word *perinatal* is unique in that it can refer to either the fetal period or the neonatal period, depending on context; specifically, whether prior to birth, or after.

In contrast to Latinate words derived from the base < **(g)n** >, the word *newborn* is of Germanic origin with a derivation of *niwe* "made or established for the first time" and *beran* "birth." *Neonate* and *newborn* have the same meaning, but different linguistic origins. In this article, the term neonate will be used as the medical lexicon is typically Latinate or Hellenic.

Definition

There is no inherent denotation or connotation of time included in the word neonate. A review of the veterinary literature reveals that the canine neonatal period is either not defined, or variably defined, depending on the reference. The neonatal period is reported to be as short as birth to 3–4 days, as long as birth to 84 days, or the time from birth to weaning.[7–10] The lack of consensus with respect to the duration of the neonatal period in the veterinary literature can be problematic when attempting to evaluate mortality rates, and may be a contributing factor to variation in reported canine neonatal mortality rates ranging from 5% to 35%.[9,11–14] Some researchers have further divided the canine as an *early neonate* or *late neonate* denoting the first 2 days of life, and 2 days of life through the end of the neonatal period respectively, which becomes especially relevant when considering disease processes and neonatal mortality rates.[13,15–17]

Recently, several authors have defined the canine neonatal period more clearly as birth to 21 days (3 weeks) of age, which is consistent with the 2012 American Animal Hospital Association (AAHA) definition of the neonatal stage extending from birth to weaning which typically starts in the canine around 3 to 4 weeks of age, and the pediatric stage, from weaning to sexual maturity.[4,12,16,18–20] In this article, the canine neonatal period will be consistent with the AAHA life stage definition; specifically, from birth to weaning.

Factors impacting

The neonatal period is a period of significant physiologic change and transition from the uterine environment to the outside world. Like other species, hypoxia and sepsis are the main causes of canine neonatal death.[10,11,21] Hypoxemia is a general term that refers to a state of oxygen deficiency which may occur from one or more of the following: a decrease in oxygen intake, hypoventilation, ventilation-perfusion mismatch, or a diffusion barrier. What becomes challenging for the veterinarian is how to objectively define pathological hypoxemia in the canine neonate, as tissue hypoxemia is a physiological condition of generally all newborns: The historic use of modifiers such as "severe" or "prolonged" to describe neonatal hypoxemia precludes succinct interpretation of risk.[22–24] In contrast, the risk of death is quantified and ninefold higher when there is a failure of passive transfer: The neonate is dependent on the intake of colostrum for local and systemic immune support.[25]

Early mortality (birth to 2 days of life) occurs in approximately 90% of all hypoxemic neonates, and 70% of septic neonates respectively.[11,14,21] suggesting that a focus on (a) the key factors impacting the canine neonatal health during parturition and initial respiration, and (b) early evaluation/identification of at-risk neonates and monitoring tools is a high priority when discussing canine neonatal health.[11,14,21]

KEY POINTS: INTRODUCTION

- Neonatal health is a continuum that starts at conception and ends when the neonatal period finishes

- The canine neonatal period is best defined as birth to weaning; birth to 3 to 4 weeks of age

- Separation of the canine neonatal prior into early (0–2 days) and late (2 days – weaning) may be helpful clinically when considering preventative care strategies for the canine neonate

- Hypoxemia and sepsis are the leading causes of death during the neonatal period and are associated with early (0–2 days) neonatal mortality

---

PRE-BREEDING SCREENING

Pre-breeding screening should at a minimum consist of a thorough physical examination well in advance of the heat cycle of breeding to identify areas of concern (*physical, conformational, behavioral, nutritional, lack of current preventative care, teratogen use*). It is medically ideal, and best practice, to include routine endocrinologic and infectious disease screening, orthopedic, ophthalmic, cardiac, and genetic screening that may impact maternal health, pregnancy, and neonatal health or be a source of zoonotic disease. Rapid expansion of the PCR market in the 1990's in conjunction with the mapping of the canine genome resulted in an increase in the availability of canine genetic disease screening over the past few decades, and normalized the use of pre-breeding genetic testing to reduce the incidence and/or eliminate specific conditions within the canine purebred population.[26–30] However, there is not a genetic test for every heritable disease in the dog. The Canine Health Information Center (CHIC) maintains a current, comprehensive, centralized, and searchable open-access canine health database that provides screening recommendations and statistics by breed (https://ofa.org) and represents the best guide for clinicians.[28] Further discussion of the impact of body condition score and fertility in the canine can be found elsewhere (see [Body Condition and Fertility in Dogs by Balogh and Sones] of this issue). Additional resources providing more in-depth information about heritable disease screening in a canine breeding program based on organ system have also been discussed in depth (see [Genetic Screening in a Canine Breeding Program by Broeckx] of this issue; [Ophthalmic Disease and Screening in Breeding Dogs by Diehl] of this issue; [Cardiac Disease and Screening in Breeding Dogs by Aherne] of this issue; and [Orthopedic Disease and Screening in Breeding Dogs by Todhunter and Hayward] of this issue).

KEY POINTS: PRE-BREEDING SCREENING

- All canines intended for reproductive use should be evaluated in advance of breeding to screen for abnormalities that may impact neonatal health
- Evaluation should include at a minimum an assessment of patient history, preventative care measures, physical examination, and temperament
- The CHIC maintains comprehensive screening recommendations for purebred dogs (https://ofa.org)

PREGNANCY

It is not uncommon for a veterinarian to commence medical management of a litter around the time of pregnancy confirmation, which may be as early as 3 to 4 weeks gestation, or as late as whelping. Although some preventative care, such as maternal vaccination, is not able to be implemented once the bitch is pregnant, it's important to educate owners regarding strategies for how to best support neonatal health in the home environment. and offer guidelines regarding what is normal, and when to seek help.

Nutrition

The ideal diet for canine pregnancy should be complete and balanced, and approved by the Association of the American Feed Control Officials (AAFCO) for growth and lactation so that it meets the nutritional demands of the growing litter, supports maternal health, and may be fed continuously through weaning. Generally, it is best to avoid supplements during canine pregnancy due to potentially negative effects on fetal, and/or neonatal health. Commercially available diets appropriate for growth and lactation are typically formulated to include nutrients, such as calcium and essential fatty acids, in appropriate amounts to support neonatal health and development; additional supplementation may be problematic.[31,32] More detailed information regarding the nutritional management of the pregnant bitch can be found elsewhere (see [Body Condition and Fertility in Dogs by Balogh and Sones] of this issue; and [Nutrition for the Pregnant Bitch and Puppies by Wakshlag and Kim] of this issue).

Drug exposure

The administration of pharmacologic or biologic agents in the pregnant bitch should be avoided where possible, except for the routine administration of heartworm prevention, anthelmintics, and flea and tick prevention as permitted based on available manufacturer and formulary guidance, and with risk: benefit consideration. This recommendation includes topical medications, as systemic absorption is possible and compounds such as glucocorticoids are associated with birth defects.

In 2015 the Federal Drug Enforcement Agency (FDA) replaced the former five pregnancy risk category system A, B, C, D, and X for people with risk summary narrative sections: pregnancy, lactation, and females and males of reproductive potential. Current veterinary formularies typically maintain a narrative section regarding reproduction/nursing safety which may sometimes reference the more familiar older letter-based system. Medical management of the pregnant bitch is further discussed elsewhere (see [Canine Pregnancy, Eutocia, and Dystocia by Davidson and Cain] of this issue).

Preparation for whelping

Preparation for whelping is an area where client education can have a profound impact on neonatal health. If the dam is presented during pregnancy, although accurate assessment of gestation age can be challenging in the dog, attempts should be made to predict the date, or anticipated time-window during which parturition is expected. As whelping typically occurs in a non-clinic setting it is vital that veterinarians educate owners about the whelping process and neonate care to facilitate early identification and intervention for at-risk neonates. Information regarding the whelping process, recommended items to have on hand, and immediate evaluation of the neonate has a positive impact on neonatal health. Clients should be given cost-effective and easy-to-implement tools. **Table 1** provides a list of items that owners may find useful when working with neonates. Additional information regarding the prediction of parturition in the dog and elective cesarean section may be found elsewhere (See [Progesterone Analysis in Canine Breeding Management by Conley and Gonzales] of this issue; and [Canine Cesarean Section: Emergency and Elective by Cain and Davidson] of this issue).

Table 1	
Useful items for owners to have in advance of whelping to improve neonatal health	
Item	**Use**
Whelping box that can be cleaned	Children's plastic swimming pool is a cost-effective solution; may be lined with newspaper for ease of cleaning
2% tincture of iodine/dental floss/scissors	Umbilical cord care
Bulb syringe/De Lee mucous trap	To safely clear neonate airway
Gram scale	Birth weight/weight gain
Non-toxic nail polish/clippers	Puppy identification
Warm blankets/towels	Puppy stimulation and warming
Gloves	Infection prevention
Thermometer, covers, and lubricant	Temperature monitoring of mum and litter
Pen/Paper	Record times of delivery, puppy weights, and APGAR scores
Canine neonate nipple, bottle, and milk replacer	Supplemental feeding

Immune support for the neonate

There are four layers to the zonary endotheliochorial placenta of the bitch, uterine endothelium on the maternal side; and chorionic epithelium, connective tissue, and fetal endothelium on the fetal side. The structure of the canine placental presents a barrier to large molecules and the canine neonate is reliant upon colostrum ingestion for the passive transfer of immunoglobulins. Failure of passive transfer is associated with neonatal mortality, but the timing and volume of ingestion appear to be limiting factors for the canine, rather than the immune quality of the colostrum itself.[33] For this reason, it is important that owners are educated regarding the importance of colostrum ingestion within 8 hours of birth. For further discussion, please see "Colostrum".

KEY POINTS: PREGNANCY

- The first opportunity for a veterinarian to commence a care plan to maximize neonatal health may be when the dam presents for pregnancy diagnosis, or whelping assistance
- Owner education regarding nutrition and medication use during pregnancy, in addition to information about what to expect and when to seek help can positively impact neonatal health
- Owners should be provided with information regarding anticipated whelping dates (if known), items to have on hand, and when to seek help
- Owners should monitor neonates after birth and make sure that colostrum is consumed within 8 hours of birth

PARTURITION

The fetus undergoes rapid change during birth as it loses maternal supports and assumes a more physiologically autonomous role as neonate *ex utero*. For the canine neonate, this transition occurs at a time when the maturation of several organ systems is still incomplete.[10]

Birth is a time during which the canine neonate is particularly vulnerable to asphyxia and hypoxemia, hypothermia, and glucose imbalance; all of which decrease survival.[34]

Minimum gestation length

The ability of a fetus to survive outside the uterine environment is dependent upon lung surfactant production and the start of respiration, without which oxygen exchange cannot occur. Prior to a gestational age of 62 days from the luteinizing hormone (LH) surge, the canine fetus lacks sufficient surfactant production for *ex utero* survival.[35] Similar to other species, it is suggested that the female canine fetus is capable of surviving earlier than her male counterpart; this sexual dimorphism is thought to be related to higher levels of Müllerian inhibiting hormone in the male impacting lung surfactant development.[35,36] In the absence of ovulation timing or known gestational age, serum progesterone may be used as a marker for fetal lung development with a serum progesterone concentration of < 2 ng/mL being associated with adequate production of lung surfactant.[37] A protocol for the direct evaluation of surfactant production using amniotic fluid and 95% ethanol to evaluate fetal maturation is described in the literature; however, due to the challenges in sampling canine amniotic fluid, this methodology is not easily clinically applicable.[35,37] Future development of a bed side surfactant screen may be useful during cesarean sections, especially when there is a need to document a lack of fetal viability versus neonatal loss from other causes. A more in-depth discussion of progesterone analysis in canine breeding management and elective cesarean sections can be found elsewhere (see [Progesterone Analysis in Canine Breeding Management by Conley and Gonzales] of this issue; and [Canine Cesarean Section: Emergency and Elective by Cain and Davidson] of this issue).

Dystocia

The duration of labor, specifically the second stage of labor (clinically identifiable as the onset of straining or discharge of fetal fluid), has been associated with an increase in neonate mortality with the most favorable outcome when it is < 12 hours duration.[3,14,38,39] Dystocia plays a significant role in canine neonatal mortality; asphyxia and hypoxia are associated with more than 60% of neonatal losses during the first 2 days of life.[14,21,40] Prompt detection of dystocia and fetal distress during parturition is a vital component of preventative neonatal care and early intervention.[41] From a practical perspective, two approaches can be used; firstly, fetal heart rate and toco-dynamic monitoring, and secondly, clinical observation of *"red flags"* that indicate further evaluation is warranted.

Tocodynamic monitoring (eg, Whelpwise Veterinary Perinatal Specialties) of the pregnant bitch in late pregnancy and during parturition provides insight regarding the identification of labor onset, monitoring of contraction strength, and response to medical interventions; it is an excellent clinical tool during the whelping process.[42–44] Tocodynamic monitoring for the canine is not always available, which necessitates the consideration of alternate clinically pragmatic options. While it is known that external abdominal contractions do not necessarily accurately reflect uterine activity, a practical and reasonable alternative option in a setting that precludes tocodynamic monitoring includes a combination of visual monitoring (behavior, external contractions, vaginal discharge), record keeping of the parturition events, and, where possible, fetal heart rate monitoring by hand-held Doppler. Handheld portable fetal heart rate Doppler units are readily available online, and with training can be utilized during pregnancy and parturition to monitor canine fetal heart rates with or without tocodynamic monitoring. Although fetal heart rate oscillation is normal during parturition during periods of uterine contraction, sustained fetal heart rates below 180 beats per minute are known to be associated with severe fetal distress and presumably greater risk to neonatal health in the first 2 days of life.[43,44] **Table 2** outlines clinical *"red flags"* during parturition and why they raise concern for neonatal health.

Hypoxemia

The normal adult dog maintains a peripheral oxygen saturation (spO2) of 96% or greater, but in the canine neonate normal spO2 values for neonates born via spontaneous vaginal delivery and elective cesarean section are approximately 90% and 80% respectively.[22] After birth, there is a period of adaptation to extra-uterine life and respiration with spO2 values stabilizing 1 hour after spontaneous vaginal delivery and 12 hours after elective cesarean section.[10,22] As published spO2 data points for the canine neonate between 1 hour and 12 hours post birth are not readily available it is difficult to define what is expected or normal during this time. What can be stated is as follows: (a) this data supports a clinical indication for repeated APGAR evaluations during the early neonatal period and (b) normal canine neonates should have an spO2 on room air within the normal adult range by 1 hour and 12 hours post birth when born by spontaneous vaginal delivery and elective cesarean section respectively.

Bradycardia, decreased lung compliance, and sepsis, are three clinically important consequences of hypoxemia in the canine neonate. During parturition, and for the first

Table 2
Clinical *"Red flags"* during parturition

Observation	Clinical Concern for Neonatal Health
Fetal heart rate < 180	Fetal distress/hypoxemia
Maternal lethargy, collapse, repeated vomiting, permanent moaning, or seizures	Fetal viability
Green or black vaginal discharge prior to delivery of the first fetus	Placental detachment without timely expulsion increasing risk fetal – neonate hypoxemia
Protrusion of fetal membranes from the vulva for 15 min or longer without delivery of the fetus	Fetal – neonate hypoxemia
Duration of stage II labor >12 h	Increased risk of neonatal distress
Time interval of more than 2 h after the delivery of the previous fetus	May indicate dystocia and thus increased risk fetal – neonate hypoxemia
Prolonged (>15 min) of ineffective abdominal contractions with no delivery of a fetus is observed	May represent physical obstruction to delivery (narrow birth cancel, malposition, malposture, large fetus, or other cause of dystocia; potential increased risk fetal – neonate hypoxemia

Adapted from Arlt SP. The bitch around parturition. *Theriogenology.* 2020;150:452 to 457. https://doi.org/10.1016/j.theriogenology.2020.02.046

few days of life, there are several factors that increase the risk of circulatory failure in the canine neonate. First, during the neonatal period, the cardiovascular system is a high volume – low-pressure circuit and cardiac output is dependent upon heart rate; second, bradycardia in the canine neonate is not vagally mediated and sympathetic innervation of the heart is incomplete; third, anoxia results in profound bradycardia (less than 45 beats per minute) and hypotension (less than 25 mm Hg).[45] Despite these risk factors, during the first days of life, it has been shown that in studies of anoxic death that circulation continues for a long time with a pulse being detected in some neonates for as long as 30 mins after the last breath.[46] The canine neonate is remarkably resistant to circulatory failure and can be resuscitated after a hypoxemic or anoxic event, providing systolic blood pressure is maintained above 8 mm Hg.[45,46]

In addition to altered cardiovascular physiology, there are important changes in the respiratory tract of the canine neonate that warrant mention. First, upper airway obstruction may occur more readily due to the relatively large tongue and less rigid airway cartilage; second, the amount of work and pressure required by a neonate to maintain breathing is increased as the ribcage is more pliable, intercostal muscles weaker, and lungs less compliant; third, the neonate is susceptible to relative hypoxemia due to a large metabolic oxygen requirement, and immature carotid chemoreceptors; and fourth, hypoxia in the canine neonate increases inspiratory resistance and decreases lung compliance.[10,47] The effect of these changes is that the canine neonate is predisposed to airway collapse, respiration fatigue, hypoxemia, and rapid oxygen desaturation.

Sepsis is an important cause of loss during the early neonatal period. Bacterial populations exist within the normal gravid canine reproductive tract, and those same bacterial isolates may be present in the dam, her colostrum, and her neonates.[48–50] As an aid in the prevention of sepsis, umbilical cords should be ligated, trimmed to approximately 0.5 to 1.0 cm from the abdominal wall and dipped in 2% tincture of iodine.[9] Aside from cardiovascular and respiratory compromise, management of hypoxia is a high priority in the canine neonate as bacterial translocation is known to occur in the absence of gastrointestinal mucosal lesions and contributes to the development of sepsis.[51]

Resuscitation

Prompt medical intervention is indicated for neonates that do not exhibit rapid spontaneous respiration regardless of birth method. As neonates are small, wet at birth, and unable to generate their own body heat, care must be taken to keep them warm during the resuscitation process. Standard approaches to resuscitation focusing on airway maintenance, breathing, and circulation are appropriate for the canine neonate; however, due to physiologic differences in the neonate, the primary focus is on support of the onset of respiration, and the maintenance of oxygenation and normal body temperature.

Hypoxemia in the canine neonate is associated with bradycardia, and decreased lung compliance. Neonates with low heart rates need an open airway, and oxygen. Parasympatholytic agents, such as atropine or glycopyrrolate, are not indicated during the resuscitation of the canine neonate because in this cohort, bradycardia is not vagally mediated.[10]

Canine neonatal airways are prone to obstruction and should always be cleared by suction rather than "swinging" due to the risk of trauma.[52] Various respiration stimulation points have been described in the literature (genital and umbilical area at birth, JenChung acupressure point) and may be considered once the airway is cleared.[9,53,54] Pharmacologic respiratory stimulants such as doxapram are controversial as carotid chemoreceptors are immature at birth in the dog, and the respiratory stimulatory effects of doxapram are obliterated during states of hypoxemia.[55,56]

For those cases where delivery involves anesthesia, it is difficult to prevent *in utero* anesthetic drug exposure as, with the exception of dexmedetomidine, induction and gaseous anesthetic agents routinely used in small animal practice cross the placenta, and epidural anesthesia alone for the canine is not practical.[57–62] A variety of anesthesia protocols for cesarean sections in the bitch are available, all of which focus on maintaining oxygenation and reducing fetal depression by using multi-modal approaches.[59,63] Neonatal resuscitation and the management of neonates born by elective cesarean section is described in more depth elsewhere (see [Canine Cesarean Section: Emergency and Elective by Cain and Davidson] of this issue). Generally, canine neonates respond well to warming, rubbing/tactile stimulation, and oxygen support.[64]

KEY POINTS: PARTURITION

- Lung surfactant production is insufficient to support life at a gestational age less than 62 days from the LH surge

- Dystocia is a significant contributor to neonatal mortality; asphyxia and hypoxemia are associated with 60% of neonatal deaths

- Tocodynamic and fetal heart rate monitoring, and observation for "red flags" during parturition can help improve neonatal health outcomes

- Sustained fetal heart rates less than 180 beats per minute are associated with fetal distress

- At birth, the normal canine neonate has a lower spO2 than the adult dog

- Neonate spO2 values increase after birth and plateau at 1 hour and 12 hours after spontaneous vaginal birth and cesarean birth respectively
- Resuscitation efforts should focus on maintaining an open airway and oxygen delivery whilst keeping neonates warm
- At birth, umbilical cords should be trimmed, ligated and 2% tincture of iodine applied to help prevent sepsis

THE NEONATE
Defining normal

Neonates are not miniature versions of the adult dog, and it is important for both veterinarians and owners to have an appreciation of what is normal at each developmental age. Suggested ambient temperature guidelines, normal vital signs, clinically relevant physiology, and developmental milestones for the canine neonate are provided in **Tables 3–6**.

The early neonate

The early canine neonate (0–2 days) has recently transitioned to *ex utero* life and the onset of respiration; these events, and the neonate's unique physiology increases susceptibility to hypoxemia, hypoglycemia, hypothermia, and dehydration. It is important to provide owners with practical and cost-effective ways for them to identify at-risk neonates as whelping typically takes place in the home environment. Separating a sick neonate from the dam and transporting it to a veterinary clinic presents a logistical challenge. Although virtual visits in veterinary medicine are more commonplace post–COVID-19 and present an option for neonatal care, depending on location virtual visits may not establish a valid client–patient relationship. Owner education plays a vital role in improving canine neonatal health outcomes.

The late neonate

The late neonatal period (3 days – weaning) is a time of rapid growth and organ maturation: The normal canine neonate will more than double its body weight during this time; eyes and ears open; more controlled ambulation and independent excretory functions begin as neurologic reflexes mature; and nephrogenesis is completed. Passive transfer of maternal immunoglobulins provides the canine neonate protection from some infectious diseases, but parasitism and sepsis remain a clinical concern through weaning.

During this period of rapid growth and maturation skeletal malformations and other abnormalities may become more apparent. Neonate survival from a nutrition lens is

Table 3	
Recommended ambient temperature guidelines for the canine neonate	
Age	**Temperature Range °C (°F)**
0–7 d	29.4–32.2 (85–90)
8–14 d	26.6 (80)
15–21 d	26.6 (80)
22–28 d	26.6 (80)

Adapted from Monson WJ. Orphan rearing of puppies and kittens. *Vet Clin North Am Small Anim Pract.* 1987;17(3):567 to 576. https://doi.org/10.1016/s0195-5616(8750054-7)

				Systolic/Diastolic
Table 4				
Normal vital signs for the canine neonate				
Age	**Heart Rate Mean (Beats/min)**	**Respiratory Rate Mean (Breaths/min)**	**Temperature Range °C (°F)**	**(Mean) Blood Pressure (mm Hg)**
0–24 h	200–250	15–35	34.4–36.0 (94–96.8)	54/30 (40)
1 wk	220		36.1–37.2 (97–99)	
2 wk	212		36.4–37.1 (97.6–98.8)	
3 wk	192		37.2–38.1 (99–100.5)	
4 wk	137–156	20–36	37.7 (100)	70/45 (60)

Adapted from Moon PF, Massat BJ, Pascoe PJ. Neonatal critical care. *Vet Clin North Am Small Anim Pract.* 2001;31(2):343 to 365. https://doi.org/10.1016/s0195-5616(0150209-0)

dependent upon adequate production and consumption of the dam's milk. Maintaining adequate nutrition planes for the dam is vital. The reader is referred elsewhere for further details (see [Nutrition for the pregnant bitch and puppies by Wakshlag and Kim] of this issue).

KEY POINTS: THE NEONATE

- The canine neonate is not just a small dog; understanding what's normal for the canine neonate helps the owner and clinician know when something is wrong
- **Tables 3–6** provide useful information regarding temperature needs, vital signs, normal physiology, and expected developmental milestones
- Health risks during the neonatal period include hypoxemia, hypoglycemia, hypothermia, and dehydration, and infectious disease

CLINICAL TOOLS

Canine neonates can be challenging to work with. Many clinicians have limited exposure to the canine neonate and are unfamiliar with their specific needs. Venous access can be more challenging, and there are not well-established guidelines regarding spO2 values requiring intervention. Even when incubators are available for use, Fi_{O_2} parameters and the maximum recommended duration of oxygen support are not well defined. Mechanical ventilatory support for the canine neonate is typically cost-prohibitive and technically challenging even in a tertiary care setting. Prevention and early detection are a central component to care and improve canine neonatal health outcomes. When the neonate is not evaluated during the early neonatal period, sepsis and other morbidities are detected later when the patient is in a more debilitated state. In this section, options for monitoring canine neonatal health will discussed, many of which can be performed by the lay person and outside of a clinic setting.

Birth weight

Across mammalian species, it is well documented that low birth weight is associated negatively with short-term survival.[65] Low birth weight neonates are physiologically at a disadvantage due to a combination of low energy reserves and high surface area to mass ratio predisposing them to hypothermia and hypoglycemia.[10,66] Hypothermic

Table 5
Clinically relevant physiology of the canine neonate

Organ System	Neonate	Clinical Implication
Ocular	• Eyelids are closed at birth • The cornea has a higher water content during the neonatal period and may appear cloudy • The iris has low pigmentation at birth and typically appears blue • Retinal vascular development is incomplete at birth	• Ocular examination is not possible in the canine neonate until the eyelids open • Pupillary light reflexes are not intact until retinal development is completed at around 2 wk of age • The normal neonate tapetum is blue-gray
Cardiovascular	• Low resistance, high flow circuit • Chronotropic responses are incomplete until 14 d of age • Bradycardia occurs in response to hypoxemia • Relative resistance to circulatory failure	• Dependent on heart rate and blood volume to maintain cardiac output • Plasma volume is expanded, and heart rate elevated • Bradycardia is not vagally mediated • Bradycardia is an indication for oxygen support
Respiratory	• Prone to upper airway obstruction (relatively large tongue, soft cartilage) • Mechanisms controlling respiratory function mature during the post-natal period • Large oxygen demand • Increased work to maintain tidal volume	• The canine neonate is susceptible to hypoxemia
Gastrointestinal	• Dentition eruption typically starts around 2–3 wk • Ileus develops at rectal temperatures of 94°F	• Hypothermia is associated with ileus which increases the risk of reflux and aspiration
Hepatobiliary	• Neonatal liver and biliary system are functionally immature at birth • Bile secretion is reduced as compared to the adult dog • Alkaline phosphatase (ALP) and gamma-glutamyl transferase (GGT) are markedly elevated at 0–2 wk • At 4 wk of age, P_{450}-specific activity is around 85% of that seen in the adult dog • Microsomal enzyme is not comparable to that of the adult dog until around 4.5 mo of age	• Serum bile acids may be used as early as 4 wk of age to detect hepatocirculatory abnormalities; a single urine bile acid to creatine ratio may be used to replace a resting or random serum bile acid concentration • Drugs requiring hepatic metabolism or excretion should be used with care

System	Characteristics	Clinical Relevance
Urinary System	• Neonatal kidney is immature and nephrogenesis continues for at least 2 wk post birth • Glomerular filtration rates are low with decreased amino acid absorption • Natriuresis in the proximal tubule is increased • Renal blood flow is best correlated to blood pressure until around 6 wk of age	• Low urine specific gravity is normal, as is the detection of protein, glucose, and various amino acids • Care should be taken to maintain fluid balance without overhydration or oncotic loading • Renally excreted or metabolized drugs should be used with care
Hematopoietic System	• Macrocytosis at birth, decreasing to that of the adult by 4 wk of age • Red blood cell counts decrease from birth to 3 wk, and then increase	• Age-based reference ranges should be used
Immune System	• At birth, the canine neonate is immunologically incompetent • Only 5%–10% canine neonate antibodies are derived from transplacental transfer; canine neonates are dependent upon the effective passive transfer of immunoglobulins • Gastrointestinal permeability is highest at birth and decreases dramatically after 8 h	• Effective passive transfer is dependent upon colostrum consumption and increased gastrointestinal permeability • Canine neonates should be monitored to ensure colostrum intake within hours of birth
Metabolism	• Normal birth weight is dependent upon breed • Growth patterns (weight gain) are typically breed independent • Canine neonates are poikilothermic and susceptible to chilling, due to a higher body surface area/mass ratio • During the first 24 h, hepatic glycogen stores decrease dramatically	• Recording neonate birth weight, and daily weight gain, is an easy way to monitor metabolic health • Neonates need access to a heat source to make sure they can maintain body temperature • Neonates require regular feeding to maintain serum glucose concentrations

Adapted from Grundy SA. Clinically relevant physiology of the neonate. *Vet Clin North Am Small Anim Pract.* 2006;36(3):443-v. https://doi.org/10.1016/j.cvsm.2005.12.002

Table 6
Developmental milestones for the canine neonate

	Development	Age of Onset (days)	Notes:
Mental State	Typically sleeping or nursing	0–14	• Normal canine neonates are typically easily roused from sleep
Gait and Posture	Righting reflex	0	• Vestibular function is present at birth, but muscle tone is lacking
	Flexion dominance	0–4	• Early movement involves a "swimming" like thoracic limb movement whilst sliding on the abdomen
	Extensor dominance	4–5	
	Stepping movements (with thoracic limb support)	5–6	
	Upright posture	10–14	• Neonates can raise their head at birth
	Pelvic limb can support body weight	14–16	• Adult posture and balance develop around 6–8 wk of age
	Uncoordinated gait	18–21	
Cranial Nerve Reflexes	Swallow reflex	0	• Eyelids open around 14 d
	Rooting Reflex	0	• Reflexes to protect the eye develop prior to the eyelids opening
	Suckling	1–2	• Ear canals open between 12 and 14 d
	Dazzle	1–2	• Rooting reflex is evoked by cupping the fingers around the muzzle and is strongest during the first 14 d, disappearing around 25 d
	Vibrissopalpebral	1–2	
	Palpebral	2–4	
	Startle response	12–14	
	Corneal	10–16	
	Pupillary Light Reflex	10–16	
	Menace response	10–28	

Adapted from Lavely JA. Pediatric neurology of the dog and cat. Vet Clin North Am Small Anim Pract. 2006;36(3):475-v. https://doi.org/10.1016/j.cvsm.2005.12.009

neonates do not have normal gastrointestinal motility or vigor, and maintenance of effective nursing is difficult.[10]

One of the challenges in veterinary medicine is the considerable breed variation in neonate size, and the lack of breed-specific data regarding critical canine neonate weight.[15,18,65,66] What is known is that lower birth weight (from the first quartile) has been associated with an increase in mortality during both the early and late neonatal period, whilst being born to a highly heterogenous litter (based on birth weight) is associated with an increase in mortality during the early neonatal period.[15] Consideration of birth weight in the context of litter weight heterogenicity, and trending of early growth rate are far more useful than birth weight alone for both the identification of the at-risk canine neonate, and for ongoing monitoring of canine neonatal health.

Weight gain

Weight loss in excess of 4% of birth weight during the first 24 hours is known to be a risk factor for mortality in the canine neonate.[67] Measurement of daily weight gain is an effective, objective, and simple way to monitor neonatal health. Growth curve analysis of multiple breeds supports that a daily weight gain of 5%–10% can be used as a marker of clinical health across all breeds and birth weight is expected to double by 7 to 10 days of age.[68] Clinical evaluation is indicated for any neonate deviating from this general rule. Assessment of maternal milk production is advised if more than one neonate is failing to thrive. Alternate nutritional support for the canine neonate is best provided by a complete and balanced canine milk replacement formula. Canine milk is 2 and 3 times more calorie dense than caprine or bovine milk, respectively, and the nutrient breakdown significantly different.[69,70] Bottle feeding using a canine neonate nipple is the preferred method. Neonates should be normothermic and the nipple aligned with the oral cavity so that the tongue forms a seal and prevents aerophagia. The stomach volume of the neonate is estimated to be 4 mLs per 100 gm body weight, and daily caloric requirements are estimated to be 200 kcal per kilogram of body weight up to 4 weeks of age.[33,71] Suggested intervals between feeding are 3–4 hours for the first week and 4–6 hours thereafter. Feeding may be extended to every 6 hours when oral feeding begins. Tube feeding may be considered for sick neonates or those with a poor suckle reflex.

APGAR (modified) score

The APGAR score is a standardized scoring system for infants based on 5 markers of health: color, heart rate, reflexes, muscle tone, and respiration. It is not a predictor of neonatal mortality; rather, by assigning a numeric value to each parameter, the APGAR score objectively quantifies both neonatal depression and response to resuscitation.[72] A modified canine APGAR scoring system was first proposed in 2009 (**Table 7**) and an alternate version by a second author in 2010.[3,14] The 2009 version has been used most consistently in the literature and provides an easily accessible objective tool that identifies the at-risk neonate: this means early intervention and need-based support for the neonates that will benefit the most.[73–78] Canine APGAR scoring can be used with equal success in the clinic and home setting.

The canine APGAR scoring system assigns a numeric value to each criterion, and the cumulative score used to categorize neonates into one of the 3 viability classes. The original cutoff values for viability class have been refined and now include consideration to the dam's breed-body-size; the updated canine neonate APGAR score cutoff values according to breed-body-size are shown in **Table 8**.

Clinically, lower APGAR scores are associated with decreased mammary gland searching as compared to the normal APGAR group, as well as an increased risk of

Table 7			
Modified canine APGAR scoring system			
	Score		
Parameter	**0**	**1**	**2**
Heart Rate	< 180 bpm	180–220 bpm	> 230 bpm
Respiratory Rate	No crying/< 6 rr	Mild crying/6–15 rr	Crying/> 15 rr
Reflex irritability	Absent	Grimace	Vigorous
Motility	Flaccid	Some flexions	Active motion
Mucous membrane color	Cyanotic	Pale	Pink

Abbreviations: bpm, beats per minute; rr, respiratory rate (breaths per minute).
From Veronesi MC, Panzani S, Faustini M, Rota A. An Apgar scoring system for routine assessment of newborn puppy viability and short-term survival prognosis. *Theriogenology.* 2009;72(3):401 to 407. https://doi.org/10.1016/j.theriogenology.2009.03.010

poor sucking reflex.[14] Neonates in the "critical" category are those with the highest risk of death despite neonatal assistance or resuscitation.[77] Specialized interventions are indicated for this group consisting of the following: immediate measures such as resuscitation and active warming, and ongoing respiratory, immunoglobulin, and nutritional support until stable. The refined canine APGAR scores in the "critical" category, those that are less than 3, are independent of breed body size at both 24 hours and 7 days.

It is worth stressing that the canine APGAR score represents the evaluation of the neonate at a single snapshot in time. A low score does not determine the prognosis for survival or predict the effectiveness of response to intervention. Rather, the canine APGAR score identifies those neonates in need of immediate intervention; subsequent APGAR scores assess the response to therapy and need for additional treatment.

Neonatal viability reflex score

The neonatal viability reflex (NVR) score is a way to evaluate canine neonate vigor, and is based on the strength of the sucking, righting, and rooting reflex as evaluated by an examiner. Effective milk consumption is difficult without the sucking, righting, and rooting reflex: A low NVR score indicates that a neonate should be further evaluated. The NVR score may be used alone, or in conjunction with the canine APGAR score when evaluating the health of the canine neonate. The NVR scoring system is shown in **Table 9**. Cumulative scores of 0 to 2 are consistent with weak vigor or vitality, 3 to 4 moderate vigor or vitality, and 5 to 6 normal vigor or vitality.[79]

Colostrum

Canine neonates are antibody deficient at birth and dependent upon effective ingestion and absorption, "passive transfer," of colostrum as a source of immunoglobulins, nutrients, microbes, and hormones, which in turn impact organ maturation, promote intestinal barrier closure, and improve nutrient absorption.[16,49,80]

During the last weeks of pregnancy, maternal IgG accumulates in mammary tissue and is subsequently released early in lactation resulting in colostrum IgG levels three to four times higher than in maternal circulation.[16,33,81] Colostrum contains both IgG, and IgA which is produced locally in the mammary gland, thus meeting both systemic and local immunity needs for the neonate.[16,33] High concentrations of IgG in colostrum results in adequate passive-transfer of immunoglobulins requiring as little as 1.3 mL of colostrum per 100-g of puppy weight but the timing is vital, and ingestion needed

Table 8
Refined canine neonate APGAR score cutoff values, and viability classes according to breed body size

	Small ≤10 kgs (≤22 Pounds)			Medium[a] 11–20 kgs (24.2–44 Pounds)			Large > 20 kgs (>44 Pounds)		
	Severe Distress "Critical"	Moderate Distress	No Distress	Severe Distress "Critical"	Moderate Distress	No Distress	Severe Distress "Critical"	Moderate Distress	No Distress
<24 h	0–3	4	5–10	0–3	4–5	6–10	0–3	4–5	6–10
24 h – 7 d	0–3	4	5–10	0–3	4–5	6–10	0–3	4–7	8–10

Abbreviation: ROC, receiver operating characteristic curve.

[a] In medium-sized neonates the newly detected viability classes were merely cautiously suggested, because they were not calculated by ROC, and data were drawn from a limited number of newborns.

Modified from Veronesi MC, Panzani S, Faustini M, Rota A. An Apgar scoring system for routine assessment of newborn puppy viability and short-term survival prognosis. Theriogenology. 2009;72(3):401-407. doi:10.1016/j.theriogenology.2009.03.010.

Table 9
Neonatal viability reflex (NVR) scoring

Parameter	Weak (0 Score)	Moderate (1 Score)	Normal (2 Score)
Suckle	Absent	Weak (>3 suckles/min)	Strong (5 suckles/min)
Rooting	Absent	Slow muzzle fitting inside circle	Immediate fitting muzzle within circle
Righting Reflex	Absent (*continues in initial position*)	Slow body repositioning	Fast body repositioning

From Vassalo FG, Simões CR, Sudano MJ, et al. Topics in the routine assessment of newborn puppy viability. *Top Companion Anim Med.* 2015;30(1):16 to 21. https://doi.org/10.1053/j.tcam.2015.02.003

within the first 8 hours.[16,33] Variation in colostrum IgG concentrations between teat pairs is normal in the bitch; however, this is clinically unimportant as canine neonates do not develop a nipple preference.[82,83]

Serum markers for colostrum consumption in the canine neonate have been evaluated; however, for intervention to be effective, blood sampling would be required prior to 8 hours of age and there is currently not a practical bedside test for this purpose. There is not a complete canine colostrum substitute currently available. When colostrum intake is known to be impaired pooled adult dog serum (2–4 mL per 100-g body weight, divided and administered subcutaneously in two sites) will raise serum IgG levels to a minimum protective level (>230 mg/dL) in colostrum deprived neonates; however, side effects include fluid pockets and/or skin necrosis.[19,84]

Hematologic and serum chemistry values

Reference ranges for the adult dog are not applicable to the canine neonate. It is important for clinicians to have access to age-based reference ranges for the dog; some analytes such as serum alkaline phosphatase, which is a marker for colostrum consumption, have a wide reference range. During the past decade, point-of-care analyzers have become standard in-practice equipment and evaluation of clinical pathology data is more readily available than ever especially when sample requirements are small. **Tables 10–12** provide hematologic and biochemical reference ranges for the canine neonate.

Future areas of research

Every clinician knows that there are few things as rewarding as saving the life of an animal, and there is a special kind of joy seeing a neonate take its first breath and cry. The development of the canine APGAR score advanced canine neonatal medicine, but there have been few additions to the clinician's toolbox since. As research in the field of canine neonatology continues, our ability to positively influence neonatal health outcomes will improve.

Biological fluids

Recently there has been an interest in evaluating neonate biological fluids including fluids such as amniotic fluid and umbilical blood with a goal of identifying objective markers that can predict neonate survival when used alone, or in conjunction with a modified canine APGAR score. Candidates have included blood gas, lactate, glucose, cortisol, urine specific gravity, cardiac troponin 1, and amniotic fluid composition in addition to serum IgG, and the ALP, and GGT as markers for evidence of colostrum consumption.[3,34,38,85–89] Further studies are needed to better define clinically useful

Table 10
Normal Hematologic values for canine neonates

Hematologic Parameter	Age				
	Birth[a]	7 d[a]	14 d[a]	21 d[a]	28 d[a]
RBC (x 10⁶/μL)	4.7–5.6 (5.1)	3.6–5.9 (4.6)	3.4–4.4 (3.9)	3.5–4.3 (3.8)	3.6–4.9 (4.1)
Hemoglobin (g/dL)	14.0–17.0 (15.2)	10.4–17.5 (12.9)	9.0–11.0 (10.0)	8.6–11.6 (9.7)	8.5–10.3 (9.5)
PCV (%)	45–52.5 (47.5)	33.0–52.0 (40.5)	29.0–34.0 (31.8)	27.0–37.0 (31.7)	27.0–33.5 (29.9)
MCV (fL)	(93.0)	(89.0)	(81.5)	(83.0)	(73.0)
MCH (pg)	(30.0)	(28.0)	(25.5)	(25.0)	(23.0)
MCHC (%)	(32.0)	(32.0)	(31.5)	(31.0)	(32.0)
nRBC/100WBC	0–13 (2.3)	0–11 (4.0)	0–6 (2.0)	0–9 (1.6)	0–4 (1.2)
Reticulocytes (%)	4.5–9.2 (6.5)	3.8–15.2 (6.9)	4.0–8.4 (6.7)	5.0–9.0 (6.9)	4.6–6.6 (5.8)
Total WBC (x 10³/μL)	6.8–18.4 (12.8)	9.0–23.0 (14.1)	8.1–15.1 (11.7)	6.7–15.1 (11.2)	8.5–16.4 (12.9)
Segmented neutrophils	4.4–15.8 (8.60)	3.8–15.2 (7.4)	3.2–10.4 (5.2)	1.4–9.4 (5.1)	3.7–12.8 (7.2)
Band neutrophils	0–1.5 (0.23)	0–4.8 (0.50)	0–1.2 (0.21)	0–0.5 (0.09)	0–0.3 (0.06)
Lymphocytes	0.5–4.2 (1.9)	1.3–9.4 (4.3)	1.5–7.4 (3.8)	2.1–10.1 (5.0)	1.0–8.4 (4.5)
Monocytes	0.2–2.2 (0.9)	0.3–2.5 (1.1)	0.2–1.4 (0.7)	0.1–1.4 (0.7)	0.3–1.5 (0.8)
Eosinophils	0–1.3 (0.4)	0.2–2.8 (0.8)	0.08–1.8 (0.6)	0.07–0.9 (0.3)	0–0.7 (0.25)
Basophils	—	0–0.2 (0.01)	—	—	0–0.15 (0.01)
Platelets (x 10³/μL)	178–465 (302)	282–560 (352)	210–352 (290)	203–370 (272)	130–360 (287)

Values in parentheses are mean values.

Abbreviations: MCH, mean corpuscular hemoglobin; MCHC, mean corpuscular hemoglobin concentration; MCV, mean corpuscular volume; nRBC/100WBC, number of nucleated red blood cells per 100 white blood cells; PCV packed cell volume, RBC red blood cell; Total WBC total white blood cell count.

[a] Normal ranges and/or mean values from Earl FL, Melveger BE, Wilson RL. The hemogram and bone marrow profile of normal neonatal and weanling beagle dogs. *Lab Anim Sci.* 1973;23(5):690 to 695.

From von Dehn B. Pediatric clinical pathology. *Vet Clin North Am Small Anim Pract.* 2014;44(2):205 to 219. https://doi.org/10.1016/j.cvsm.2013.10.003

diagnostic criteria for biological fluids and proteomics as for the early identification of the at-risk canine neonate.

Microbiome

Advances in molecular biology have improved our ability to evaluate biological samples for not only the presence of bacteria using 16S ribosomal RNA as a marker, but also rapidly sequence bacterial populations, identify species, resistance patterns, and more using techniques such as matrix-assisted laser desorption/ionization time-of-flight (MALDI-TOF) and next generation sequencing. As more biological samples are evaluated across species, historical medical concepts such as the "sterile womb" are being challenged and further defined. We are just beginning to discover the complex relationship between microbial populations and canine reproductive and neonatal health.

There appear to be species differences, but for the canine, current research supports that microbial colonization begins prior to birth and that amniotic fluid, the placenta, uterus, and fetal gastrointestinal tract are not sterile environments.[48,50,90,91] For the canine, similar to humans, there is evidence that delivery type alters canine neonate microbiome colonization patterns and colostrum microbiota composition, and that in turn neonate microbiota populations influence neonate growth rates.[48–50] Canine microbial biodiversity is noted to be lowest in colostrum and neonates of dams post emergency cesarean section.[49] Canine neonates with culturable placental or meconium microbiota exhibit higher relative weight gains during the first few days of life when neonatal mortality rates are known to be higher; however, these benefits were short term and not found to be correlated with survival or long term weight gain.[48] It's an exciting area of research with vast and far reaching clinical implications for both the reproductive management of the bitch, and neonatal medicine.

Immunoglobulin Y

IgY is the main immunoglobulin produced by chickens. Inoculating hens with canine pathogens results in the presence of IgY for those specific pathogens in the yolk of her eggs, which can subsequently be harvested and dried for oral administration to puppies.[19,92] Products containing immunoglogulin Y (IgY) are available for use in the dog and there is evidence to support improved weight gain in colostrum fed neonates receiving IgY supplementation during the first 8 hours of life. Further studies are needed to define the therapeutic role of IgY when there is a failure of passive transfer.

KEY POINTS: CLINICAL MONITORING TOOLS

- A variety of clinical tools for monitoring the neonate are available; many of which can be performed in the home environment, and by the lay person
- Birth weight and weight gain, especially for the first 7 to 10 days of life, is an excellent marker of canine neonatal health
- Modified canine APGAR and neonatal viability reflex (NVR) scores can be used to identify neonates that benefit from assistance and monitor response to intervention
- Neonates should be monitored to ensure colostrum ingestion within the first 8 hours of life
- Reference ranges for the canine neonate should be used when interpreting hematologic and biochemical data

• Biological fluids, the microbiome, and IgY administration are current areas of research with respect to neonatal health

THE NEONATAL TRIAD

The neonatal triad is an elegant term that refers to 3 clinical signs often associated with sepsis and clinical demise in canine neonates: hypothermia, hypoglycemia, and dehydration. The normal canine neonate is active, vocal, and vigorously seeks to nurse. Sick canine neonates have low vigor and do not nurse robustly or seek out warmth; without nutritional support and warming, the neonatal triad develops placing neonates at great risk for sepsis and demise. Although not pathognomonic for neonatal sepsis, diarrhea is known to be present in 93% of canine neonates with sepsis; for this reason, the perineal area should be closely monitored for signs of diarrhea such as wetness, staining, proctitis, or erythema.[11] Changes to mucous membrane color, swelling or erythema of the umbilicus or abdomen, extremity changes such as sloughing, and the failure to gain weight, are other clinician signs associated with canine neonatal sepsis.[9–11]

Hypothermia

The canine neonate is poikilothermic (lacks the ability to generate heat). Shivering and vasoconstrictive reflexes are not functional in the newborn.[93] Body temperature is known to have a dramatic effect on gastrointestinal movement, and at rectal temperatures less than 94° F (34.4°C), ileus occurs, which increases the risk of aspiration pneumonia. Hypothermic neonates are at increased risk of infection.[93] Well-established heat-seeking behavior in the neonate is typically able to maintain a stable rectal temperature providing there is access to available heat sources. The risk of hypothermia is greater for low-birth-weight neonates due to a higher body surface area-to-mass ratio. For this reason, neonates with lower birth weights (lower quartile), and/or neonates born to litters with high birth-weight variability, should be provided with supplemental heat forms.[10,15,64] To decrease the risk of thermal burns, direct contact with any heat source should be avoided; heating pads (whether electronic or microwavable gel) should always be covered. Maintenance of a temperature gradient in the nursery

Table 11
Reference intervals for the canine neonate using a point-of-care analyzer and whole blood

Analyte	Age			
	4 d	**10–12 d**	**16 d**	**28 d**
pH	7.36–7.60	7.39–7.52	7.34–7.53	7.36–7.50
Na (mmol/L)	136.1–148.9	138.8–146.0	140.9–145.6	141.3–145.6
K (mmol/L)	3.90–5.20	4.10–5.30	4.40–5.80	4.10–5.70
Cl (mmol/L	101.1–107.5	105.2–110.8	105.8–111.9	105.5–112.1
iCa (mmol/L)	1.31–1.61	1.42–1.59	1.45–1.61	1.46–1.59
Glucose (mg/dL)	70.9–136.2	94.2–148.0	107/9–144.9	118.4–147.2
BUN (mg/dL)	10.1–26.8	13.6–24.5	8.7–18.6	0.0–16.2
HCO_3 (mmol/L)	26.1–33.6	24.2–29.9	23.8–31.5	21.9–31.5

From O'Brien MA, McMichael MA, Le Boedec K, Lees G. Reference intervals and age-related changes for venous biochemical, hematological, electrolytic, and blood gas variables using a point of care analyzer in 68 puppies. *J Vet Emerg Crit Care (San Antonio).* 2014;24(3):291 to 301. https://doi.org/10.1111/vec.12162

Table 12
Normal biochemical chemistry values for canine neonates

	Age		
Biochemical Parameter	0–3 d	8–10 d	28–33 d
Albumin (g/dL)	1.76–2.75	1.71–2.5	2.17–2.97
ALP (U/L)	452–6358	195–768	153–490
ALT (U/L)	9.1–42.2	4.1–21.4	4.3–17.4
Bilirubin (mg/dL)	0.04–0.38	0.01–0.18	0.02–0.15
BUN (mg/dL)	29.5–118	29.1–66.7	13.1–46.2
Total Ca (mg/dL)	10.4–13.6	11.2–13.2	10.4–13.2
Cholesterol (mg/dL)	90–234	158–340	177–392
Creatinine (mg/dL)	0.37–1.06	0.28–0.42	0.25–0.83
GGT (U/L)	163–3558	–	–
GLDH (U/L)	1.8–17.0	0.2–17.7	1.2–9.0
Glucose (mg/dL)	76–155	101–161	121–158
Total protein (g/dL)	3.7–5.77	3.26–4.37	3.71–4.81
Triglycerides (mg/dL)	45–248	52–220	36–149
Phosphorous (mg/dL)	5.26–10.83	8.35–11.14	8.66–11.45

From von Dehn B. Pediatric clinical pathology.Vet Clin North Am Small Anim Pract. 2014;44(2):205 to 219. https://doi.org/10.1016/j.cvsm.2013.10.003

area is advantageous as it allows neonates to move as needed and can help reduce over-heating; this can be difficult to achieve if using heated air for thermal support. Ambient temperature can rise quickly in contained environments and judicious temperature monitoring at the level of the neonate is advised.

Hypoglycemia

At birth, placental glucose support is terminated, and the neonate is reliant on endogenous food stores for glucose production. Colostrum provides a calorie dense initial energy source for the neonate (1400–1800 kcal/L).[94] The canine neonate is capable of glycogenolysis and gluconeogenesis but has limited glycogen stores and ability to maintain serum glucose concentrations as compared to the adult: normal serum glucose concentrations are lower than the adult and neonates require regular feeding to maintain blood glucose concentrations.[93,95,96] Nutritional requirements in the dam must be met as energy deficits in the dam will negatively impact glucose production in the neonate.[95]

From a clinical lens, prolonged hypoglycemia in the early neonate should raise concern for sepsis, and the underlying cause treated.[11] Other differentials include juvenile hypoglycemia in toy breeds, hepatic vascular anomalies, and storage diseases. Oral glucose supplementation may be considered for non-nursing or symptomatic neonates short-term; high concentrations of dextrose can cause phlebitis, and intravenous access can be challenging. More complete nutritional support such as frozen-thawed canine milk or milk replacer is advised longer term. Feeding guidelines may be found in section 6.2 of this article, and [Nutrition for the Pregnant Bitch and Puppies by Wakshlag and Kim] of this issue).

Dehydration

Neonates are predisposed to dehydration as compared to the adult dog for several reasons; they have a high surface area to body weight ratio, inability to concentrate urine, and increased skin permeability.[7] Hydration is difficult to evaluate in the canine neonate as skin turgor is unreliable, and mucous membranes may be tacky from dried milk.[93] As red blood cell concentration is higher in the neonate, measurement of packed cell volume is not also particularly clinically useful. Daily fluid requirements for the canine neonate are best via oral liquid nutrition; gastric volume may be estimated based on body weight at 4 mL per 100-g body weight.[33] If intravenous fluid therapy is needed, fluids should be warmed to body temperature prior to administration to avoid contributing to hypothermia. Daily fluid requirements are higher in the early neonate (80–120 mLs/kg/d or 4–5 mLs/kg/h) and decrease to that of an adult dog by around 4 months of age.[97]

KEY POINTS: THE NEONATAL TRIAD

The neonatal triad refers to three clinical signs associated with clinical demise in the neonate: hypothermia, hypoglycemia, and dehydration.

INFECTIOUS DISEASE

Effective passive transfer of immunoglobins plays an important role in the prevention of infectious disease in the neonate; but not all infections, for example, internal and external parasites, are able to be prevented this way. The use of preventative care measures such as heartworm prophylaxis, basic hygiene, and environmental barriers such as outside shoe removal in the nursery area can minimize neonate exposure.

When losses do occur, it's helpful to have tissue samples for analysis. The placenta, which is often discarded after delivery, represents the maternal – fetal interface and can be used to problem solve causes of reproductive and neonatal loss. Placental tissue can be stored chilled for 1 to 3 days post-partum and submitted for histology, PCR, and/or culture. As zoonotic diseases such as *Brucella canis* can concentrate in the placenta, risk: benefit assessment and strict handling guidelines should be communicated to owners to prevent the transmission of zoonotic disease. Canine tissue should never be stored in a cooling unit or container used to store items for human consumption. The reader is referred elsewhere for additional recommendations and further discussion (see [Pathology of Neonatal Disorders by Agnew and Wiliams] in this issue).

Sepsis and canine herpesvirus are 2 diagnoses associated with neonatal loss: For both conditions, early monitoring and preventative measures improve canine neonatal health outcomes.

Sepsis

Sepsis in the canine neonate presents differently as compared to the adult dog. Successful treatment is dependent upon early identification and appropriate treatment. Clinical signs consistent with canine neonatal sepsis include: the neonatal triad, low NVR scores, diarrhea, proctitis, cyanotic mucous membranes or extremities, necrosis of the extremities, omphalitis/omphalophlebitis, weight loss, and lethargy.[11] **Table 13** provides further detail regarding the frequency of clinical signs associated with neonatal sepsis.

In one study, *Escherichia coli* was noted to be the most common bacterial agent associated with sepsis. Treatment of consists of antimicrobial and fluid support, thermoregulatory support, and maintenance of nutrition. Broad-spectrum beta-lactams such as potentiated amoxicillin, ceftriaxone, or ceftiofur are appropriate for use in

Table 13
Frequency of clinical signs presented by neonates with sepsis

Clinical signs	N	(%)
Hypothermia	(65/113)	57.5%
Hypoglycemia	(74/113)	65.5%
Dehydration	(72/113)	63.7%
Apathy	(52/113)	46%
Reduced muscle tone	(56/113)	49.5%
Reduced sucking reflex	(70/113)	62%
Reduced rooting reflex	(67/113)	59.2%
Reduced vestibular righting	(55/113)	48.6%
Vocalization	(17/113)	15%
Failure to gain weight[a]	(37/113)	32.7%
Hyperthermia	(8/113)	7%
Congested or cyanotic mucous membranes	(59/113)	52.2%
Diarrhea	(105/113)	93%
Bloody diarrhea	(18/113)	16%
Hematuria	(26/113)	23%
Vomiting	(5/113)	4.4%
Procitis	(32/113)	28.3%
Abdominal/body erythema	(77/113)	68.1%
Omphalitis/omphalophlebitis	(29/113)	25.6%
Neonatal conjunctivitis/opthalmia	(12/113)	10.6%
Mucopurulent nasal discharge/pneumonia	(4/113)	3.5%
Skin desquamation (scaled skin syndrome)	(5/113)	4.4%
Abscesses	(9/113)	8%
Seizures	(5/113)	4.4%
Abdominal bruises or hematomas	(16/113)	14.1%
Violaceous (cyanotic) extremities of limbs, tail, or ears	(33/113)	29.2%
Tissue necrosis in limbs, pads and other body extremities	(15/113)	13.2%
Bradycardia	(62/113)	54.8%
Dyspnea	(22/113)	19.4%
Bradypnea	(19/113)	16.8%
Agonal breathing	(19/113)	16.8%
Epistaxis	(7/113)	6.2%
Pale mucous membranes	(16/113)	14.1%
Oliguria/anuria	(19/113)	16.8%
Reduced peripheral So_2	(31/113)	27.4%

[a] Failure to gain weight was described only in litters whose weight was recorded daily by owners.
From Nobre Pacifico Pereira KH, Fuchs KDM, Hibaru VY, et al. Neonatal sepsis in dogs: Incidence, clinical aspects and mortality. *Theriogenology*. 2022;177:103 to 115. https://doi.org/10.1016/j.theriogenology.2021.10.015

the neonate. Administration of subcutaneous or oral medication, fluid support, and nutrients may be sufficient for some cases of sepsis; however, for those patients presenting moribund or in septic shock, intravenous access is advised. Clinical markers delineating sepsis from septic shock are shown in **Table 14**. Intravenous drug

Table 14			
Useful clinical markers for the differentiation of sepsis versus septic shock in the canine neonate. Values listed are mean and standard deviation			
Parameter	Healthy	Sepsis	Septic Shock
HR (bpm)	238 ± 19.5[a]	200 ± 7.68[b]	110 ± 44.3[c]
Blood glucose (mg/dL)	125.4 ± 22.6[a]	81 ± 36.5[b]	37.6 ± 32.3[c]
Temperature (°C)	36 ± 0.61[a]	34 ± 1.6[b]	32.5 ± 0.85[c]
Peripheral spO2 (%)	99 ± 0[a]	98.6 ± 0.65[a]	66.2 ± 19.8[b]
Reflex Score	5.9 ± 0.44[a]	3.9 ± 0.40[b]	0.4 ± 0.46[c]

Abbreviations: HR heart rate, bpm beats per minute.
[a] Means followed by different letter indicate significant differences among the evaluated groups (*P* < .05).
[b] Means followed by different letter indicate significant differences among the evaluated groups (*P* < .05).
[c] Means followed by different letter indicate significant differences among the evaluated groups (*P* < .05).
From Nobre Pacifico Pereira KH, Fuchs KDM, Hibaru VY, et al. Neonatal sepsis in dogs: Incidence, clinical aspects and mortality. *Theriogenology.* 2022;177:103 to 115. https://doi.org/10.1016/j.theriogenology.2021.10.015

administration should be considered until clinical improvement is noted. Depending on the body-weight and physiological status of the canine neonate, standard peripheral venous access may be possible; however, for some patients, the use of jugular or intra-osseous routes may be required. **Tables 15** and **16** provide information regarding fluid rates, and antimicrobial dosing for the neonate.

Herpesvirus

Canine herpesvirus (CHV-1) is an alpha herpesvirus capable of causing disease in a variety of organ systems.[98] Neonatal losses occur when an immunologically naïve bitch is infected for the first time during the last 3 weeks of pregnancy, or when neonates born to an immunologically naïve bitch are infected during the first weeks of life. Two strategies can be implemented to minimize this risk: (a) pre-breeding screening to identify seronegative females so that they may be isolated during pregnancy and for 6 weeks post-partum, as discussed in this issue (see [Canine pregnancy, eutocia, and dystocia by Davidson and Cain] in this issue) (b) vaccination of the bitch prior after breeding, and 6 weeks later if canine CHV-1 vaccination is available. Biosecurity

Table 15	
Fluid bolus rates for the canine neonate	
Fluid	Rate
Bolus: Hypovolemia	3–4 mL/100 gm body weight
Bolus: Hypoglycemia	1 mL to 3 mL of 12.5% dextrose[a]
Bolus: Colloid	2 mL/kg to 5 mL/kg, followed by 1 mL/kg/h as needed[b]
Whole blood (*for anemia correction*)	10–20 mL/kg

[a] 1:3 dilution of 50% dextrose with sterile water.
[b] After crystalloid boluses have failed.
Adapted from Lee JA, Cohn LA. Fluid Therapy for Pediatric Patients. *Vet Clin North Am Small Anim Pract.* 2017;47(2):373 to 382. https://doi.org/10.1016/j.cvsm.2016.09.010

Table 16
Select drug dosing for the canine neonate

Class	Drug	Dose	Notes:
Antimicrobial[a]	Amoxicillin/Clavulanic acid	20 mg/kg PO q 12 hr	• The author prefers Ceftiofur 2.5 mg/kg SC q 12 h for no more than 5 consecutive days
	Ceftiofur	2.2–4.4 mg/kg SC q 12 hr	
Analgesic[b]	Buprenorphine	0.005–0.010 mg/kg SC q 6 hr	• Pediatric dose is shown; lower doses are advised in the neonate and dosing should be titrated up to effect
	Butorphanol	0.1–0.2 mg/kg SC q 1–4 hr	• Naloxone should always be available when using an opioid in a canine neonate
	Hydromorphone	0.05–0.1 mg/kg SC q 2–4 hr	• SC dosing is advised for the canine neonate, but listed doses may be administered IM, or slow IV
	Methadone	0.1–0.5 mg/kg SC q 1–4 hr	
	Morphine	0.1–0.5 mg/kg SC q 1–4 hr	

Abbreviations: hr hour, IM intramuscular; IV intravenous, kg kg; mg mg, PO per esophagus/by mouth; SC subcutaneous.

[a] *From* Nobre Pacifico Pereira KH, Fuchs KDM, Hibaru VY, et al. Neonatal sepsis in dogs: Incidence, clinical aspects and mortality. *Theriogenology.* 2022;177:103 to 115. https://doi.org/10.1016/j.theriogenology.2021.10.015.
[b] *Adapted from* Mathews KA. pain management for the pregnant, lactating, and neonatal to pediatric cat and dog. *Vet Clin North Am Small Anim Pract.* 2008;38(6):1291-vii. https://doi.org/10.1016/j.cvsm.2008.07.001.

measures are an important preventative management strategy for kennels within the United States where vaccination is not possible, as the introduction of new breeding stock presents a risk for both CHV-1, and other infectious disease.[99]

The clinical course of CHV-1 infection in the canine neonate varies depending on when infection occurs. Transplacental infection generally results in *in utero* death; specifically, mummification or stillbirth or neonatal infection. As the incubation period is 6 to 10 days, neonates infected with CHV-1 during the first week of life were most likely infected *in utero*. Post-natal transmission occurs via contact with mucosal secretions; both vaginal and oro-nasal secretions from the dam and infected littermates are potential sources. Clinical disease in the neonate is typically fatal despite intervention.

The most frequently observed clinical signs include: poor weight gain; abdominal pain; dyspnea; diarrhea; nasal discharge; and petechiation or echymosis. Treatment options are limited. Antiviral therapy has been described (oral acyclovir solution at 10 mg/kg PO q 6 hr for 5–7 days).[100] Although not frequently discussed, neonates do feel pain and analgesia may be warranted. **Table 16** provides analgesia options for the canine neonate.CHV-1 replication is supported at temperature ranges between 91.4 and 85°F (33–35°C): Anti-viral treatment in conjunction with increased ambient temperatures is currently the best option to decrease mortality especially if implemented prior to exposure. Necropsy of affected puppies, and/or PCR screening confirms the diagnosis (see [Pathology of Neonatal Disorders by Agnew and Wiliams] in this issue). Once a bitch has been exposed, subsequent immune response and passive transfer of anti-CHV-1 immunogluobulins is expected. Where available, the administration of CHV-1 booster vaccination is advised for each breeding cycle.

KEY POINTS: INFECTIOUS DISEASE

- The clinical signs of sepsis are different for the canine neonate as compared to the adult dog
- The frequency of clinical signs associated with neonatal sepsis may be found in **Table 13**, and septic shock in **Table 14**
- Broad-spectrum beta-lactams are the antimicrobial of choice for the septic neonate
- The breeding bitch should be screened for antibodies to CHV-1 and vaccinated where possible prior to breeding
- Neonatal infection with CHV-1 is typically fatal; treatment options are limited to supportive care, acyclovir, and increased ambient temperature

CLINICAL APPROACH TO THE NEONATE

The 2 most important components of health for the early neonate are oxygenation and temperature. Hypoxemia and hypothermia, especially during the first 2 days of life, trigger a cascade of physiological events that ultimately threaten life. As neonates are typically in the home environment during this life-phase, and owners sometimes reluctant to separate them from the bitch and transport them to a veterinary clinic, owner education becomes a major factor in the ability of a veterinarian to influence neonatal health outcomes. Essential components of care include the following: umbilical cord care; neonate identification for weight monitoring; initial birth weight and daily weight recording for at least the first 10 days; APGAR score assignment at birth; and use of correct resuscitation methods such as airway suctiion and warming.

The late neonate (3 days – weaning) experiences dramatic growth, and continued organ development. During this time developmental abnormalities may become more apparent. Infectious diseases continue to be a risk during as the canine neonate's immune system is immature, and environmental exposure to pathogens increases along with the ability to ambulate. Essential components of care include the following: hygiene maintenance; daily weight recording for at least the first 10 days; 7-day APGAR score evaluation; monitoring for clinical signs of sepsis; and maintenance of an adequate plane of nutrition for the dam.

CLINICS CARE POINTS

- History Taking
  When evaluating a neonate, it's important to obtain as much information as possible from the owner. For the canine neonate, detailed history taking can help clinicians make diagnoses such as failure of passive transfer (*lack of colostrum intake at birth*), Brucella Canis (*intermittent litter losses*), or aspiration secondary to hyperthermia and ileus (*outside housing*).
- Clinical Tools (Dam)
  - Progesterone: For the normal canine pregnancy, a maternal serum progesterone concentration less than 2 ng/mL is a clinical marker of adequate fetal lung development.
  - Labor: More favorable neonate outcomes are associated with stage II labor less than 12 hours in duration.
- Clinical Tools (Neonate)
  - Birth Weight: At birth, neonates should be individually identified, and their body weight recorded. This forms a baseline for weight gain/loss in the first week of life.
  - APGAR scores: A neonate with an initial APGAR score less than 3 is considered "critical": these neonates should receive resuscitation efforts, active warming, and nutritional support. Subsequent APGAR scores are used to assess the response to intervention.
  - Colostrum Ingestion: Passive transfer is dependent upon the ingestion of 1.3 mLs colostrum per 100-g body weight by mouth during the first 8 hours of life. When intake is impaired, 2 to 4 mL per 100-g body weight may give given subcutaneously, divided between two sites.
  - Weight Gain/Loss: Weight loss greater than 4% of birth weight in the first 24 hours is a risk factor for mortality and evaluation by a veterinarian is indicated. Expected daily weight gain is 5% to 10% for the first week, with birth weight doubling by 7 to 10 days of age.
  - Daily Caloric Requirement: Neonate caloric requirements are estimated to be 200 kcal per kilogram of body weight up to 4 weeks of age.

DISCLOSURE

The Author is currently employed by Banfield Pet Hospital. The views expressed do not necessarily represent those of Banfield.

ACKNOWLEDGMENTS

Gina Cooke, PhD and Autumn Davidson, DVM, DACVIM.

REFERENCES

1. Brown CR, Garrett LD, Gilles WK, et al. Spectrum of care: more than treatment options. J Am Vet Med Assoc 2021;259(7):712–7.
2. Mackenzie JS, Jeggo M. The One Health Approach-Why Is It So Important? Trop Med Infect Dis 2019;4(2):88.

3. Groppetti D, Pecile A, Del Carro AP, et al. Evaluation of newborn canine viability by means of umbilical vein lactate measurement, apgar score and uterine tocodynamometry. Theriogenology 2010;74(7):1187–96.
4. Mila H, Guerard C, Raymond-Letron I. Guidelines for *postmortem* examination of newborn dogs. Anim Health Res Rev 2021;22(2):109–19.
5. Uchańska O, Ochota M, Eberhardt M, et al. Dead or Alive? A Review of Perinatal Factors That Determine Canine Neonatal Viability. Animals (Basel) 2022;12(11):1402.
6. Lewis C, Short C, Freund W. A new Latin dictionary: founded on the translation of freund's Latin-German lexicon. Harper; 1891. https://archive.org/details/LewisShortLatnDiccionary.
7. Lawler DF. Neonatal and pediatric care of the puppy and kitten. Theriogenology 2008;70(3):384–92.
8. Papich MG, Davis LE. Drug therapy during pregnancy and in the neonate. Vet Clin North Am Small Anim Pract 1986;16(3):525–38.
9. Davidson AP. Neonatal resuscitation: improving the outcome. Vet Clin North Am Small Anim Pract 2014;44(2):191–204.
10. Grundy SA. Clinically relevant physiology of the neonate. Vet Clin North Am Small Anim Pract 2006;36(3):443.
11. Nobre Pacifico Pereira KH, Fuchs KDM, Hibaru VY, et al. Neonatal sepsis in dogs: Incidence, clinical aspects and mortality. Theriogenology 2022;177:103–15.
12. Gill MA. Perinatal and late neonatal mortality in the dog. PhD Thesis. 2001. Faculty of Veterinary Science, University of Sydney, Australia. http://hdl.handle.net/2123/4137
13. Chastant-Maillard S, Guillemot C, Feugier A, et al. Reproductive performance and pre-weaning mortality: Preliminary analysis of 27,221 purebred female dogs and 204,537 puppies in France. Reprod Domest Anim 2017;52(Suppl 2):158–62.
14. Veronesi MC, Panzani S, Faustini M, et al. An Apgar scoring system for routine assessment of newborn puppy viability and short-term survival prognosis. Theriogenology 2009;72(3):401–7.
15. Mugnier A, Mila H, Guiraud F, et al. Birth weight as a risk factor for neonatal mortality: Breed-specific approach to identify at-risk puppies. Prev Vet Med 2019;171:104746.
16. Chastant-Maillard S, Aggouni C, Albaret A, et al. Canine and feline colostrum. Reprod Domest Anim 2017;52(Suppl 2):148–52.
17. Mila H. Neonatal Period In The Dog: Immunological And Nutritional Determinants For Survival. Sciences Ecologiques, Vétérinaires, Agronomiques et Bioingénieries (SEVAB), Université du Toulouse, September 2015. https://oatao.univ-toulouse.fr/15972/1/Mila.pdf
18. Mugnier A, Chastant S, Saegerman C, et al. Management of Low Birth Weight in Canine and Feline Species: Breeder Profiling. Animals (Basel) 2021;11(10):2953.
19. Mila H, Grellet A, Mariani C, et al. Natural and artificial hyperimmune solutions: Impact on health in puppies. Reprod Domest Anim 2017;52(Suppl 2):163–9.
20. Bartges J, Boynton B, Vogt AH, et al. AAHA canine life stage guidelines. J Am Anim Hosp Assoc 2012;48(1):1–11.
21. Münnich A, Küchenmeister U. Causes, diagnosis and therapy of common diseases in neonatal puppies in the first days of life: cornerstones of practical approach. Reprod Domest Anim 2014;49(Suppl 2):64–74.

22. de Almeida LL, Abreu RA, Brito MM, et al. Both spontaneous vaginal delivery and elective caesarean section influence neonatal redox status in dogs. Vet Rec 2022;190(5):e1082.
23. Rishniw M, Freeman KP. Clinical pathologists should limit modifier terms used to denote probability of a diagnosis: a survey-based study [published online ahead of print, 2023 Feb 2]. J Am Vet Med Assoc 2023;1–8. https://doi.org/10.2460/javma.22.11.0488.
24. Pereira KHNP, Fuchs KDM, Corrêa JV, et al. Neonatology: Topics on Puppies and Kittens Neonatal Management to Improve Neonatal Outcome. Animals (Basel) 2022;12(23):3426.
25. Mila H, Feugier A, Grellet A, et al. Inadequate passive immune transfer in puppies: definition, risk factors and prevention in a large multi-breed kennel. Prev Vet Med 2014;116(1–2):209–13.
26. Fore J Jr, Wiechers IR, Cook-Deegan R. The effects of business practices, licensing, and intellectual property on development and dissemination of the polymerase chain reaction: case study. J Biomed Discov Collab 2006;1:7.
27. Olson PN, Hall MF, Peterson JK, et al. Using genetic technologies for promoting canine health and temperament. Anim Reprod Sci 2004;82-83:225–30.
28. Dziuk E. CHIC–the Canine Health Information Center. Theriogenology 2007;68(3):375–7.
29. Traas AM, Casal M, Haskins M, et al. Genetic counseling in the era of molecular diagnostics. Theriogenology 2006;66(3):599–605.
30. Goldstein RE, Atwater DZ, Cazolli DM, et al. Inheritance, mode of inheritance, and candidate genes for primary hyperparathyroidism in Keeshonden. J Vet Intern Med 2007;21(1):199–203.
31. Greco DS. Nutritional supplements for pregnant and lactating bitches. Theriogenology 2008;70(3):393–6.
32. Oberbauer AM, Daniels R, Levy K, et al. Maternal omega-3 polyunsaturated fatty acid supplementation on offspring hip joint conformation. PLoS One 2018;13(8):e0202157.
33. Chastant S, Mila H. Passive immune transfer in puppies. Anim Reprod Sci 2019;207:162–70.
34. Veronesi MC, Fusi J. Biochemical factors affecting newborn survival in dogs and cats. Theriogenology 2023;197:150–8.
35. Kutzler M, Volkmann D. Fetal lung development and surfactant production in the dog. In: Proceedings of the 6th ISCFR symposium. Vienna, Austria: University of Veterinary Sciences; 2008. p. 13–5.
36. Catlin EA, Powell SM, Manganaro TF, et al. Sex-specific fetal lung development and müllerian inhibiting substance. Am Rev Respir Dis 1990;141(2):466–70.
37. Suprith D, Unnikrishnan M, Kurien M, et al. Assessment of foetal lung surfactant in amniotic fluid of dogs by bubble test, to evaluate foetal maturity. J Vet Anim Sci 2020;51(2):128–31.
38. Groppetti D, Martino PA, Ravasio G, et al. Prognostic potential of amniotic fluid analysis at birth on canine neonatal outcomes. Vet J 2015;206(3):423–5.
39. Arlt SP. The bitch around parturition. Theriogenology 2020;150:452–7.
40. Münnich A. The pathological newborn in small animals: the neonate is not a small adult. Vet Res Commun 2008;32(Suppl 1):S81–5.
41. Tønnessen R, Borge KS, Nødtvedt A, et al. Canine perinatal mortality: a cohort study of 224 breeds. Theriogenology 2012;77(9):1788–801.
42. Davidson AP. Uterine and fetal monitoring in the bitch. Vet Clin North Am Small Anim Pract 2001;31(2):305–13.

43. Gil EM, Garcia DA, Giannico AT, et al. Canine fetal heart rate: do accelerations or decelerations predict the parturition day in bitches? Theriogenology 2014; 82(7):933–41.
44. Zone MA, Wanke MM. Diagnosis of canine fetal health by ultrasonography. J Reprod Fertil Suppl 2001;57:215–9.
45. Swann HG, Christian JJ, Hamilton C. The process of anoxic death in newborn pups. Surg Gynecol Obstet 1954;99(1):5–8.
46. Cassin S, Swann HG, Cassin B. Respiratory and cardiovascular alterations during the process of anoxic death in the newborn. J Appl Physiol 1960;15:249–52.
47. Goodwin W. Anesthesia for Pediatric Patients. Today's Veterinary Technician 2017;39–46. https://todaysveterinarynurse.com/wp-content/uploads/sites/3/2017/09/FarryGoodwin_PediatricAnesthesia_TVTechSepOct2017.pdf.
48. Zakošek Pipan M, Kajdič L, Kalin A, et al. Do newborn puppies have their own microbiota at birth? Influence of type of birth on newborn puppy microbiota. Theriogenology 2020;152:18–28.
49. Kajdič L, Plavec T, Zdovc I, et al. Impact of Type of Parturition on Colostrum Microbiota Composition and Puppy Survival. Animals (Basel) 2021;11(7):1897.
50. Del Carro A, Corrò M, Bertero A, et al. The evolution of dam-litter microbial flora from birth to 60 days of age. BMC Vet Res 2022;18(1):95.
51. Lelli JL Jr, Drongowski RA, Coran AG, et al. Hypoxia-induced bacterial translocation in the puppy. J Pediatr Surg 1992;27(8):974–82.
52. Grundy SA, Liu SM, Davidson AP. Intracranial trauma in a dog due to being "swung" at birth. Top Companion Anim Med 2009;24(2):100–3.
53. Fox M. The ontogeny of behaviour and neurologic responses in the dog. Anim Behav 1964;12:301–10.
54. Skarda RT. Anesthesia case of the month. Dystocia, cesarean section and acupuncture resuscitation of newborn kittens. J Am Vet Med Assoc 1999; 214(1):37–9.
55. Haddad GG, Mellins RB. Hypoxia and respiratory control in early life. Annu Rev Physiol 1984;46:629–43.
56. Kruszynski S, Stanaitis K, Brandes J, et al. Doxapram stimulates respiratory activity through distinct activation of neurons in the nucleus hypoglossus and the pre-Bötzinger complex. J Neurophysiol 2019;121(4):1102–10.
57. De Cramer KGM, Joubert KE, Nöthling JO. Puppy survival and vigor associated with the use of low dose medetomidine premedication, propofol induction and maintenance of anesthesia using sevoflurane gas-inhalation for cesarean section in the bitch. Theriogenology 2017;96:10–5.
58. Vilar JM, Batista M, Pérez R, et al. Comparison of 3 anesthetic protocols for the elective cesarean-section in the dog: Effects on the bitch and the newborn puppies. Anim Reprod Sci 2018;190:53–62.
59. Schmidt K, Feng C, Wu T, et al. Influence of maternal, anesthetic, and surgical factors on neonatal survival after emergency cesarean section in 78 dogs: A retrospective study (2002 to 2020). Can Vet J 2021;62(9):961–8.
60. Melandri M, Alonge S, Peric T, et al. Effects of Alfaxalone or Propofol on Giant-Breed Dog Neonates Viability During Elective Caesarean Sections. Animals (Basel) 2019;9(11):962.
61. Roos J, Maenhoudt C, Zilberstein L, et al. Neonatal puppy survival after planned caesarean section in the bitch using aglepristone as a primer: A retrospective study on 74 cases. Reprod Domest Anim 2018;53(Suppl 3):85–95.
62. Groppetti D, Di Cesare F, Pecile A, et al. Maternal and neonatal wellbeing during elective C-section induced with a combination of propofol and

dexmedetomidine: How effective is the placental barrier in dogs? Theriogenology 2019;129:90–8.

63. Antończyk A, Ochota M. Is an epidural component during general anaesthesia for caesarean section beneficial for neonatal puppies' health and vitality? Theriogenology 2022;187:1–8.

64. Traas AM. Resuscitation of canine and feline neonates. Theriogenology 2008; 70(3):343–8.

65. Mugnier A, Chastant S, Lyazrhi F, et al. Definition of low birth weight in domestic mammals: a scoping review [published online ahead of print, 2023 Jan 13]. Anim Health Res Rev 2023;1–8. https://doi.org/10.1017/S146625232200007X.

66. Mugnier A, Chastant-Maillard S, Mila H, et al. Low and very low birth weight in puppies: definitions, risk factors and survival in a large-scale population. BMC Vet Res 2020;16(1):354.

67. Wilsman NJ, Van Sickle DC. Weight change patterns as a basis for predicting survival of newborn Pointer pups. J Am Vet Med Assoc 1973;163(8):971–5.

68. Alves I. A model of puppy growth during the first three weeks. Vet Med Sci 2020; 6(4):946–57.

69. Heinze CR, Freeman LM, Martin CR, et al. Comparison of the nutrient composition of commercial dog milk replacers with that of dog milk. J Am Vet Med Assoc 2014;244(12):1413–22.

70. Prosser CG. Compositional and functional characteristics of goat milk and relevance as a base for infant formula. J Food Sci 2021;86(2):257–65.

71. Kirk CA. New concepts in pediatric nutrition. Vet Clin North Am Small Anim Pract 2001;31(2):369–92.

72. Committee Opinion No. 644: The Apgar Score. Obstet Gynecol 2015;126(4): e52–5.

73. Veronesi MC. Assessment of canine neonatal viability-the Apgar score. Reprod Domest Anim 2016;51(Suppl 1):46–50.

74. Titkova R, Fialkovicova M, Karasova M, et al. Puppy Apgar scores after vaginal delivery and caesarean section. Vet Med (Praha) 2017;62(9):488–92.

75. Doebeli A, Michel E, Bettschart R, et al. Apgar score after induction of anesthesia for canine cesarean section with alfaxalone versus propofol. Theriogenology 2013;80(8):850–4.

76. Antończyk A, Ochota M, Niżański W. Umbilical Cord Blood Gas Parameters and Apgar Scoring in Assessment of New-Born Dogs Delivered by Cesarean Section. Animals (Basel) 2021;11(3):685.

77. Veronesi MC, Faustini M, Probo M, et al. Refining the APGAR Score Cutoff Values and Viability Classes According to Breed Body Size in Newborn Dogs. Animals (Basel) 2022;12(13):1664.

78. Batista M, Moreno C, Vilar J, et al. Neonatal viability evaluation by Apgar score in puppies delivered by cesarean section in two brachycephalic breeds (English and French bulldog). Anim Reprod Sci 2014;146(3–4):218–26.

79. Vassalo FG, Simões CR, Sudano MJ, et al. Topics in the routine assessment of newborn puppy viability. Top Companion Anim Med 2015;30(1):16–21.

80. Heird WC, Schwarz SM, Hansen IH. Colostrum-induced enteric mucosal growth in beagle puppies. Pediatr Res 1984;18(6):512–5.

81. Mila H, Feugier A, Grellet A, et al. Immunoglobulin G concentration in canine colostrum: Evaluation and variability. J Reprod Immunol 2015;112:24–8.

82. Arteaga L, Rödel H, Elizalde M, et al. The Pattern of Nipple Use Before Weaning Among Littermates of the Domestic Dog. Ethology 2013;119(1):12–9.

83. Viaud, Camille. Le Comportement de Tetee Du Chiot et Son Implication Dans Le Transfert Passif de l'immunite. Theeee d'exercice. Ecole Nationale Veterinaire de Toulouse - ENVT; 2018. http://oatao.univ-toulouse.fr/

84. Bouchard G, Plata-Madrid H, Youngquist RS, et al. Absorption of an alternate source of immunoglobulin in pups. Am J Vet Res 1992;53(2):230–3.

85. Veronesi MC, Bolis B, Faustini M, et al. Biochemical composition of fetal fluids in at term, normal developed, healthy, viable dogs and preliminary data from pathologic littermates. Theriogenology 2018;108:277–83.

86. Bolis B, Prandi A, Rota A, et al. Cortisol fetal fluid concentrations in term pregnancy of small-sized purebred dogs and its preliminary relation to first 24 hours survival of newborns. Theriogenology 2017;88:264–9.

87. Bolis B, Scarpa P, Rota A, et al. Association of amniotic uric acid, glucose, lactate and creatinine concentrations and lactate/creatinine ratio with newborn survival in small-sized dogs - preliminary results. Acta Vet Hung 2018;66(1):125–36.

88. Miller I, Schlosser S, Palazzolo L, et al. Some more about dogs: Proteomics of neglected biological fluids. J Proteomics 2020;218:103724.

89. Groppetti D, Meazzi S, Filipe JFS, et al. Maternal and neonatal canine cortisol measurement in multiple matrices during the perinatal period: A pilot study. PLoS One 2021;16(7):e0254842.

90. Wang H, Yang GX, Hu Y, et al. Comprehensive human amniotic fluid metagenomics supports the sterile womb hypothesis. Sci Rep 2022;12(1):6875.

91. Rota A, Del Carro A, Bertero A, et al. Does Bacteria Colonization of Canine Newborns Start in the Uterus? Animals (Basel) 2021;11(5):1415.

92. Van Nguyen S, Umeda K, Yokoyama H, et al. Passive protection of dogs against clinical disease due to Canine parvovirus-2 by specific antibody from chicken egg yolk. Can J Vet Res 2006;70(1):62–4.

93. The neonate—from birth to weaning. In: Johnston SD, Root Kustritz MV, Olson PNS, editors. Canine and feline theriogenology. 1st edition. Philadelphia: WB Saunders; 2001. p. 146–67.

94. Adkins Y, Lepine AJ, Lönnerdal B. Changes in protein and nutrient composition of milk throughout lactation in dogs. Am J Vet Res 2001;62(8):1266–72.

95. Kliegman RM, Miettinen EL, Adam PA. Fetal and neonatal responses to maternal canine starvation: circulating fuels and neonatal glucose production. Pediatr Res 1981;15(6):945–51.

96. Kliegman RM, Morton S. The metabolic response of the canine neonate to twenty-four hours of fasting. Metabolism 1987;36(6):521–6.

97. Lee JA, Cohn LA. Fluid Therapy for Pediatric Patients. Vet Clin North Am Small Anim Pract 2017;47(2):373–82.

98. Evermann JF, Ledbetter EC, Maes RK. Canine reproductive, respiratory, and ocular diseases due to canine herpesvirus. Vet Clin North Am Small Anim Pract 2011;41(6):1097–120.

99. Farrell J, Douglas J, Johnson A, et al. Canine herpes virus in a breeding kennel of Wirehaired Dachshund. Clinical Theriogenology 2020;12(3):431.

100. Davidson AP, Grundy SA, Foley JE. Successful medical management of neonatal canine herpesvirus: a case report. Commun Therio 2003;3:1–5.

Early Puppy Behavior
Tools for Later Success

Ericka Mendez, DVM

KEYWORDS

- Puppy • Behavior • Socialization • Bite prevention • Anxiety • Aggression
- Housetraining

KEY POINTS

- Early behavior strategies can positively influence a dog's life.
- Emotional stability can be fostered with early socialization and by building frustration tolerance.
- Good toileting habits can be formed by taking special care to keep the nest clean, by providing a toileting area within the play area, and by engaging in early potty training.
- Bite prevention training involves body handling exercises, food bowl exercises, and object exchange exercises.
- Early life skill training that teaches puppies how to rest calmly in a crate, come when called, and to sit politely when they want something can make puppyhood and adolescence easier for new puppy owners.

INTRODUCTION

The goals of reproductive medicine are to successfully manage the conception, pregnancy, and birth of healthy small animal pets. However, one should not forget that along with this goal comes an equally important goal, which is to create physically and emotionally healthy small animal companions that are capable of forging an unbreakable human-animal bond.

Veterinarians have the unique opportunity to guide and educate breeders with simple, yet effective early behavior strategies that encourage the creation of emotionally balanced adult pets. These pets will not only have a greater chance of experiencing an overall higher quality of life, they will also receive better and more extensive health care over the course of their lives, because they are better patients.

The 2-, 4-, 6-, and 8-week deworming schedule recommended for neonates gives veterinarians and their teams an opportunity to implement an educational program to help breeders learn about and incorporate these early behavior tools and strategies into their breeding and puppy raising practices (**Table 1**). There are advantages to

PO Box 15073, Daytona Beach, FL 32115, USA
E-mail address: erickamendezdvm@gmail.com

Vet Clin Small Anim 53 (2023) 1195–1207
https://doi.org/10.1016/j.cvsm.2023.05.009
0195-5616/23/© 2023 Elsevier Inc. All rights reserved.

Table 1
In-clinic early behavior program

Visit	Questions to Ask	Talking Points
Prenatal/puppy count visit	What does your whelping box look like? What is your birthing plan? Have you ever performed early neurological stimulation (ENS), Bio Sensor or Super Dog training with your litters?	Puppy hygiene Decreasing stress and anxiety in mother ENS and body handling
Neonatal examination and deworming week 2	How is nursing going? What kind of potty set up do you have? Do you have a relatively quiet or noisy household?	Frustration tolerance and fostering good mother-pup relationship Early housetraining set up Emotional resilience and the startle recovery cycle
Deworming week 4	How is weaning going? How is mealtime going? How is potty time going? What kind of things do you have in your puppy pen? Do the puppies ever spend time by themselves?	Fostering good mother-pup relationship Building frustration tolerance with obstacles, food bowl exercises, and recall Early housetraining skills Early socialization to objects Crate training
Deworming week 6	How is housetraining going? Have the puppies met any people or animals yet? How do the puppies behave when you try to take things away from them? How are the puppies behaving when it is time to be let out of their pen? What kind of games do you play with the puppies?	Early housetraining skills Early socialization to people and animals and how to do so safely Object exchange exercises Sit to say please Positive reward marker Learn to offer behavior
First vaccines and deworming week 8	How is housetraining going? What age are you planning on sending the puppies home? Do you know of a local trainer who has good puppy classes? What are the classes like?	Early housetraining skills Optimal go home age and go home routine Good puppy class guidelines

both parties when this type of behavior program is implemented. The breeder is creating puppies that have a greater chance of being well cared for and staying in their homes permanently, which fosters good word of mouth for buyers and potentially increasing value of the puppies because of the extra training and socialization. The veterinary team is not only helping to create better future patients, but they are also increasing revenue and becoming a valuable source of information for the breeder.

With a strong human animal bond in place, these dogs are more likely to be treated as beloved family members and can be potentially safeguarded from some of the more devastating behaviors that can weaken or destroy the human-animal bond, which can lead to neglect, abuse, abandonment, or euthanasia (**Table 2**).

DISCUSSION
Goals of Early Behavior Strategies

There are 4 key components to creating a companion animal that is capable of forming and sustaining a strong human-animal bond:

- Physical stability
- Emotional stability
- Good toileting habits
- Early life skill training

When speaking to breeders, it may become evident that some of them are already using some of these strategies. The goal, however, is for them to develop a process that works for them that they can then standardize to use in every litter so that it becomes a matter of procedure and planning instead of happenstance.

Physical stability
When considering physical stability, good breeding practices that create physically healthy offspring are essential. However, emotional stability should not be overlooked. Behavior tendencies such as fearfulness and anxiety have some degree of genetic heritability that can predispose offspring to nervous-type temperaments.[1]

Table 2	
Behaviors that can weaken the human-animal bond	
Aggression	• Family members • Strangers • Animals in household • Animals outside of household
Poor toileting habits	• Inappropriate elimination • Coprophagia
Destructive and unruly habits	• Excessive and inappropriate chewing • Jumping • Chasing • Barking • Hyperactivity
Anxiety	• Generalized anxiety • Separation anxiety • Thunderstorm anxiety • Noise phobias • Situational anxiety • Novel situations

Prenatal care of the dam should include prenatal veterinary care, good nutrition, low-stress handling, and emotional support in the form of petting and attention. A whelping plan should be formulated in an attempt to minimize trauma and stress to the dam as well as the offspring (see Autumn Davidson and Janis Cain's article, "Canine Pregnancy, Eutocia and Dystocia," in this issue).

Once the offspring are born, ENS can be started on day 3 of life. ENS is a technique originally developed and popularized by Carmen Battaglia, who was an American Kennel Club (AKC) judge and breeder.[2] It is also known as Bio Sensor or Super Dog Training. The technique was originally developed for military working dogs as a way of creating increased physical resiliency (**Box 1**). Anecdotal support for this technique is strong, while scientific research suggests that there is some evidence that ENS may help dogs cope better with stress later in life as long as the stress created with ENS is not excessive.[3]

To perform ENS, there are 5 exercises that are performed on each neonate starting on day 3, until day 16.

- Stimulate the area between the toe pads with a cotton swab (**Fig. 1**).
- Hold the puppy head up (**Fig. 2**).
- Hold the puppy head down (**Fig. 3**).
- Hold the puppy supine or on its back (**Fig. 4**).
- Place the puppy on a cool washcloth on a flat safe surface and allow it to crawl off if desired (**Fig. 5**).

Multiple online video examples exist demonstrating the exercises. Each exercise is to be done once daily for only 3 to 5 seconds and no more.

In a large and robust litter of offspring, ENS may be unnecessary, as these positions and circumstances would happen organically. However, in a smaller, less active litter or in the case of a singleton, ENS would be more beneficial.

It is important to note that more is not better, as too much stress could cause more harm than good. Each exercise should only be done once a day and for only 3 to 5 seconds each. If the litter is already under some kind of stress from illness or tail docking/ dewclaw removal, then a grace period should be given before starting ENS.

ENS is not a substitution for the regular daily handling of neonates but is to be done in addition to the regular handling of puppies and kittens in their neonatal period. Regular gentle handling, stroking, carrying, and touching of all body areas should be done with all neonates during their awake cycle after the mother has been given the opportunity to stimulate elimination.

Emotional stability

The goal of employing emotional stability behavior strategies is to produce small animal companions that are even-tempered and well-socialized. This helps to safeguard these pets from suffering from many kinds of anxieties and aggression.

Box 1
Benefits of early neurologic stimulation

- Increase tolerance of stress
- Promote a stronger heartbeat
- Faster response from adrenal glands
- Increased resistance to disease

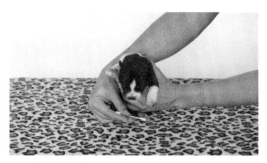

Fig. 1. Toe stimulation. Photo credit to Diane Zahorodny, World Ready Pets.

Neonatal period 0 to 2 weeks. Creating emotional stability begins in the neonatal period from 0 to 14 days, and it begins with the relationship the offspring has with its mother. It is important for the mother to be an attentive and calm mother.[4,5] One way to facilitate this is the simple act of increasing her comfort during nursing by trimming the offspring's toenails. Stress can also be reduced by keeping the nest area clean and avoiding any unnecessary stressors for the mother during this neonatal period.

Emotional stability training continues throughout this period through the daily struggle of nursing. Not only do neonates have to navigate their way to the dam using only the senses of touch and smell, but they also must compete with other offspring for their position at the teat. This daily stress not only helps them with muscle formation and coordination but is also their first opportunity to learn frustration tolerance. Neonates should be allowed to experience this struggle without intervention unless they are not growing at a normal rate or have a medical disadvantage.

Socialization period 3 to 12 weeks. Once the puppy's eyes and ears open, they move into the socialization period, in which they begin to explore and learn about the world around them. Puppies have 2 worlds that they need to learn about at an early age. One world is the world of people and everything that comes with them, and the other world is the world of animals. It is important that when this early socialization is performed that both of these worlds are kept in consideration.

Animal world Socialization to the animal world began with the mother-offspring relationship and continues to evolve as the offspring matures. As weaning approaches, this adds a new dimension to this relationship, as the mother will begin to limit access to herself as weaning progresses. It is important that during this period

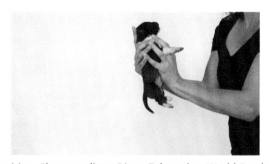

Fig. 2. Head up position. Photo credit to Diane Zahorodny, World Ready Pets.

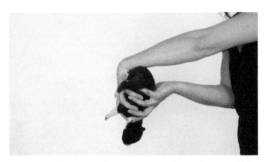

Fig. 3. Head down position. Photo credit to Diane Zahorodny, World Ready Pets.

the mother has an easy way to limit access to herself (usually by jumping up onto an elevated platform/bed/couch) so that she does not have to resort to confrontational techniques such as growling or snapping.

When socializing these young animals to adult animals, it is important to avoid negative experiences. The animals that they are to be interacting with should be known well, be kind and gentle, and have a good play history with young animals. These may be the other animals in the household at first and as the puppies approach 5 weeks, then animals from outside of the household can begin to enter the environment.

The introduction area should be large and provide high places for the adult animals to escape, as well as low places for the puppies to hide. Various animals should visit, some big, some small, some with short hair, some with long hair, some with stand-up ears, and some with floppy ears. A concerted effort should be made to introduce puppies to dogs of different breeds in order to generalize their acceptance of other dogs.

If the puppies are reluctant to engage, sometimes petting the adult animal and offering praise is all that is needed to encourage a hesitant youngster to interact. These sessions should be short, between 15 and 30 minutes, and the animals they are visiting with should all be healthy, vaccinated, and without any recent travel or show history.

People world When considering socialization to people a lot of the same rules apply. As the puppies are not yet fully vaccinated, safety should be a priority, and people should be instructed to take off their shoes before entering the play area and wash their hands. If they have been at a veterinary clinic, shelter, grooming salon, or show, be sure to provide a clean change of clothes. These sessions should also be short, no

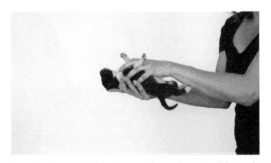

Fig. 4. Supine position. Photo credit to Diane Zahorodny, World Ready Pets.

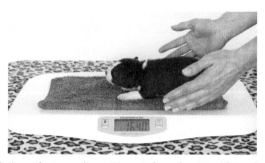

Fig. 5. Cold stimulation. Photo credit to Diane Zahorodny, World Ready Pets.

more than 15 to 30 minutes, and positive with lots of attention, pets, and praise, as well as some treats.

Various people should be introduced: young people, older people, children of varying ages, different races, men with beards, people with sunglasses, people wearing hats, people in uniform, and people carrying things. It can be helpful to keep various wigs, props, hats, and costumes for this purpose so that the puppies can experience several different-looking people even if you have just a trusted few.

Emotional resilience and environmental enrichment. When discussing emotional stability, it is important to note that socialization is not the only thing to do during this life stage. One also needs to consider emotional resilience as well as providing an enriched environment.

Emotional resilience is the ability to recover from frustration or fear in a timely manner. This resilience can be strengthened by triggering the startle recovery cycle.[6] At 3 to 4 weeks of age, puppies have no real fear response. They will, however, be startled. To trigger the startle recovery cycle, loud and sudden noises can be made in the puppies' vicinity 1 to 3 times a day. This can be in the form of doors slamming shut a few rooms away, dropped metal dishes, vacuum cleaners running, or dropped books. When first introducing these sounds, it is best to begin a few rooms away and decrease the distance as time allows. If the mother is likely to react or become frightened of these noises, then it is best to do this when she is not in the room.

To help puppies continue their frustration tolerance training, novel challenges can be created in their home environment. These challenges can be as simple as putting them in a box and letting them figure out a way to navigate themselves out of the box. Other challenges can include creating an obstacle course between them and their meals that they then have to navigate over, under, or around. Items such as a rolled-up yoga mat to go over, a table to go under, and a gate or pen to go around are useful for setting up such obstacles. Again, multiple instructive examples of puppy obstacle courses exist online.

Environmental enrichment using food is another way to challenge puppies so that they continue to learn frustration tolerance along with flexing and developing their problem-solving skills. Examples of this can include an ice cube tray filled with food, a food-filled Kong toy, a towel sprinkled with kibbles and rolled up, or a snuffle mat.

Toys are yet another way of enriching the environment as long as the toys are of various materials and are rotated frequently to preserve the novelty of the toys. However, toys can be somewhat limiting and other objects should be brought into the daily space. This includes all varieties of everyday items such as umbrellas (have them watch you open and close them), strollers, skateboards, big crinkly bags, garden hoses, helium balloons, tools, tarps, chairs tilted over, tunnels, teeter boards, baskets, chutes, boxes, trash can lids, statues, etc.

Good elimination habits

Early toilet training for puppies is a simple and effective way to prevent inappropriate house soiling as adults. It also keeps the puppies clean and healthy and decreases the likelihood of coprophagia by preventing the experimentation with stool left in a soiled environment. Puppies are born with a natural aversion to fecal matter, however, if fecal matter is something that is ubiquitous in their environment, they will lose that natural aversion, which will make house training much more difficult. By engaging in early toilet training, the natural aversion to excrement is preserved, which is ideal in a pet dog.

Early toilet training has several phases that correspond with the puppies' physical abilities and maturity level.

Phase 1: birth to 3 weeks. At this stage, it is up to the caretaker and the dam to keep the nest clean. Frequent changing of the bedding material is recommended to ensure a clean nest.

Phase 2: 3 weeks. From the time the puppies open their eyes around week 3, they will begin to naturally move away from the nest to urinate and defecate. It is at this time that a litter pan can be introduced with pellet newspaper litter. This should be placed in an area where the puppies naturally gravitate to when they eliminate. The pan should be shallow to ease their ability to enter and exit and the pan should not be located near the entry or exit of the nest.

Phase 3: weeks 4 to 6. At this stage, the puppies are ready to be moved to a larger area consisting of a large play area and a smaller potty area. Again, ensure that the potty area is away from the door to the pen so that the dam and the puppies do not have to walk through it to get out of their pen. This potty area should be kept as clean as possible.

Phase 4: week 6 and up. By week 6, the puppies can begin to be taken outside during key toileting times such as: when they wake up, immediately after eating, and 5 minutes into playtime. The puppies should be positively reinforced for eliminating outside with a high-reward food treat within 5 seconds of elimination or praise. Playtime outside can begin once the puppies have eliminated.

During early toilet training and socialization, puppies should also be exposed to a variety of substrates to eliminate upon (ie, grass, artificial grass, gravel, sand, dirt, and concrete).

Early training

The goals of performing early training with puppies is twofold. The first goal is to begin bite prevention training, and this training includes body handling training, object exchanges, food bowl exercises, and resting place training.

The second goal is to begin training that makes life with puppies and adolescents easier for new puppy owners by teaching and reinforcing early life skills. This training includes crate training, installing a recall, creating a positive reward marker, learning to offer behavior, and saying please.

Bite prevention training. Body handling training is the process of getting puppies accustomed to being touched in a gentle yet purposeful way. From the moment of birth, puppies should be touched by people. Starting at 3 weeks puppies should be examined in a deliberate yet gentle way. Eyes, ears, nose, mouth, toes, and the peri-anal area should all be gently touched and as the puppy ages, treats can be paired with the body handling sessions.

Object exchanges are used to teach puppies that having objects taken from them is a positive experience. This is important to do, as guarding objects is a normal puppy behavior when directed at other puppies in their litter. However, when they direct this behavior to people, it can become problematic.

Here is the sequence of an object exchange:[7]

1. Give the puppy a high-value object to chew on.
2. Leave the puppy to chew for 3 to 5 minutes uninterrupted.
3. Approach the puppy.
4. Touch the puppy.
5. Say "thank you."
6. Take the object from the puppy (even if growling).
7. Reward the puppy once you have the object with a tasty treat.
8. Give the object back.

When performing these exercises, it is best to keep the treat out of view when approaching the puppy and only offer the treat after the object has been taken. This ensures that the puppy associates the object being taken with the treat instead of being distracted by the treat. If the treat is offered before the object is taken, this qualifies as a bribe and does not create the desired positive emotional response that would be created if the treat were given after the object is taken. Bribes can be employed if the object the puppy is chewing on is dangerous as the goal at that moment is to distract the puppy.

The goal of object exchanges is to create a "this is no big deal" or "this is great" feeling when people take their favorite chewing objects. Repetition of object exchanges is key to creating a solid emotional foundation, and these exercises can be done once every few days starting at 4 weeks, although some puppies will only need this performed once to get the idea.

There are 2 food bowl exercises that can be done to accustom puppies to people around the food bowl:

The first is the bad waiter routine.[8] In this exercise, the puppies are called and only one-fourth of their usual meal is placed in the dish. When the puppies have finished the food, the food bowl is picked up, and another one-fourth of their meal is put down. This is repeated until the entire meal is fed.

The second is the *special treat delivery routine*.[8] As the puppies are eating their meal, they are gently pushed aside, and a special tasty treat is deposited into the dish in front of them. The puppies should be touched while they are eating for a few minutes and then left alone for a few more minutes before repeating the process. This can be done at every other meal.

The methodology of this training can also be carried over to get puppies accustomed to being disturbed while sleeping, as well as for puppies that are up in arms or on laps, which can be especially important for small breeds.

For puppies resting,

- Approach a sleeping pup
- Rouse the pup gently
- Offer a treat
- Retreat

For puppies up in arms or on laps,

- Approach pup in arms or on a lap
- Offer a treat
- Touch pup
- Offer a treat
- Retreat

Early life skill training. Crate training is begun by providing an open crate in the weaning pen with the door removed. At 4 to 5 weeks, the puppies can be removed from the litter and placed in a crate with a high-value chew object or special treat. Monitor the youngster in the crate and let it out before it becomes distressed. Short car rides in the crate with litter mates for company can also be started to prepare them for departure day.

Installing a good recall is started at mealtime by choosing a recall phrase and using it every time the puppies are fed. Young animals respond best to higher-pitched fast sounds such as "puppy puppy puppy." It is best to think of this as a musical note or song as opposed to a word. Every time the puppies are fed, this song is used to call them to the mealtime area. Once they are responding to this call readily, it can then be used outside of the context of mealtime with food rewards, attention, praise, or toys for responding. It is important not to use this recall to end outside time or end playtime as that would weaken the cue. This recall song can be taught to the new owners at pick-up so that they can continue to use it at home.

A positive reward marker is a useful tool to teach puppies as a means of communication. It lets the puppy know that the behavior they just performed is about to be rewarded and is a way of introducing the game of training to them in a positive way. The positive reward marker is a bridge that links a sound to positive reinforcement (most often food) so that the dog feels good when it hears the marker.

The sequence for installing a reward marker is

- Give the marker (a word like "yes" or "yup").
- Present a food treat within 1 second.

The sequence should be repeated for 30 to 60 seconds, and then the training session should end. The training sessions should be short, 1 to 3 minutes for pups under 12 weeks, and no more than 15 minutes for pups 12 to 20 weeks. A rest period of 15 to 30 minutes should be given if attempting multiple training sessions per day.

Once the puppies have an installed positive reward marker (PRM), then the puppies can be taught to offer behavior. By teaching them to offer behavior they are encouraged to problem solve, to experiment with their behaviors and their environment, and opens the door to the game of training. This method of training can be empowering to puppies and helps them to stay encouraged while training. The sequence to teach is

- Present the puppy with a box.
- Mark and reward any interaction with the box.

The end result of this training is not a specific behavior; it is an opportunity to see what the puppy comes up with on its own. In this instance, it may paw at the box, they might crawl into the box, nudge the box with its nose, or bite the box. With each interaction, the puppy is rewarded for whatever the behavior it chooses to do. The puppy can then make the decision to do it again and again, to continue getting the rewards. The goal of this training is to teach the puppy that training is a fun and rewarding game and helps it to understand that actions can lead to positive reinforcement. The training sessions should be kept short, 1 to 3 minutes each, and should end on a positive note.

The last early training technique is to teach the puppy to say please. The goal of this training is to create a default behavior that the puppy will offer when it wants something. For most pet dogs, the default behavior that is most helpful is sitting. For puppies that will one day enter the show ring, the default behavior can be "four on the floor" or stand/stay.

By creating a desired default behavior that the puppy displays when it wants something, it is automatically avoiding more rambunctious attention-seeking behaviors such as barking, pawing, biting, or jumping. This is achieved by reinforcing the puppy when it naturally offers the default behavior during interactions. When teaching this tool, the caregiver is not asking the puppy or cueing the puppy to sit or stand/stay. They are simply in possession of something the puppy wants and then gives it to the puppy when it offers the default behavior. This can be opening the exercise pen door to play, opening the door to go outside, food bowls, treats, toys, engaging with a toy (throwing it or playing tug), petting, or attention.

The sequence to teach say please

- Sit or stand in the puppy's presence with something it wants (the puppy should know that you have the item).
- Wait until the puppy "says please" (ie, offers the desired default behavior [sitting or stand/stay]).
- As soon as the puppy "says please," give the reward marker and follow with the thing it wants.

Again, you need to keep the sessions short, 1 to 3 minutes. You can do this outside of the puppy pen and reward all the pups that "say please" instead of jumping. This is a great way to give puppies a way of politely asking for what they want and establishing a means of communication.

Going Home

The general consensus is for puppies to go to their new homes between 8 and 12 weeks of age. This age range allows them to go to their new homes after their first vaccinations.

Fear periods should also be taken into consideration. This is typically a brief period in which the puppy begins to show fear in situations or around objects that they had previously felt comfortable around. In puppies, these generally happen around 8 weeks of age and again at 20 weeks of age. A fear period can last a few hours, a day, or as long as a week. If puppies must be taken to a veterinarian during this time period, it is important that low stress handling techniques are used to minimize negative interactions that can leave a lasting impression.

If the new owners live close enough, then they should be encouraged to visit their puppy before go home day so that they can become acquainted with their puppy and they can begin to learn about the early training that has been started. If they do not live close by, then time should be allowed to show the new owners the early training exercises and instruct them on how to continue the training and socialization in a safe manner. They should also be encouraged to attend well-run puppy classes. Good puppy classes should follow these 10 guidelines:

1. Off-leash play that is managed (puppies are separated by temperament and play style, not necessarily by size)
2. No physical punishments
3. Nothing scary (meaning no shaker cans or water bottles)
4. Places for pups to hide

5. No prong or choke collars
6. No verbal corrections
7. No stopping behavior (owners should be coached to teach puppies what to do instead of stopping what they do not want them to do)
8. Building good behaviors
9. Good instructor-to-puppy ratio, 1 instructor per 2 to 3 pups
10. Behavior and puppy-rearing help (so that owners have someone to answer their housetraining questions and other behavior questions)

Summary

Veterinarians are duty-bound to be advocates for patients and a champion for their physical and mental well-being. These early behavior strategies are preventative medicine for behavior problems much like deworming and vaccinations are preventatives for disease and are just as essential. Like most diseases, prevention is much easier, and requires much less money, time, and effort than treatment. This is especially true when it comes to behavior problems, as treatment failure can often result in behavioral euthanasia, which contributes to the moral distress that veterinarians and their teams face.[9] Incorporating the education of early behavior strategies to breeders and puppy owners into daily practice can not only greatly benefit the puppies, but also benefits the entire veterinary team by creating future patients that have a strong human-animal bond with their owners, and are a joy to interact with and care for.

CLINICS CARE POINTS

- During prenatal visits and litter deworming visits, time should be allotted to educate breeders about early behavior strategies, specifically
  - Early neurologic stimulation and body handling
  - Early toileting training
  - Early socialization (and how to do so safely)
  - Early food bowl and object exchange training

- During the first puppy visit, time should be allotted to educate new puppy owners regarding
  - Continuing socialization safely
  - Food bowl and object exchange training
  - Toilet training
  - Enrolling in a good puppy class

- Low stress handling techniques should be used with all puppies, but especially puppies around 8 and 20 weeks of age, when they may be in their fear period. Invasive procedures or handling may leave lasting negative associations to veterinary care.

DISCLOSURE

The author has nothing to disclose.

REFERENCES

1. University of Helsinki. Fearful Great Danes provide new insights to genetic causes of fear. ScienceDaily 2020. Available at: http://www.sciencedaily.com/releases/2020/05/200529150627.htm. Accessed November 2, 2022.
2. Battaglia CL. Periods of early development and the effects of stimulation and social experiences in the canine. J Vet Behav Clin Appl Res 2009;4(5):203–10.

3. Boone G, Romaniuk A, Croney C. Early neurological stimulation (ENS): implications for canine welfare and management In: Purdue College of Veterinary Medicine - Purdue Extension. 2020. Available at: https://www.extension.purdue.edu/extmedia/VA/VA-24-W.pdf. Accessed November 2, 2022.
4. Guardini G, Bowen J, Mariti C, et al. Influence of maternal care on behavioural development of domestic Dogs (Canis familiaris) Living in a home environment. Animals (Basel) 2017;7(12):93.
5. Foyer P, Wilsson E, Jensen P. Levels of maternal care in dogs affect adult offspring temperament. Sci Rep 2016;6:19253.
6. Stolzlechner L, Bonorand A, Riemer S. Optimising puppy socialisation–short- and long-term effects of a training programme during the early socialisation period. Animals 2022;12(22):3067.
7. Donaldson J. Mine! A practical guide to resource guarding in dogs. Wenatchee: Dogwise Publishing; 2002.
8. Dunbar I. After you get your puppy. Berkeley (CA): James & Kenneth Publishers; 2001.
9. Yu Y, Wilson B, Masters S, et al. Mortality resulting from undesirable behaviours in dogs aged three years and under attending primary-care veterinary practices in Australia. Animals (Basel) 2021;11(2):493.

Decision-Making on Recommended Age of Spay/ Neuter for a Specific Dog

General Principles and Cultural Complexities

Lynette A. Hart, MA, PhD[a],*, Benjamin L. Hart, DVM, PhD[b], Abigail P. Thigpen, BS[a]

KEYWORDS

- Aggression • Behavior • Body weight • Dog breed • Sex • Vasectomy
- Hysterectomy

KEY POINTS

- Age of neutering plays a role in risks of joint disorders or cancers for some breeds of dogs, but smaller breeds usually are spared the joint disorders.
- Some larger breeds suffer heightened likelihood of joint disorders if neutered before 1, or sometimes 2, years of age.
- Shelters can perform very early neutering on dogs that will remain small without fear of elevating the risks of joint disorders.
- For mixed-breed dogs expected to weigh more than 20 kg in adulthood, waiting until 1 year of age for neutering avoids the elevated risks for joint disorders of early neutering.
- A personalized assessment of the entire living situation of the dog, as well as its breed, gender, and adult body weight, can yield the best decision for age of neutering of a particular dog.

INTRODUCTION

Castrating a male dog or spaying a female dog is a common practice with puppies, generally referred to as neutering. Offering a foolproof method to avoid reproduction, the practice of early neutering of young pups, often before 6 months of age, became

[a] Department of Population Health and Reproduction, School of Veterinary Medicine, University of California, Davis, 1079 Veterinary Medicine Drive, Davis, CA 95616, USA; [b] Department of Anatomy, Physiology, and Cell Biology, School of Veterinary Medicine, University of California, Davis, 1 Shields Avenue, Davis, CA 95616, USA
* Corresponding author.
E-mail address: lahart@ucdavis.edu

Vet Clin Small Anim 53 (2023) 1209–1221
https://doi.org/10.1016/j.cvsm.2023.05.005
0195-5616/23/© 2023 Elsevier Inc. All rights reserved.
vetsmall.theclinics.com

standard practice in the United States in recent decades, although in many countries in Europe neutering is discouraged, if not illegal. In the United States, animal shelters often had legal requirements for neutering before adoption and typically neutered very young pups. It is sometimes suggested that the decline in the number of dogs euthanized in animal shelters and humane societies resulted from increased neutering before adoption. But another consideration in addressing the historic pet overpopulation is that the decline in euthanasia of dogs preceded the widespread onset of early neutering methods and practice[1-4]—perhaps reflecting a general increase in responsible dog ownership.

In 2002, a study of New York state veterinarians reported their strong support for early neutering of dogs and cats, where the median earliest age recommended for neutering both male and female client–owned dogs was 5 months, and the median earliest age veterinarians favored for male and female shelter animals was 3 months.[5] In addition to pet population control, early neutering of females was effective in preventing mammary cancer and pyometra.

The tide has turned by now in availability of dogs for adoption, with some concerns that there is a scarcity of dogs. The USDA reports that more than one million dogs are now imported into the United States each year.[6] Most of these imports qualify as pets of the people bringing them into the country. The 2019 report described that only 3000 dogs were imported for resale in the previous year, but this was a sharp increase from the previous year, and continued increases seem likely in the future. Further, it is possible that a greater number of the million imported dogs actually were being brought in for resale or to stock the supply of dogs for adoption at shelters.

In recent years, deciding when to neuter a specific dog has become more complicated. Neutering at an early age, such as younger than 6 months, or before 1 year of age, for some breeds is associated with an increase in risks of one or more joint disorders or some cancers[7]; this creates a major complication for the veterinary profession and pet owners: no longer does a universal rule hold for an optimal age of neutering all dogs. Particularly with some breeds of large dogs, early neutering can sharply increase the risks of the dog suffering from hip dysplasia, cranial cruciate ligament tear or rupture, or elbow dysplasia. In addition, some breeds show heightened risks of one or more cancers with early neutering, or in a few cases even neutering as late as 2 years is associated with heightened risks. For those that feel it is important to neuter before sexual maturity because of a risk of mammary cancer or to reduce problem behaviors, our paper on 35 breeds lays out the breed-specific risks of mammary cancers with neutering after 1 year. The data indicate that the risk of mammary cancer in females left gonadally intact in the breeds analyzed is generally low and rarely exceeds 6%. These data align with an extensive meta-analysis of mammary cancers and neutering from the United Kingdom.[8] Further, mammary cancer usually is a late-onset disease of older dogs, whereas the joint diseases often affect young dogs.

The argument for early neutering is strengthened in communities with numerous street dogs and/or where large numbers of dogs are in shelters. In these communities, preventing unwanted litters of puppies is paramount to the long-term adverse health effects associated with delaying neutering until after puberty. Yet, as mentioned earlier, more than one million dogs are brought into the United States,[6] partially to address a shortfall in available dogs for adoption. Some authorities have argued that a shortage of adoptable dogs could be addressed by encouraging the breeding of healthy dogs likely to have good behavior, for example, the National Animal Interest Alliance.[9]

Seeking desirable behavior in their dog, some people may be tempted to neuter a young male pup to reduce the onset of male sexual behaviors. Aggression, which is not a male sexual behavior, may be reduced after neutering, whether the neutering occurs before or after the onset of aggressive behavior. However, aggression toward other dogs is diminished by castration only in a minority of male dogs[10,11] and may affect aggression to dogs more than aggression to people.[12] It is important to mention that in several instances, aggression toward humans can be increased after neutering, especially if the dog is already displaying aggressive behaviors at the time it is neutered.

Currently in the United States when making decisions on when to neuter a specific dog, it is advisable to evaluate the varied circumstances of each specific situation, as well as the dog's genetics and likely body size in adulthood. This paper examines in more detail some general principles regarding neutering ages for dogs of various breeds and body weights. It then discusses some of the cultural considerations that play a role in neutering decisions. And it provides reminders of alternatives to consider when delaying neutering that can make the delay easier to manage.

GENERAL PRINCIPLES FOR EFFECTS OF AGE OF NEUTERING

In several open-access research papers published over the past decade, our team has investigated the impacts of neutering at different ages in increasing the risks of one or more joint disorders and some cancers with regard to breed, sex, and age at neutering. The 3 initial papers examined Golden Retrievers,[13] Labrador Retrievers,[14] and German Shepherd Dogs.[15] These breeds contribute in working roles as police canines and assistance/service dogs.[16] For these 3 breeds, the risks of a joint disorder, including hip dysplasia, cranial cruciate ligament tear or rupture, and elbow dysplasia, were increased several-fold by neutering before 1 year of age compared with that of gonadally intact dogs. In the case of female Golden Retrievers, risks of a cancer were increased by neutering at any age.

Disease patterns in dogs affected by neutering differ with breed, sex, and age of neutering. In an examination of 35 breeds (including the 3 mentioned earlier), neutering did not increase the incidence of joint disorders or cancers over that of dogs left intact in most breeds[7]; this was especially true in the smaller breeds, except for increased cancers in the Boston Terrier and Shih Tzu breeds. Only some of the larger breeds were affected. Increasing attention focused on the physiologic effects of neutering: something that was an ancient practice with long-known effects.[17]

Specific Breeds

As mentioned, the published data revealed heightened risks of joint disorders or cancers based on the age of neutering in only a minority of breeds examined: for males, 14 out of 35 breeds; for females, 13 out of 35 breeds.[7] For joint disorders and cancers, the increased risks occurred about equally often, and this was true for both males and females. Generally, the enhanced risks of joint disorders befell some of the larger breeds, yet male Beagles, Cocker Spaniels, and Miniature Poodles were smallish dogs that had elevated joint disorders associated with early neutering. Very early neutering for male Corgis was associated with elevated risks for an intervertebral disc disorder.

Because of elevated cancer risks with neutering at any age, it was recommended that male Dobermans be left intact, and a similar recommendation was made for female Golden Retrievers. Male Golden Retrievers suffered both increased joint diseases and cancer risks with neutering before 1 year of age. Delays in neutering were suggested for female Shetland Sheepdogs, Collies, and German Shepherd Dogs, due to marked increases in urinary incontinence with early neutering. Male and female German Shepherds had heightened risks of joint disorders with neutering before 2 years of age. Male Bernese Mountain Dogs, Labrador Retrievers, and Rottweilers also experienced heightened risks for joint disorders with early neutering, as well as female Australian Cattle Dogs, Dobermans, Labrador Retrievers, Rottweilers, and St. Bernards. Elevated risks of one or more cancers were found in male Border Collies, Boston Terriers, Boxers, Irish Wolfhounds, and Standard Poodles, as well as in female Border Collies, Boxers, Cocker Spaniels, Collies, and Shih Tzus.

Some further information is now available on German Shorthaired Pointer, Mastiff, Newfoundland, Rhodesian Ridgeback, and Siberian Husky. To obtain the ages of neutering of these dogs, it was usually necessary to telephone referring veterinarians, and then, records could not be obtained for all patients. The percentages of neutered males and females in our samples are included for each breed. The actual percentages of neutered dogs among all patients would be higher for each breed if complete neutering information had been available for all neutered dogs. The data suggest that neutering may be less frequent for German Shorthaired Pointer, Newfoundland, and Mastiff males, as compared with Rhodesian Ridgeback and Siberian Husky males. Newfoundland females in our sample had the lowest rate of neutering for females among these 5 breeds.

German Shorthaired Pointer

Body weights are as follows: 55 to 70 lbs., 25 to 32 kg males; 45 to 60 lbs., 20 to 27 kg females (**Fig. 1**). This favored hunting breed is highly active and trainable. These

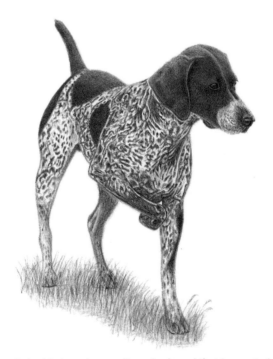

Fig. 1. German Shorthaired Pointer is a medium-size breed that is very trainable and used in hunting. Delaying neutering until 1 year of age is recommended for males and is a cautionary suggestion for females due to their incidences of cancers.

Pointers were brought to the United States almost 100 years ago and were recognized as a breed by the AKC in the 1930s. Among males in our sample (n = 200+), only 31% were neutered and 46% of females (n = 150+). For males, numbers of cancer cases are a bit concerning despite not being statistically significantly elevated; it could be cautionary to delay neutering to 1 year of age. Females neutered before 1 year of age showed significantly elevated cancers; a neutering guideline for females is to wait for 1 year of age.

Mastiff

Body weights are as follows: 160 to 230 lbs., 73 to 105 kg males; 120 to 170 lbs., 55 to 77 kg females (**Fig. 2**). This giant breed has ancient origins for use in hunting, warfare, and guarding, such as in Babylon, Greece, Rome, and England. They can be aggressive, have very low activity, and do not bark excessively, only barking as watchdogs. Fortunately, they are moderately trainable. Only 28% of males in this sample were neutered (n ∼ 200) and 49% of females (n = 125+). Mastiff males neutered before 1 year had significantly elevated joint disorders due to cranial cruciate ligament tear, and females, although results were nonsignificant, may have done better for joint disorders and cancers if left intact. Possibly females would show effects of neutering with larger numbers. A guideline if the male or female dog is being neutered is to wait until after 1 year of age.

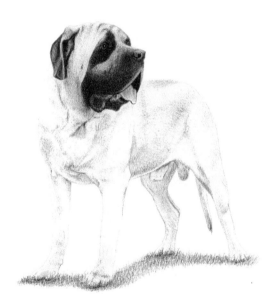

Fig. 2. Mastiff is a giant breed with an aggressive temperament sometimes used for guarding. Although the surgery and recovery are more difficult when delayed, waiting at least a year to neuter a Mastiff can reduce the risk of a joint disorder.

Newfoundland

Body weights are as follows: 130 to 150 lbs., 59 to 68 kg males; 100 to 120 lbs., 45 to 55 kg females (**Fig. 3**). Coming from the island of Newfoundland, this giant breed assisted in maritime tasks. Perhaps it was derived from Mastiffs breeding with local dogs on the island. Among males in this sample (n ~ 100), only 31% were neutered and 36% of females (n ~ 90). The nonsignificant effects on joint disorders nonetheless appeared elevated in males and females neutered before 1 year, suggesting a cautious strategy of neutering after 1 year of age.

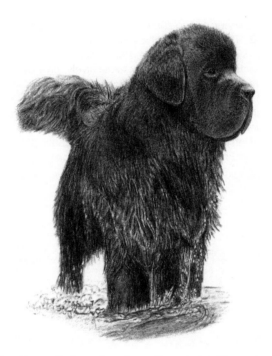

Fig. 3. Newfoundland is a quite large breed sometimes trained to work with people in marine settings. Waiting until 1 year for neutering may reduce risks for a joint disorder. However, the elevated results of these disorders for early neutered dogs were not statistically significant.

Rhodesian Ridgeback

Body weights are as follows: 80 to 90 lbs., 36 to 41 kg males; 65 to 75 lbs., 30 to 34 kg females (**Fig. 4**). This somewhat aggressive and unaffectionate breed was generated from a mixture of European breeds brought to Rhodesia (now Zimbabwe) and bred with the local ridgeback, resulting in a trainable, healthy hunting breed. Among males in this sample (n = 100+), 48% were neutered and 55% of females (n = 60+). Ridgebacks had extremely low numbers of joint disorders overall and low numbers of cancer cases; a current guideline would be neutering after 6 months.

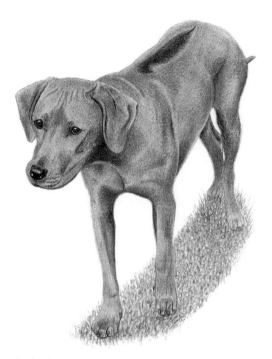

Fig. 4. Rhodesian Ridgeback is a large breed that can be aggressive. With its very low incidence of joint disorders and cancers, young dogs from 6 months of age can be neutered without increasing risks for the diseases studied.

Siberian Husky

Body weights are as follows: 45 to 60 lbs., 20 to 27 kg males; 35 to 50 lbs., 16 to 23 kg females (**Fig. 5**). This rugged, aggressive, and barky breed provided essential support to the Siberian Chukchi and Alaskan Inuit peoples before becoming known as the fastest sled dogs. Once a dogsled team of Huskies delivered diphtheria antitoxin 600 miles away during a 1925 diphtheria epidemic, the development of the Iditarod race and 1930 AKC recognition followed. Among males in this sample (n = 125+), 50% were neutered and 58% of females (n = 110+). This breed had very low, nonsignificant incidences of joint disorders and cancers, so neutering at 6 months is a reasonable choice.

Effects of Bodyweight for Mixed Breeds

In an additional research paper, data on mixed breed dogs were evaluated, with separate analyses for mixed breed dogs weighing less than 10 kg, 10 to 19 kg, 20 to 29 kg, 30 to 39 kg, and more than 40 kg.[18] Heavier mixed breed dogs, both males and females weighing at least 20 kg, were at elevated risks for joint disorders when neutered before 1 year of age. This result gives reason for heightened concern when deciding to neuter pups destined to be large. Mixed breed dogs weighing less than 20 kg were at no elevated risk for joint disorders. Neutered dogs of mixed breeds in the various weight categories were not at elevated risks for cancers when comparing neutered with intact mixed breed dogs.

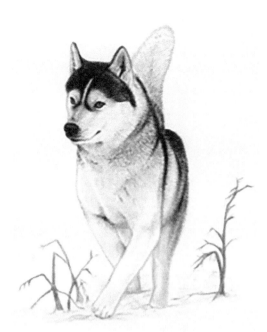

Fig. 5. Siberian Husky is a medium-sized breed tending to be aggressive. With very low incidences of the studied joint disorders and cancers, neutering can be scheduled soon after the puppy is 6 months of age with no increased risks of these conditions.

General Guidelines

General guidelines for 40 breeds of dogs and mixed breeds based on their body weights are provided in **Table 1**.

CULTURAL CONTEXTS

The discussion so far has provided information that is useful to a responsible dog owner who not only wants to prevent the dog from producing unwanted litters of puppies but who, above all, especially wants to optimize the dog's lifelong health. Decisions on neutering are made with consideration of the dog's future health but also must address challenges with dogs in the local community who are not responsibly owned. Virtually all shelters require that dogs be neutered before adoption. The state of California has such a requirement for adoptions of dogs from animal control.

ALTERNATIVE METHODS OF PREVENTING REPRODUCTION DUE TO THE PHYSIOLOGIC EFFECTS OF NEUTERING

Removal of gonadal hormones by spay/neuter surgery can predispose a dog to various adverse health effects, including various cancers.[19] Removing gonads results in extremely elevated luteinizing hormone (LH) for the animal—chronic levels that are more than 30-fold.[20] The elevated LH may sensitize some receptor sites to developing cancers.

Vasectomy of male dogs is a simple surgical procedure, more straightforward with an easier recovery than with standard castration. For female dogs, hysterectomy,

Table 1
Suggested guidelines by breed or mixed breed weight group for ages of neutering

Suggested Guidelines for Age of Neutering: 40 Breeds and Mixed Breed Weight Groups

	Males				Females			
	Leave intact	Beyond 6 mo	Beyond 11 mo	Beyond 23 mo	Leave intact	Beyond 6 mo	Beyond 11 mo	Beyond 23 mo
Australian Cattle Dog	✔					✔		
Australian Shepherd	✔						✔	
Beagle			✔			✔		
Bernese Mountain Dog				✔		✔		
Border Collie			✔				✔	
Boston Terrier			✔			✔		
Boxer				✔				✔
Bulldog		✔				✔		
Cavalier King Charles Spaniel		✔				✔		
Chihuahua		✔				✔		
Cocker Spaniel		✔						✔
Collie		✔					✔	
Corgi		✔				✔		
Dachshund		✔					✔	
Doberman Pinscher	c						✔	
English Springer Spaniel		✔					✔	
German Shepherd				✔			✔	
German Shorthaired Pointer			✔					✔
Golden Retriever			✔		✔			
Great Dane		✔				✔		
Irish Wolfhound				✔		✔		
Jack Russell Terrier		✔				✔		

(continued on next page)

Table 1
(continued)

	Suggested Guidelines for Age of Neutering: 40 Breeds and Mixed Breed Weight Groups					
Labrador Retriever	✓				✓	
Maltese	✓			✓		
Mastiff		✓			✓	
Miniature Schnauzer	✓			✓		
Newfoundland	✓				✓	
Pomeranian	✓			✓		
Poodle (Toy)	✓			✓		
Poodle (Miniature)		✓		✓		
Poodle (Standard)			✓	✓		
Pug	✓				✓	
Rhodesian Ridgeback	✓			✓		
Rottweiler		✓		✓		
Saint Bernard	✓			✓		
Shetland Sheepdog	✓			✓		
Shih Tzu	✓					✓
Siberian Husky	✓			✓		
West Highland White Terrier	✓			✓		
Yorkshire Terrier	✓			✓		
Mixed Breed < 20 kg Small and Medium	✓			✓		
Mixed Breed 20–39 kg Standard and Large	✓				✓	
Mixed Breed 40+ kg Giant		✓			✓	

Summary of spaying and neutering guidelines based on findings regarding joint disorders and cancers.

which is more complicated than vasectomy of a male, can prevent pregnancy without altering gonadal hormone production. Specific methods for gonad-sparing surgical sterilization in male and female dogs are becoming more available.[21] When vasectomy or hysterectomy is performed, it has been suggested as useful to provide a standard mark to avoid a subsequent neutering surgery; a green tattoo could be used, with an X for hysterectomy and a V for vasectomy.[22] Nonsurgical methods of contraception also are of increasing interest and available, using hormonal treatments with progestins, androgens, or gonadotropin releasing hormone analogues, or vaccines, or other methods.[23]

Gonadal hormones play an important role in growth and development as is well known in human medicine. With depletion of the gonadal hormones, one can expect some effects. Gonadal hormones play a role in the closure of long bone growth plates as the animal approaches maturity. Neutering allows the long bones to grow a little longer, possibly altering the joint alignment in some neutered dogs and leading to a clinically apparent joint disorder.[7] With regard to the occurrence of cancers, we have presented the perspective that gonadal hormones are protective against some metastatic cells in sensitive tissues, and when removed it allows the cancer cells to reproduce.[7]

Discussion

Given the important physiologic effects of gonadal hormones, one should expect consequences when they are removed from animals, especially early in the animal's life. For dogs, having such a broad and differing range of breed-specific anatomic and physiologic characteristics, it is not surprising to find major breed and gender differences in the effects of removal of gonadal hormones. The authors of this chapter started this 10-year project to explore breed and sex differences in disease responses to neutering at various ages. Initially there was understandable resistance to accepting the data in our papers on Golden Retrievers and Labrador Retrievers because the field of small animal medicine had become so accustomed to the 6-month spay/neuter paradigm. This dialogue has now changed. Based on our 10-year experience in researching this topic, the authors have proposed a new paradigm shift for veterinarians working with clients to arrive at an age for neutering for the individual dog in consideration: a personalized decision for the dog. This shift should benefit the long-term health and welfare of the dog and set the stage for an ongoing dialogue between the dog's caregiver and their veterinarian.

SUMMARY

An early age of neutering for some breeds of dogs is associated with adverse heightened risks of one or more joint disorders or some cancers, with different effects for males and females. These 5 open-access papers have been heavily viewed by a wide range of readers,[7,11–13,16] reflecting that dog owners are highly motivated to assure the health of their dogs. Although these elevated risks are found in a minority of the breeds studied, the impacts are significant for the affected dog breeds and should be considered when making decisions on age of neutering for a specific dog. For dogs of mixed breed or a breed not covered in the data analyses, some conjectures regarding joint disorders can be drawn from closely related breeds or by taking into account the body size of the dog. A personalized assessment that considers the lifestyle and situation of the dog involved, as well as the breed, gender, and body weight, can yield the best overall outcomes.

CLINICS CARE POINTS

- When adopting a mixed-breed dog likely to reach more than 20 kg, consider delaying neutering until the dog is at least 1 year of age to avoid increasing the risk of a joint disorder.
- When adopting a purebred dog at increased risk of a joint disorder or cancer with early neutering, negotiate with the breeder for a delay in neutering.
- For a dog neutered at a young age that has an elevated risk of a joint disorder or a cancer, monitor the dog more carefully for those conditions.
- Engage the client of an unneutered puppy and advise concerning the appropriate age of neutering to avoid heightened risk of a joint disorder or a cancer.
- Considering small breed dogs, advise clients that these dogs are not vulnerable to early neutering, with only a couple exceptions.
- Include discussions of neutering effects in consultation with clients.

ACKNOWLEDGMENTS

The authors acknowledge the generous support of the American Kennel Club and the UC Davis Center for Companion Health that made possible the extensive work involved in studying the effects of age of neutring for forty dog breeds and five weight classes of mixed breed dogs. The authors very much appreciate the ongoing research teams of undergraduate students who have assisted in this project for over a decade. Emma Mooring once again has provided exceptional artwork.

DISCLOSURE

The authors have nothing to disclose.

REFERENCES

1. Zawistowski S, Morris J, Salman MD, et al. Population dynamics, overpopulation, and the welfare of companion animals: new insights on old and new data. J Appl Animal Welfare Science 1998;1(3):193–206. https://www.tandfonline.com/doi/abs/10.1207/s15327604jaws0103_1.
2. Aronsohn MG, Faggella AM. Surgical techniques for neutering 6- to 14-week-old kittens. J Am Vet Med Assoc 1993;202:53–5.
3. Faggella AM, Aronsohn MG. Anesthetic techniques for neutering 6- to 14-week-old kittens. J Am Vet Med Assoc 1993;202:56–62.
4. Howe LM. Short-term results and complications of prepubertal gonadectomy in cats and dogs. J Am Vet Med Assoc 1997;211:57–62.
5. Spain CV, Scarlett JM, Cully SM. When to neuter dogs and cats: a survey of New York state veterinarians' practices and beliefs. J Amer Anim Hosp Assn 2002;38:482–8.
6. United States Department of Agriculture. Report on the importation of live dogs into the United States. 2019. https://www.naiaonline.org/uploads/WhitePapers/USDA_DogImportReport6-25-2019.pdf.
7. Hart BL, Hart LA, Thigpen AP, et al. Assisting decision-making on age of neutering for 35 breeds of dogs: associated joint disorders, cancers, and urinary incontinence. Front Vet Sci 2020. https://doi.org/10.3389/fvets.2020.00388. Sec. Animal Reproduction - Theriogenology.

8. Beauvais W, Cardwell JM, Brodbelt DC. The effect of neutering on the risk of mammary tumours in dogs – a systematic review. J Small Anim Pract 2012;53: 314–22.
9. National Animal Interest Alliance. Website accessed February 20, 2023: https://www.naiaonline.org/about-ux/position-statement/dogs.
10. Hart BL, Eckstein RA. The role of gonadal hormones in the occurrence of objectionable behaviours in dog and cats. Appl Anim Behav Sci 1997;52:331–44.
11. Neilson JC, Eckstein RA, Hart BL. Effects of castration on problem behaviors of male dogs with reference to the role of age and experience. J Am Vet Med Assoc 1997;211:180–2.
12. Kriese M, Kufniewska E, Gugolek A, et al. Reasons for and behavioral consequences of male dog castration—A questionnaire study in Poland. Animals 2022;12:1883.
13. Torres de la Riva G, Hart BL, Farver TB, et al. Neutering dogs: effects on joint disorders and cancers in Golden Retrievers. PLoS One 2013. https://doi.org/10.1371/journal.pone.0055937.
14. Hart BL, Hart LA, Thigpen AP, et al. Long-term health effects of neutering dogs: comparison of Labrador Retrievers with Golden Retrievers. PLoS One 2014;9: e102241.
15. Hart BL, Hart LA, Thigpen AP, et al. Neutering of German Shepherd Dogs: associated joint disorders, cancers and urinary incontinence. Veterinary Medicine and Science 2016;2:191–9.
16. Walther S, Yamamoto M, Thigpen AP, et al. Assistance dogs: historic patterns and roles of dogs placed by ADI or IGDF accredited facilities and non-accredited facilities. Front Vet Sci 2017. https://doi.org/10.3389/fvets.2017.00001.
17. Hart LA, Hart BL. An ancient practice but a new paradigm: personal choice for the age to spay or neuter a dog. Front Vet Sci 2021. https://doi.org/10.3389/fvets.2021.603257.
18. Hart BL, Hart LA, Thigpen AP, et al. Assisting decision-making on age of neutering for 5 weight categories of mixed breeds of dogs: associated joint disorders, cancers, and urinary incontinence. Front Vet Sci 2020;7:388.
19. Kutzler MA. Possible relationship between long-term adverse health effects of gonad-removing surgical sterilization and luteinizing hormone in dogs. Animals 2020;10:599.
20. Zwida K, Kutzler M. Non-reproductive long-term health complications of gonad removal in dogs as well as possible causal relationships with post-gonadectomy elevated luteinizing hormone (LH) concentrations. J Etiol Anim Health 2016;1:002.
21. Kutzler MA. Gonad-sparing surgical sterilization in dogs. Front Vet Sci 2020; 7:342.
22. Brent L. Growing interest in hormone sparing dog sterilization and recommendations for standard identification methods. Clinical Theriogenology 2019;11(3): 247–53.
23. Kutzler M, Wood A. Non-surgical methods of contraception and sterilization. Theriogenology 2006;66(3):514–25.

Pyometra in Small Animals 3.0

Ragnvi Hagman, DVM, PhD

KEYWORDS

- Endometritis • Cystic endometrial hyperplasia • Sepsis • Aglepristone
- Prostaglandin • Cabergoline • Bromocriptine • Epidemiology

KEY POINTS

- Pyometra is a potentially life-threatening illness in female pets. It is common in middle- to older aged bitches and queens, and usually diagnosed within 4 months of estrus. Hormones and bacteria are involved in the disease development, and progesterone plays a key role. Disorders of the endometrium such as cystic endometrial hyperplasia (CEH) are considered predisposing factors but pyometra and CEH can develop independently.
- There are considerable age-related and breed-related differences in the occurrence of pyometra, and genetic factors may contribute to an increased vulnerability in high-risk breeds.
- The diagnosis is based on case history, clinical signs, and findings on physical examination, hematology and biochemistry laboratory tests, and diagnostic imaging identifying intrauterine fluid.
- Peritonitis, endotoxemia, and systemic inflammatory response syndrome are common complications of pyometra and are associated with more severe illness. Several biomarkers and inflammatory variables have been identified that may be valuable for diagnosis, prognostication, and treatment follow-up.
- The safest and most effective treatment of pyometra is ovariohysterectomy, which directly removes the source of infection and prevents recurrence. Purely medical (pharmacologic) treatment can be an alternative in younger and otherwise healthy breeding animals with open cervix pyometra and without other uterine or ovarian pathologic conditions.

 Video content accompanies this article at http://www.vetsmall.theclinics.com.

INTRODUCTION

Pyometra, literally meaning "pus-filled uterus", is a common illness in adult intact female dogs and cats and a less-frequent diagnosis in other small animal species.[1,2] The disease is characterized by an acute or chronic suppurative bacterial infection of the uterus postestrus with the accumulation of inflammatory exudate in the uterine

Department of Clinical Sciences, Swedish University of Agricultural Sciences, PO Box 7054, Uppsala SE-75007, Sweden
E-mail address: Ragnvi.Hagman@slu.se

Vet Clin Small Anim 53 (2023) 1223–1254
https://doi.org/10.1016/j.cvsm.2023.04.009
0195-5616/23/© 2023 Elsevier Inc. All rights reserved.

lumen and a variety of clinical and pathologic manifestations, locally and systemically.[3] The disease develops during the luteal phase, and progesterone plays a key role for the establishment of infection with ascending opportunistic bacteria. The pathogen most often isolated from pyometra uteri is *Escherichia coli*.[4–6] A wide range of clinical signs is associated with the disease, which can be life-threatening in severe cases. It is important to seek immediate veterinary care when pyometra is suspected because a patient's status may deteriorate rapidly and early intervention increases chances of survival. The diagnosis is generally straightforward but can be challenging when there is no vaginal discharge and obscure clinical signs. Surgical ovariohysterectomy (OHE) is the safest and most efficient treatment but purely medical alternatives may be an option in some cases.

EPIDEMIOLOGY AND RISK FACTORS

Pyometra is an important disease, particularly in show dogs or in countries where elective neutering of healthy dogs and cats is not generally performed.[1,2,7] In Sweden, in average 20% of all bitches are diagnosed before 10 years of age and more than 50% in certain high-risk breeds. The disease generally affects middle-aged to older bitches, with a mean age at diagnosis of 7 years, and has been reported in dogs from 3 months to 18 years of age.[8] The overall incidence rate is 199 per 10,000 dog-years at risk.[7] In cats, pyometra is not as common, which is thought to depend on less progesterone dominance due to seasonality and induced ovulation. In queens, 2.2% are diagnosed with the disease before 13 years of age, with an incidence rate of 17 cats per 10,000 cat-years at risk.[2] The mean age at diagnosis is 5.6 years, with an age range of 10 months to 20 years, and the incidence increases with age and markedly greater than 7 years of age.[2,9,10] There are age-related and breed-related differences in the occurrence of pyometra in dogs, that is, some breeds develop the illness at an earlier age and in a larger proportion than other breeds.[1,7] Breed differences have also been reported in cats diagnosed with pyometra.[2] The clear breed predisposition suggests that genetic risk factors are involved in disease development (**Tables 1** and **2**).[1,2,7,10–13] In the golden retriever, a breed that has an increased risk of pyometra, a genome-wide significant association to a region on chromosome 22, localized in the *ABCC4* gene, was recently identified.[11] The findings suggested a potential causal function of this gene, which encodes a prostaglandin transporter, to the development of pyometra but implicated that the complex disease likely is promoted by several genetic risk factors.

Exogenous treatment with steroid hormones, such as progestogens, or estrogen compounds that increase the response to progesterone, are associated with increased risk of the disease.[13,14]

Pregnancy is slightly protective in dogs, an effect that is also influenced by breed.[15] Cystic endometrial hyperplasia (CEH) and pseudoplacentational endometrial hyperplasia (PEH) are thought to increase the uterine susceptibility for infection.[16–18] In cats, less is known about risk factors and protective factors but previous hormone therapy (ie, exogenous progesterone) is associated with an increased risk.[19]

ETIOLOGY AND PATHOGENESIS

The complex pathogenesis of pyometra is not yet completely understood but involves both hormonal and bacterial factors. Although most studies have been done in dogs, the development is thought to be similar in cats. The uterine environment during the luteal phase is suitable for pregnancy but also for microbial growth. Progesterone stimulates growth and proliferation of endometrial glands, increased secretion, cervical closure, and suppression of myometrial contractions.[16] The local leukocyte

Table 1
The 10 dog breeds with highest and lowest risk of developing pyometra, expressed as proportion of bitches per breed that had developed the disease before 10 y of age, out of the total number of bitches in that breed

	Proportion (%)
Dog breed at high risk at < 10 y of age	
Bernese Mountain Dog	66
Great Dane	62
Leonberger	61
Rottweiler	58
Irish Wolfhound	58
Staffordshire Bull Terrier	54
Keeshond	52
Bull Terrier	52
Bouvier des Flandres	50
Newfoundland	50
Dog breed at low risk at < 10 y of age	
Finnish Spitz	3
Norrbotten Spitz	4
Coton de Tulear	5
Maltese	8
Gordon Setter	8
Laika	8
Saluki	10
Tibetan Terrier	10
Lancashire Bull Terrier	10
Norwich Terrier	11

As investigated in Swedish insurance data, adapted with permission from Jitpean and colleagues 2012.

response and uterine resistance to bacterial infection also become decreased.[20–22] Circulating concentrations of estrogen and progesterone are not usually abnormally elevated in pyometra, and increased numbers and sensitivity of hormone receptors are thought to initiate an amplified response.[23,24] Simultaneous corpora lutea and

Table 2
Proportion of queens diagnosed with pyometra before 10 y of age in different breeds, as investigated in Swedish insurance data

Cat Breed/Breed Group and Risk at <10 y of Age	Pyometra (%)
All breeds	2.2
Norwegian Forest cat	14.8
Birman	3.1
Persian group	3.4
Siamese group	8.8
Domestic cat	0.9

Adapted with permission from Hagman and colleagues 2014.

follicular cysts are more often found in bitches with pyometra, supporting a synergistic hormonal effect.[25]

Progesterone-mediated pathologic proliferation and growth of endometrial glands and formation of cysts (ie, CEH) is thought to predispose for pyometra but the 2 disorders can develop independently (**Fig. 1**).[26] With increasing age, CEH is more common and is associated with inadequate endometrial regeneration, which may predispose for pyometra.[27,28] Sterile fluid may accumulate in the uterine lumen, with or without CEH, which is defined as hydrometra or mucometra or, more rarely, hematometra, depending on the type of fluid and its mucin content. Clinical signs are generally subclinical or mild when there is no bacterial infection of the uterus.[3,29,30] PEH, a noninflammatory proliferative lesion in which the endometrium becomes organized in a placental-like pattern, has been associated with pyometra but its role in the development is not precisely determined.[18,31]

Escherichia coli is the predominant pathogen isolated from pyometra uteri but other species also occur (**Table 3**).[4,32,33,40,41] Dysbacteriosis may be a contributing factor because the uterine microbiome is less rich in pyometra, with greater quantity of the certain bacterial genera.[42] *Pseudomonas aeruginosa* sp *and Mycoplasma, Enterococcus*, and *Hemophilus* genera were suggested as potential biomarkers for the disease.[42] *Brucella abortus* has been isolated from a dog and cat with pyometra.[43] More than one bacterial species can be involved, and cultures are sometimes negative.[33,41] Emphysematous pyometra is caused by gas-producing bacteria.[34] A healthy uterus eliminates bacteria that have entered during cervical opening but the clearance capacity varies depending on the estrus cycle stage.[44] Experimental *E coli* infection during the luteal phase more often leads to CEH/pyometra compared with other estrus cycle stages.[45] The infection is most likely ascending because the same strains are present in the gastrointestinal tract but hematogenic spread could possibly also occur.[6,46,47] Transfer of a pyometra-causing *E coli* strain to another susceptible/predisposed individual in the same household cannot be completely ruled out, although the fecal microbiome at diagnosis generally is similar in pyometra and in healthy dogs.[48,49] The same bacterial clone can frequently be isolated from the uterus and

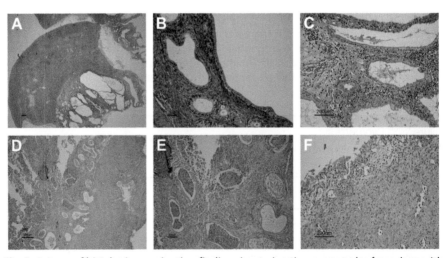

Fig. 1. Images of histologic examination findings in uterine tissues examples from dogs with CEH/pyometra. (*A*) CEH; (*B*) larger magnification of (*A*); (*C*) CEH-endometritis; (*D*) pyometra; (*E*) larger magnification of (*D*); (*F*) pyometra-atrophic endometrium.

Table 3
Bacterial species isolated from the uterus in bitches with pyometra

Organism	Proportion in Bitches (%)
Escherichia coli	30–90
Staphylococcus spp	2–15
Streptococcus spp	4–23
Pseudomonas spp	1–8
Proteus spp	1–4
Enterobacter spp	1–3
Enterococcus spp,	<1–3
Citrobacter spp	<1–3
Salmonella spp	0–2
Pasteurella spp	1–2
Klebsiella spp	2–14
Mixed culture	4–16
No growth	10–26
Mycoplasma spp, *Nocardia* spp, *Enterococcus* spp, *Clostridium perfringens*, *Corynebacterium* spp, *Moraxella* spp, *Edwardsiella* spp, Salmonella spp, *M. morganii*, *Hafnia paraalvei*, and others	

Data from Refs.[4,5,8–10,12,32–39]

the urinary bladder in pyometra but the initial site of infection is not yet known.[5,6,47] Positive urine bacterial culture can be obtained in 30% to 70% of pyometra cases.[5,50]

E.coli is a natural inhabitant of the vaginal flora and has an increased ability to adhere to specific receptors in a progesterone-stimulated endometrium.[5] The glycosylation of the endometrium may also facilitate bacterial attachment.[51] Certain serotypes and phylotypes of *E coli* are more common and often exhibit the same virulence traits as isolates from urinary tract infections.[52–54] Presence of *E coli* in the uterus is associated with severe endometrial damage.[53–55] The ability to produce biofilm, extracellular matrix, toxins, and adhesion and invasion are likely important for *E coli* in pyometra.[55–57]

Bacteria and bacterial products are potent inducers of local and systemic inflammation.[58–60] Endotoxin, lipopolysaccharide components of Gram-negative bacteria, such as *E coli*, are released into the circulation during bacterial disintegration and induces fever, lethargy, tachycardia, and tachypnea.[60–62] Higher endotoxin concentrations may cause fatal shock, disseminated intravascular coagulation, and generalized organ failure.[63,64] Pyometra has been associated with endotoxemia[64,65] and bacteremia,[66] and disseminated infection may affect various organs.[67,68] Approximately 60% of bitches and 86% of queens with pyometra suffer from sepsis (ie, life-threatening organ dysfunction caused by a dysregulated host response to an infectious process).[69,70] The illness is considered a medical emergency and it is important to seek immediate veterinary care because a patient's health status may deteriorate rapidly.

CLINICAL PRESENTATION

Typically, middle-aged to older animals are presented up to 2 months to 4 months after estrus with a history of various signs associated with the genital tract and systemic illness (**Tables 4** and **5**). A continuous or intermittent mucopurulent to hemorrhagic vaginal discharge is often present but can be absent if the cervix is closed.[35] The systemic illness is often more severe if the cervix is closed, and the uterus may become severely distended.[71] Classic systemic signs are anorexia, depression/lethargy, polydipsia, polyuria, tachycardia, tachypnea, weak pulse quality, and abnormal visible mucous membranes. Fever, dehydration, vomiting, abdominal pain on palpation, anorexia, gait abnormalities, and diarrhea are present in approximately 15% to 30% of bitches with the disease.[35,72] Cardiac arrhythmias are common in pyometra-induced sepsis.[80] The most common clinical signs in queens are vaginal discharge, lethargy, and gastrointestinal disturbances, such as anorexia, vomiting, and diarrhea (**Fig. 2**).[9,10,74–77,81] Vaginal discharge may either be absent or be concealed by fastidious cleaning habits in up to 40% of affected queens.[9,74] Weight loss, dehydration, polydipsia/polyuria, tachycardia, tachypnea, abdominal pain on palpation, abnormal mucous membranes (pale, hyperemic, or toxic), and unkept appearance are other findings associated with feline pyometra.[9–11,74–76,81]

DIAGNOSIS

The disease is easy to recognize in classic cases but can be more challenging when there is no vaginal discharge (ie, closed cervix), and the history and clinical picture are obscure. Pyometra should be a differential diagnosis in bitches and queens admitted with signs of illness after estrus but the disease can occur at any time during the estrus cycle. The preliminary diagnosis is based on history and findings on physical and gynecologic examinations, hematology and blood biochemistry analyses, and ultrasonography and/or radiography of the abdomen. Bacterial growth in cultures from the vaginal discharge alone is not diagnostically helpful because the same microbes are

Table 4 History data and clinical signs in bitches with pyometra	
Case History and Clinical Signs	**In Percentage (%)**
Vaginal discharge[a]	57–88
Lethargy/depression[a]	63–100
Inappetence/anorexia[a]	42–87
Polydipsia[a]	28–89
Polyuria[a]	34–73
Vomiting	13–38
Diarrhea	0–27
Abnormal mucous membranes	16–76
Dehydration	15–94
Palpable enlarged uterus	19–40
Pain on abdominal palpation	23–80
Lameness	16
Distended abdomen	5
Fever	32–50
Hypothermia	3–10
Tachycardia	23–28
Tachypnea	32–40
Systemic inflammatory response syndrome	57–61

[a] Usually in greater than 50% of the bitches.
Data from Refs.[29,30,37,39,71–73]

Table 5
History data and clinical signs in queens with pyometra

Case History and Clinical Signs	In Percentage (%)
Vaginal discharge	40–100
Lethargy/depression	24–100
Inappetence/anorexia	24–100
Licking of the vulva	>20
Painful abdomen on palpation	38–57
Polydipsia[a]	9–100
Polyuria[a]	9–100
Vomiting	16–100
Diarrhea	9
Dehydration	33–75
Palpable uterus	28–100
Distended abdomen	17–40
Fever	8–66
Hypothermia	25
Tachycardia	19
Tachypnea	1–42
Bradycardia	2
Systemic inflammatory response syndrome	60
Postoperative hospitalization ≥2 d or increased	27–100
Uterine rupture	3,8–4
Peritonitis	3,8–12
Mortality	3–10
Weight loss	3–14
Unkept appearance	9
Abnormal mucous membranes	75

[a] Usually in greater than 50% of the bitches.
Data from Refs.[9,10,65,74–79]

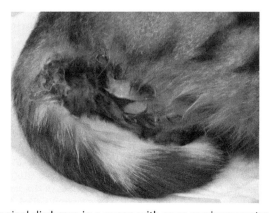

Fig. 2. Purulent vaginal discharge in a queen with open cervix pyometra.

present in the vaginal flora in healthy animals but in pyometra, the isolates are generally the same in the uterus as in the vagina.[44] Careful abdominal palpation, to avoid rupture of a fragile uterus, may identify an enlarged uterus. Diagnostic imaging is valuable for determining the uterine size and to rule out other causes of uterine enlargement (**Fig. 3**A–G). Radiography frequently identifies a large tubular structure in the caudoventral abdomen. Ultrasonography, with or without contrast enhancement, has the advantage of detecting intrauterine fluid, even when the uterine diameter is within the normal range and of revealing additional pathologic changes of the uterine tissue and ovaries, such as ovarian cysts or CEH, which may affect the outcome of medical treatment negatively (**Fig. 4**, Video 1). In emphysematous pyometra, the gas-filled uterus is visible on diagnostic imaging (**Fig. 5**A, B).[34,82] More advanced diagnostic imaging techniques are seldom necessary. Differential diagnoses include mucometra, hydrometra, and hematometra that may have similar clinical presentation and ultrasonography findings.[83] Vaginal cytology usually shows severe leukocyte

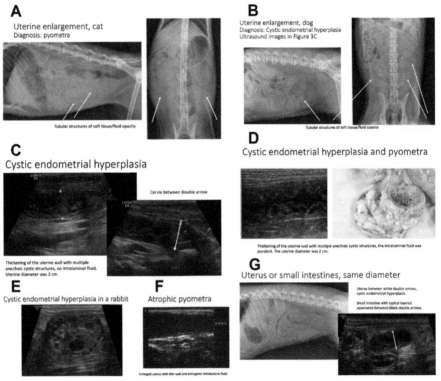

Fig. 3. (*A*) Uterine enlargement in a cat; diagnosis: pyometra. Tubular structures of soft tissue/fluid opacity (*arrows*). (*B*) Uterine enlargement in a dog; diagnosis: CEH. Tubular structures of soft tissue/fluid opacity (*arrows*). (*C*) Ultrasound images of CEH in a dog. Thickening of the uterine wall with multiple anechoic cystic structures, no intraluminal fluid. Uterine diameter was 2 cm. Cervix located between double-headed arrow. (*D*) CEH and pyometra—thickening of the uterine wall with multiple anechoic cystic structures; the intraluminal fluid was purulent. Both images in (*D*) are of the same uterus. The uterine diameter was 2 cm. (*E*) CEH in a rabbit. (*F*) Atrophic wall pyometra: enlarged uterus with a thin wall and echogenic intraluminal fluid. (*G*) Uterus or small intestines of the same diameter (radiograph to the left). Uterus between white double-headed arrows, CEH. Small intestine with typical layered appearance between black double-headed arrows.

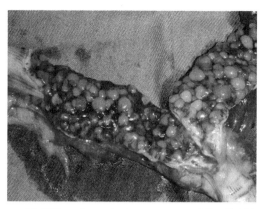

Fig. 4. Canine uterus with CEH and purulent appearance of the fluid in some cysts.

degeneration, neutrophils, and some macrophages, plasmacytes, and lymphocytes but bacterial phagocytosis is not always visible.[36] Vaginoscopy is helpful for determining the origin of a vaginal discharge and to exclude other pathologic conditions but is usually not performed in the emergent clinical setting. The diagnosis pyometra is verified by postoperative macroscopic and histologic examination of the uterus and ovaries, and microbiological examination of the uterine content (see **Fig. 4**).

CLINICOPATHOLOGIC TESTING—LABORATORY PARAMETERS

Hematology and biochemistry parameter abnormalities are generally investigated,[35,37,68,69] with additional tests performed depending on the health status (**Tables 6** and **7**). Leukocytosis, with neutrophilia and left shift and monocytosis are characteristic findings in pyometra together with normocytic, normochromic regenerative anemia. Renal dysfunction is common, to which endotoxemia, glomerular dysfunction, renal tubular damage, and decreased response to antidiuretic hormone contribute.[38,84–86] Concomitant cystitis and proteinuria usually resolve after treatment of the pyometra but severe proteinuria that remains may predispose for renal failure.[38,86] Insulin resistance and glucose sensitivity are reversibly decreased.[87] Circulating inflammatory

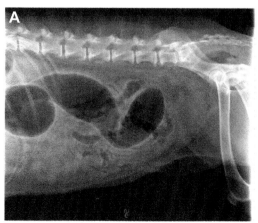
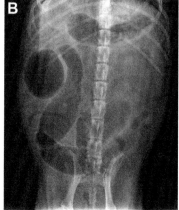

Fig. 5. (*A, B*). Canine emphysematous pyometra, radiography images.

Table 6
Laboratory findings in bitches with pyometra

Abnormality	In proportion of Bitches (%)
Leukopenia	4
Leukocytosis	61
Neutropenia	4
Neutrophilia	55
Monocytopenia	3
Monocytosis	60
Anemia	55
Band neutrophils	40
Band neutrophils >3%	83
Trombocytopenia	37
Toxic changes present	9
Increased ALAT	22
Hypoalbuminemia	33
Decreased ALP	49
Increased ALP	37
Increased AST	64
Cholesterolemia	74
Hypernatremia	29
Hypochloremia	2
Hypochloremia	33
Azotemia	5
BUN decreased	10
BUN increased	5
Bile acids increased	21
Hypoglycemia	6
Hyperglycemia	4
Hypokalemia	4
Hypercalcemia	6
Hypokalemia	25
Hyperlactatemia	10
Urine enzymes increased	42
Bacteriuria	25

Abbreviations: ALAT, alanine aminotransferase; ALP, alkaline phosphatase; AST, aspartate transaminase; BUN, blood urea nitrogen.
Data from Refs.[29,30,37,39,71–73]

mediators and acute phase proteins are generally increased.[81,88] A hypercoagulable state is usually present.[89]

TREATMENT ALTERNATIVES

Surgical treatment, OHE, is safest and most effective because the source of infection and bacterial products are removed and recurrence prevented.[37,74] Laparoscopically assisted techniques have been developed but are not commonly used and used only

Table 7
Laboratory findings in queens with pyometra

Abnormality	In proportion of Queens (%)
Leukopenia	4–5
Leukocytosis	56–100
Neutrophilia	83–100
High percentage neutrophils	45–100
Monocytosis	62
Anemia	4–40
Low packed cell volume	7
High packed cell volume	9
Trombocytopenia	56
Toxic changes present	50
Increased ALAT	7
Decreased creatinine	50
Increased creatinine	6
Hyperproteinemia	30–79
Hyperglobuinemia	50–60
Increased ionized calcium	45
Increased ionized calcium	7
Azotemia	12–20
BUN decreased	9
BUN increased	18
Bilirubinemia	2
Hypoglycemia	0
Hyperglycemia	40
Hypokalemia	10

Abbreviations: ALAT, alanine aminotransferase; ALP, alkaline phosphatase; AST, aspartate transaminase; BUN, blood urea nitrogen.
Data from Refs.[9,10,12,74–76,78,79]

in mild cases.[90] Medical management (solely pharmacologic) may be possible in young and otherwise healthy breeding animals or in a patient for which anesthesia and surgery is hazardous. In patients with serious illness or when complications, such as peritonitis or organ dysfunctions, are present or the cervix is closed, medical treatment is not recommended and surgery is the treatment of choice. Candidates for medical treatment need to be carefully selected for best prognosis for recovery and subsequent fertility.[91] Microbiological culturing and sensitivity testing are prerequisites for the optimal selection of antimicrobial therapy, for which samples are obtained either from the cranial vagina or postoperatively from the uterus.

SURGICAL TREATMENT

Before surgery, the patient is stabilized with adequate intravenous fluid therapy to correct hypotension, hypoperfusion, shock, dehydration, acid–base balance and electrolyte abnormalities, coagulation disturbances, and organ dysfunctions.[92] Monitoring and intervention in critically ill patients following parameters according to the "rule of 20" is recommended.[93] In moderately to severely and severely ill patients, or if sepsis or serious complications are identified, intravenous broad-spectrum bacteri-cidal antimicrobials are administered in addition to supportive therapy, to prevent sys-temic effects of bacteremia and sepsis.[94] The initial choice of antimicrobial drug should be effective against the most common pathogen *E coli* and adjusted after cul-ture and sensitivity results to a narrow-spectrum alternative.[94] The drug should not be nephrotoxic, and the dose, route, and frequency of administration adjusted to ascer-tain optimal effect. In one study, 90% of Swedish *E coli* pyometra isolates were sen-sitive to ampicillin.[4] However, the same proportion is considerably higher in some other countries.[8,95,96] Multiresistant bacteria (ie, resistant to 2 or more drugs) have been reported.[4,8,95,96] The frequency of antimicrobial resistance may differ greatly by geographic location, which needs to be considered, and national regulations con-cerning restriction of antimicrobial usage in pets should be followed.[4,8,32,46] In life-threatening peritonitis, severe sepsis, or septic shock, a combination of antimicrobials is usually recommended for covering a wider range of pathogens.[94,97] If the health sta-tus is close to normal or only mildly depressed and without complications or concur-rent diseases, OHE is curative for pyometra *per se*, and antimicrobials not necessary to include in the perioperative supportive treatment. When following the Swedish Na-tional recommendations for antimicrobial therapy, perioperative antimicrobials were not administered in nearly 45% of 776 bitches that were surgically treated at a Univer-sity animal hospital. None of these bitches that did not receive antimicrobials died or suffered from severe complications.[98] In another Swedish report of 140 surgically treated bitches with pyometra, nearly 60% of the bitches did not recieve perioperative antimicrobial therapy.[99] This points to the possibility of limiting unnecessary use of an-timicrobials in less severely affected bitches with pyometra that are surgically treated.

Removal of the infection is key, and surgery should not be unnecessarily delayed due to the risk of endotoxemia and sepsis when the uterus remains in situ. Anesthesia and perioperative management are focused on maintaining hemodynamic function, gastrointestinal function and protection, pain management, cellular oxygenation, nutrition, and nursing care. Certain drugs may alleviate the inflammatory response.[100] A standard OHE is performed with some modifications.[19,101] The uterus may be large, friable, and prone to rupture, and it is important to handle the tissues carefully (**Figs. 6–11**). The abdominal cavity should be protected from accidental leakage of purulent material via uterine laceration or the fallopian tubes/ovarian bursa opening by packing off the uterus with moistened laparotomy swabs (see **Fig. 11**). Vessels in the broad lig-ament are usually ligated. Purulent material is completely removed from the remaining

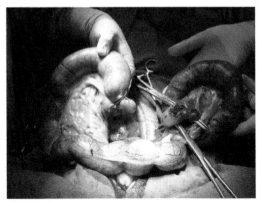

Fig. 6. Canine pyometra uterus.

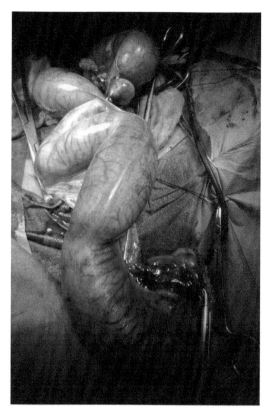

Fig. 7. Canine pyometra uterus.

cervical tissue stump, which is not oversewn. Urine for bacterial culturing can be obtained by cystocentesis when the bladder is exposed. The abdomen is routinely closed but if contaminated with purulent material, this should be removed and the abdomen rinsed with several liters of warmed physiologic saline solution and a closed suction (or open) drainage considered.[97,101] Samples for bacterial culturing are

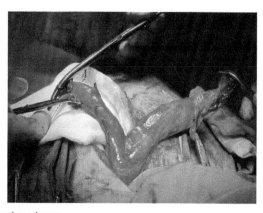

Fig. 8. Feline pyometra uterus.

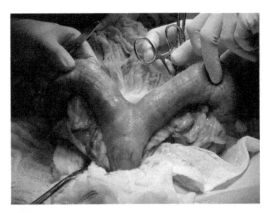

Fig. 9. Canine pyometra uterus.

acquired before abdominal closure if needed. For verification of the diagnosis, macroscopic and histopathologic examination of the uterus and ovaries is performed.

Intensive postoperative monitoring is essential, and in uncomplicated cases, 1 day to 2 days of postoperative hospitalization is usually sufficient. The need for continued supportive care and antimicrobial therapy is evaluated several times daily on a case-by-case basis.[88] Hypothermia, for up to 48 hours postoperatively is expected and may be unresponsive to normal warming therapies.[102] Antimicrobial therapy is discontinued as soon as possible. The overall health status and most laboratory abnormalities improve rapidly after surgery and often normalize within 2 weeks.[88,103]

Considering the seriousness of pyometra, the prognosis for survival is good and mortality rates relatively low, 3% to 20%.[1,10,72,74,104] If more severe systemic illness or complications, such as uterine rupture, peritonitis, or septic shock, develop, however, mortality rates can be considerably higher.[10,94,105] In queens with pyometra and uterine rupture, a mortality rate of 57% has been reported.[9,10] Complications develop in approximately 20% of pyometra patients, the most common being peritonitis (12% of the patients).[10,67,68,72,75,106] Other reported complications include uveitis, urinary tract infection, intracranial thromboemboli, bacterial osteomyelitis, pericarditis, myocarditis, septic arthritis, incisional swelling, dehiscence, urethral trauma, recurrent estrus, uterine stump pyometra, fistulous tracts, and urinary incontinence.[38,67,68,70]

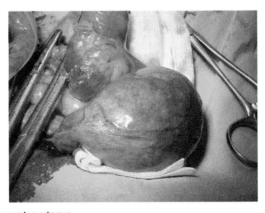

Fig. 10. Canine pyometra uterus.

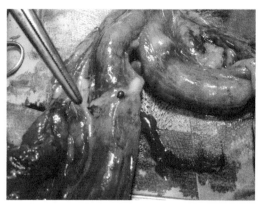

Fig. 11. Canine pyometra uterus with rupture and leakage of pus showing at the tip of the clamp.

In queens, adenocarcinoma may be concominant in pyometra, which needs to be considered.[81]

MEDICAL (NONSURGICAL) TREATMENT

For purely medical (pharmacologic) management, careful patient selection is central to ensure the best possible outcome (ie, resolution of clinical illness and maintained fertility). Suitable candidates are young and otherwise healthy breeding bitches and queens with open cervix and that have no ovarian cysts. It is important that the patients are stable and not critically ill because it may take up to 48 hours until treatment effect for some drugs used.[107] Contraindications include systemic illness, fever or hypothermia, intrauterine fetal remains, organ dysfunctions, or complications, such as peritonitis or sepsis. Adverse drug effects may occur, and endotoxemia and sepsis can quickly transform a clinically stable pyometra to an emergency. Hospitalization is therefore recommended to allow close monitoring, supportive treatments, and rapid intervention. Clinical signs, reduction, and clearing of the vaginal discharge, the uterine size, and laboratory abnormalities gradually normalize in 1 week to 3 weeks.[108] OHE may be necessary without delay if complications arise or the general health status deteriorates and in refractory cases. Antimicrobials alone for the treatment of pyometra may reduce the disease and prevent its progression but does not result in uterine healing.

The strategies of medical treatment are to minimize effects of progesterone by preventing its production and/or action, eliminate the uterine infection, promote relaxation of the cervix and expulsion of the intraluminal purulent material, and facilitate uterine healing. Commonly used drugs are natural prostaglandin $F_{2\alpha}$, ($PGF_{2\alpha}$; ie, dinoprost tromethamine) or its synthetic analog cloprostenol, dopamine agonists (cabergoline and bromocriptine), or progesterone receptor blockers (aglepristone).[109] (**Tables 8** and **9**) The available protocols for purely medical treatment of pyometra include systemic antimicrobial therapy often recommended for 2 weeks or more.[120] The shortest effective duration of adjunctive antimicrobial therapy, however, has not been determined, and 5 days and 6 days were sufficient in 2 studies using aglepristone.[107,114] The antimicrobial drug and administration protocol should be based on bacterial culturing, sensitivity tests, and pharmacokinetics/pharmacodynamics for achieving optimal effect. Additional supportive treatment, including intravenous fluids and electrolyte

Table 8
Examples of studies of medical treatment protocols for open cervix pyometra in dogs

Drug	N	Protocol and Dosage	Outcome and Side Effects	Reference
Aglepristone	24	Aglepristone 10 mg/kg SC q 24 h on day 2, 7, and 14	Recovery in 100%; recurrence after up to 54 mo 12%; fertility in 12% of 17 bitches mated	Jurka et al,[110] 2010
Aglepristone	28	Aglepristone 10 mg/kg SC q 24 h on days 1, 2, 7, 15, and 23, 29 if not cured	Recovery in 75% (resolution of clinical signs); recurrence: 48% after up to 6 y; fertility in 69% of 13 mated bitches	Ros et al,[111] 2014
Aglepristone	52	Aglepristone 10 mg/kg SC q 24 h on days 1, 2, and 7	Recovery in 92%; recurrence: 10% after 3 mo, 19% in 37 bitches followed-up to 1 y; fertility in 83% (5/6 mated bitches)	Trasch et al,[112] 2003
Aglepristone	13	Aglepristone 10 mg/kg SC q 24 h on days 1, 2, 7, and 14	Recovery in 46%	Gurbulak et al,[113] 2005
Aglepristone	20	Aglepristone 10 mg/kg SC q 24 h on days 1, 2, and 8 and if not cured on day 15	Recovery in 60%	Fieni,[107] 2006
Aglepristone + cloprostenol	32	Aglepristone 10 mg/kg SC q 24 h on days 1, 2, and 8 and if not cured on days 14 and 28 + cloprostenol: 1 μg/kg SC q 24 h on days 3–7	Recovery in 84%; no side effect of cloprostenol in 45% of the bitches; in 56% some side effects were noted: loss of appetite, lethargy, vomiting, nausea; 19% recurrence; in closed cervix pyometra cases: recovery in 76.5%, in open cervix pyometra recovery in 74.3%; 1 euthanasia due to declining health, 1 death; Follow-up time: 90 d and up to 2 y in 23 bitches; fertility in 80% (4/5 mated bitches)	Fieni,[107] 2006
Aglepristone	73	Traditional protocol: aglepristone 10 mg/kg SC q 24 h on days 1, 2, and 7 (N = 26) Modified protocol: aglepristone 10 mg/kg SC q 24 h on days 1, 3, 6, and 9 (N = 47)	Recovery with traditional protocol in 88%; recurrence: 17%; fertility in 86% Resolution of clinical signs of pyometra with modified protocol, in 100%; recurrence: 0%; fertility in 78% Follow-up after 2 y	Contri et al,[114] 2015

Protocol	N	Details	Outcome	Reference
Aglepristone + cloprostenol	174	Traditional protocol: aglepristone 10 mg/kg SC q 24 h on days 1, 2, and 8 and every 7 d until low blood progesterone levels/recovery; cloprostenol: 1 µg/kg SC q 24 h on days 3–5	Resolution of clinical signs of pyometra in 100%; recurrence: 8.6%; fertility in 92.1%; no side effects reported. Follow-up after 3 y	Melandri et al,[115] 2019
Aglepristone + cloprostenol	15	Aglepristone 10 mg/kg SC q 24 h on days 1, 3, 8, and 15 (if not cured) + cloprostenol: 1 µg/kg SC q 24 h on days 3 and 8 (N = 8) 1 µg/kg, SC q 24 h on days 3, 5, 8 10, 12, and 15 (N = 7)	Recovery in 100%, recurrence: 20% by the next estrus cycle (in all 15 bitches); fertility in 100% (1 bitch mated); no side effects reported	Gobello et al,[116] 2003
Aglepristone	5	Aglepristone 10 mg/kg SC q 24 h on days 1, 2, 8, and 15 (if not cured)	Resolution of clinical signs of pyometra in 100%, uterine endometrium not fully restored (CEH, endometritis); no side effects reported	Da Rosa Filho et al,[117] 2020
Aglepristone + cloprostenol	5	Aglepristone as above + cloprostenol: 1 µg/kg SC q 24 h on days 1–7 (N = 8) 1 µg/kg, SC q 24 h on days 3, 5, 8 10, 12, and 15 (N = 7)	Resolution of clinical signs of pyometra in 100%, uterine endometrium not fully restored (CEH, endometritis); side effects tachypnea up to 60 min, emesis, hypersalivation, diarrhea, mydriasis, or miosis	Da Rosa Filho et al,[117] 2020
Cabergoline + cloprostenol	29	Cabergoline 5 µg/kg PO q 24 h 1 cloprostenol 1 µg/kg SC q 24 h for 7–14 d	Recovery in 83% by day 14, recurrence: 21%; fertility in 1 out of 2 mated bitches. Mild side effects noted	Corrada et al,[118] 2006
Cabergoline + cloprostenol	22	Cabergoline 5 µg/kg PO q 24 h + cloprostenol 5 µg/kg every third day SC for 7–13 d	Recovery in 90.5% by day 13; recurrence: 20%; fertility in 64% of 11 bitches mated; side effects: retching, vomiting, mild abdominal straining, diarrhea, and panting up to 60 min after administration	England et al,[108] 2007

All protocols combined with and systemic antimicrobial therapy. See the original reference for the most accurate information and more details.
Abbreviations: CEH, cystic endometrial hyperplasia; N, number of bitches; PG, prostaglandin; PO, per os; recovey, resolution of pyometra; SC, subcutaneous.

Table 9
Selected studies of medical treatment protocols for open cervix pyometra in cats

Drug	N	Protocol and Dosage	Outcome and Side Effects	Reference
PGF$_{2\alpha}$ (natural)	21	0.1 mg/kg SC q 12–24 h for 3–5 d (6 queens); 0.25 mg/kg was used in 15 queens but was not more effective	Resolution of signs of pyometra and return to cyclicity in 95%; treatment was repeated in 1 queen; fertility in 81%; no difference between the 2 different dosages (ie, the lower dosage recommended); transient side effects observed in 76%: vocalization, panting, restlessness, grooming, tenesmus, salivation, diarrhea, kneading, mydriasis, emesis, urination, and lordosis lasting up to 60 min. Recurrence of pyometra in 14% (3 cats)	Davidson et al,[9] 1992
Prostaglandin F$_{2\alpha}$ (synthetic analog cloprostenol)	5	5 µg/kg SC q 24 h for 3 consecutive days	Resolution of signs of pyometra in 100%; no recurrence after 1 y; fertility in 40%; transient side effects: diarrhea, vomiting, vocalization	Garcia Mitacek et al,[79] 2014
Progesterone receptor blocker (aglepristone)	10	10 mg/kg SC q 24 h on days 1, 2, and 7 and on day 14 (if not cured)	Resolution of signs of pyometra in 90%; no recurrence after 2-y follow-up; no side effects observed	Nak et al,[78] 2009
Progesterone receptor blocker (aglepristone)	5	15 mg/kg SC q 24 h on days 0, 2, 5 and 8.	Resolution of signs of pyometra in 100%; no side effect but early new estrus; fertility and kittens in 75%	Attard et al,[119] 2020

See the original reference for the most accurate information and more details.
Abbreviations: IM, intramuscular administration; N, number of cats; PO, oral administration; q, every; SC, subcutaneous administration.

supplementation, is provided depending on physical examinations and laboratory tests results.

PGF$_{2\alpha}$ is luteolytic and uterotonic and stimulates smooth musculature. Side effects, such as hypothermia, frequent defecation, diarrhea, salivation, vomiting, restlessness, shivering, and depression, are common and dose-dependent and may last for approximately 1 hour after administration.[121] PGF$_{2a}$ should be administrated far from feeding to reduce the risk of vomiting.[115] Treatment with metoclopramide or walking the bitch for 15 minutes to 20 minutes after administration has been suggested to lessen nausea and vomiting.[109] Serious adverse effects of PGF$_{2\alpha}$, such as death, shock, and ventricular tachycardia, have been reported and the therapeutic window is narrow, which is why dosage calculations should be done meticulously. It is therefore very important to choose the lowest possible effective dose and hospitalize patients during the treatment of monitoring and immediate intervention if severe side effects develop. Brachycephalic breeds may be predisposed to bronchospasm, making PGF$_{2\alpha}$ contraindicated.[120,122] Owner consent, with information of potential risks, is necessary to obtain before extralabel drug usage. Several protocols are considered experimental because efficiency and optimal dosages have not yet been established. For natural PGF$_{2\alpha}$, subcutaneous administration of 0.1 mg/kg every 12 hours to 24 hours until resolution is the dose generally recommended in bitches and queens. Despite at the lower end of the recommended range and administered once daily, this dose is associated with many undesired side effects (the recommended range includes higher doses, following evaluation of the effect of a lower dose), which is why other lower dose alternatives and drug combinations are becoming more commonly used.[121,123] Other authors suggest starting by giving 10 µg/kg subcutaneously 5 times on the first day, gradually increasing the dose to 25 µg/kg 5 times on the second day, and reaching 50 µg/kg by day 3. Doses of 50 µg/kg were then given 3 times to 5 times daily from day 3 and onward during the treatment period, a regime resulting in side effects in 15% of treated bitches.[109] A dose of 100 µg/kg natural PGF$_{2\alpha}$ administered subcutaneously once daily for 7 days resulted in clinical recovery in 7 bitches but many side effects were observed and lower doses are preferable.[124] Natural PGF$_{2\alpha}$, 20 µg/kg, was given intramuscularly 3 times daily on up to 8 consecutive days in 1 study, and 30 µg/kg was given subcutaneously twice daily for 8 days in another study, resulting in the resolution of the illness in 70% of 10 bitches and in 100% of 7 bitches, respectively, and no side effects.[125,126] More recent low-dose protocols recommend subcutaneous administration of natural PGF$_{2\alpha}$ at a dose of 10 to 50 µg/kg every 4 to 6 hours.[120] The synthetic PGF$_{2\alpha}$ analog cloprostenol is administered at a notably lower dose than for natural PGF$_{2\alpha}$,[124] and accurate calculations are crucial to avoid serious side effects or fatalities. For cloprostenol, subcutaneous administration of 1 µg/kg to 3 µg/kg every 12 hours to 24 hours to resolution/effect is the recommended dose for bitches and queens.[121] Subcutaneous administration of low-dose cloprostenol, 1 µg/kg, once daily was effective in 100% of 7 bitches in 1 study but with a high recurrence rate, 85%, and subsequent fertility rate of 14%.[124]

The dopamine agonists cabergoline and bromocriptine are effectively luteolytic from day 25 after estrus because of their antiprolactin effects and have been used together with PGF$_{2\alpha}$ for augmented treatment of pyometra.[108,109] Cabergoline has the advantages of usually causing less vomiting than bromocriptine and is administered once daily compared with 3 to 4 times daily for bromocriptine.[108,109,122] Cabergoline combined with a low dose of cloprostenol led to resolution of the illness in 90.5% of 22 treated bitches with pyometra in one study.[108] In another study using cabergoline and cloprostenol, 83% of 29 bitches recovered from the illness.[118] This combination was also shown the most effective compared with only low-dose cloprostenol or natural $PGF_{2\alpha}$.[123] For treatment of pyometra in cats, no clinical studies have been published on cabergoline and bromocriptine but similar doses and regimes as for dogs have been suggested.[19]

The progesterone blocker aglepristone is commonly used in Europe for the treatment of pyometra (see) but is not currently approved for use in North America. Aglepristone binds to progesterone receptors effectively and competitively and without stimulating any of the hormone's effects. Side effects are usually rare and not severe, and cervical relaxation induced within 48 hours.[78,107,110–114,117,119,127] According to the recommended traditional protocol, 10 mg/kg aglepristone is administered subcutaneously once daily on days 1, 2, and 7 or 8, and on days 14 and 28 if not yet cured. This protocol results in success rates of 46% to 100%, recurrence rates 0% to 48% and subsequent fertility rates of 69% to 85%.[127] Aglepristone was administered more frequently (on days 1, 3, 6, and 9) in a modified protocol, which resulted in resolution of the illness in all 47 treated bitches and with no reported recurrence for up to 2 years.[114] The traditional aglepristone protocol in combination with cloprostenol 1 μg/kg subcutaneously on days 3 to 5 was used in a study of 32 bitches and resulted in 76%, 5% to 84% recovery, 19% recurrence rate and reported fertility 80%, that is, 4 of 5 mated bitches. However, one death and one euthanasia due to declining health were also reported.[107] In a recent larger study of 174 bitches, the same protocol resulted in 100% recovery, a recurrence rate of 8.6%, and fertility rate of 92.1%.[115] In this latter study, cloprostenol was administered far from feeding and no side effects were reported.[115] Treatment with aglepristone resulted in the resolution of pyometra in 9 of 10 queens, with no recurrence reported after 2 years and no side effects observed (see **Table 8**).[78] A modified protocol, in which aglepristone was administered at a dose of 15 mg/kg, on days 0, 2, 5, and 8, was studied in 5 queens with pyometra but very few or no signs of illness. In all 5 queens, clinical resolution was achieved after 10 days, a new estrus cycle started 6 to 11 days after treatment start, and temporarily postponed using melatonin. Four queens were mated, where of 3 (75%) became pregnant at the first mating, with uneventful birth of live kittens (see **Table 8**).[119] Prostaglandin and antigestagen have been shown to have somewhat different local effects on the endometrium, which may contribute to differences in treatment results.[117]

Local treatment methods of pyometra have been shown effective but are not yet commonly used in clinical practice in bitches or queens.[128,129] Intravaginal infusion of prostaglandins and antimicrobials yielded successful result in 15 of 17 treated bitches, without side effects or recurrence after 12 months.[130] Aglepristone in combination with intrauterine antimicrobials was successful in 9 of 11 bitches.[113] Intrauterine drainage through transcervical catheters may facilitate recovery in refractory cases.[128,129] Surgical drainage and intrauterine lavage resulted in fertility in 100% of 8 treated bitches.[131] Whether prostaglandin E_2, administered intravaginally or orally, and the associated cervical relaxation is beneficial in medical treatment protocols remains to be studied.[120,122]

PROGNOSIS AFTER MEDICAL TREATMENT

The prognosis for survival after purely pharmacologic treatment is good, provided the right patient selection. Breeding on the subsequent estrus cycle is consistently recommended after medical treatment, to avoid recurrence. The mean reported long-term success (resolution of clinical illness) of medical treatment is approximately 87% (range 46%–100%) in dogs[104,107,108,111–114,116,118,124] and 95% (range 90%–100%) in cats[8,78,79] (see **Tables 8** and **9**). The prognosis for fertility after medical treatment is generally considered good, with a mean fertility rate of 70% (range 14%–100%) reported in dogs and of 78% in cats. The mean recurrence rate reported in dogs is

18.5% (range 0%–48%), and 0% to 14% in cats. Fertility rates after aglepristone treatment are higher in younger (<5 years) bitches and those that have no other uterine or ovarian pathologic condition.[110,111]

PREDICTIVE MARKERS

Of clinical and laboratory parameters investigated, leukopenia has been associated with both presence of peritonitis and increased postoperative hospitalization in surgically treated bitches with pyometra.[72] Uterine rupture, inappetence, high blood urea nitrogen concentrations or creatinine, low packed cell volume and dehydration were associated with increased postoperative hospitalization.[132,133] Concentrations of acute-phase proteins such as C-reactive protein and serum amyloid A are increased in sepsis.[39,106] Increased white blood cell count, lymphocytes, monocytes, neutrophils, alanine aminotransferase concentrations, neutrophil/leukocyte ratio, monocyte/lymphocyte ratio, percentage band neutrophils/albumin ration was higher in pyometra-induced SIRS (systemic inflammatory response syndrome), compared with non-SIRS cases. However, white blood cell count was included in the SIRS-criteria applied.[134] Concentrations of C-reactive protein and $PGF_{2\alpha}$ have been linked with length of postoperative hospitalization.[29,30] Acute-phase proteins concentrations and inflammatory mediators decrease gradually during postoperative recovery, and maintained or increased concentrations may indicate complications.[81,88] Persistent proteinuria, increased urinary to protein-creatinine ratio greater than 1.0 and concentrations of renal biomarkers after treatment, indicate renal disease that requires special attention.[38,85,86] Central venous oxygen saturation and base-deficit and lactate levels were valuable for determining outcome in bitches with pyometra and sepsis.[135] A quick-sepsis-related organ failure assessment score (qSOFA) of 2 or above was linked with in-hospital mortality and length of hospitalization in dogs with pyometra and sepsis.[136] Band neutrophil concentrations, lymphopenia and monocytosis, blood urea nitrogen greater than 30 mg/dL, and creatinine concentrations greater than 1.5 mg/dL have been associated with death.[137] Certain inflammatory variables, proteins, and measurement of cell-free DNA may be clinically useful for prognostication provided that cage-side tests become available.[39,133,138,139] In queens, white blood cell counts, neutrophils, band neutrophils, monocytes, and the percentage band neutrophils were positively, and albumin concentrations negatively, associated with postoperative hospitalization.[12] Depressed mentation, abnormal ionized calcium blood levels were associated with increased postoperative hospitalization, and fever, absence of vaginal discharge, and heart murmur may indicate a more severe illness.[74]

Salivary variables are currently investigated for diagnostic and prognostic purposes, as a noninvasive sampling method.[140–142] Plasma and salivary proteomics, and metabolomics studies have identified future potential diagnostic and prognostic biomarkers if tests become clinically available.[139–143]

DIFFERENTIATION OF PYOMETRA AND MUCOMETRA OR HYDROMETRA

Fluid in the uterine lumen is present in both pyometra and mucometra/hydrometra, and their clinical manifestations can be similar. In pyometra, however, life-threatening complications may develop because of the bacterial infection, and differentiation of these disorders is thus important to optimize treatments. In mucometra/hydrometra, there is no bacterial infection of the uterus, and thus no risk of subsequent endotoxemia. As long as pyometra is not looming or there are additional ovarian or uterine tissue disorders, patients with mucometra or hydrometra could be candidates for purely pharmacologic therapy, or ovary-sparing surgery in case there are high-risk for side effects of

OHE.[144–147] However, if any undetected pathologic condition remains, the susceptibility to infection may be increased.[17,28] Ultrasonographic examination of the uterus illustrating the fluid echogenicity and hemodynamic parameters may be helpful to differentiate pyometra from mucometra/hydrometra in some cases but is not diagnostic.[83] The health status is more depressed and lethargy and gastrointestinal disturbances more frequently observed in pyometra than in mucometra/hydrometra. More than 3 clinical signs of illness and a more pronounced inflammatory response are also indicative of pyometra as opposed to mucometra/hydrometra.[29,30] Possible circulating biomarkers to differentiate pyometra from CEH are C-reactive protein, $PGF_{2\alpha}$-metabolite, percentage band neutrophils, interleukin (IL)-6, secretory leukocyte protease inhibitor, and IL-10.[29,30,148]

PREVENTION

To diagnose and treat CEH and pyometra early is favorable, and noninvasive diagnostic methods are warranted.[149,150] Elective spaying has the advantage of being performed in a healthy animal and preventing the development of pyometra and other uterine diseases (provided the uterus is removed). Because there are many negative side effects of spaying, all pros and cons of such intervention, need to be thoroughly evaluated in each individual.[7,144–147,151–154] In dogs with high risk of debilitating side effects of reproductive hormone loss after spaying, ovary-sparing surgical options may be considered.[146] If breeding on the first estrus after medical treatment of pyometra is not possible, close monitoring is advisable to rule out abnormalities that may emerge during the following luteal phase because there might be a predisposing factor for the development of pyometra. Progesterone receptor blockers or prostaglandins may prevent the development of pyometra in high-risk patients.[149] Some investigators recommend postponing the subsequent estrus after medical treatment of pyometra to promote uterine healing.[109,119,153,154]

STUMP PYOMETRA

A stump pyometra is when pyometra develops in residual uterine tissue in incompletely spayed bitches and queens, most often because of hormone-producing ovarian remnants or after an incomplete hysterectomy.[155,156] The clinical presentation is similar, except for a history of previous spay. Ultrasonography usually shows areas of local fluid accumulation at the tissue stump but it may be difficult to localize the ovarian remnant tissue unless follicles are present (**Fig. 12**). Incomplete ovarian resection

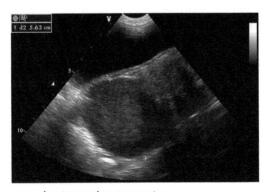

Fig. 12. Stump pyometra due to ovarian remnant.

during an OHE is the leading cause but ectopic or revascularized ovarian tissue separated from the ovary during surgery has also been proposed.[155] Estrogen receptor modulating drugs such as tamoxifen, or topical estrogen compounds prescribed to the owner, have also been associated with the development of stump pyometra.[157–159] Treatment includes surgical resection of remaining uterine and ovarian tissue, in combination with supportive treatments and antimicrobials, if indicated.

In addition to dogs and cats, pyometra has been described in many small animals such as rabbits (see **Fig. 3**), rodents, guinea pigs, hamsters, gerbils, ferrets, and chipmunks.[73,160–163] In other pets, the causative microbes often differ from the bacteria isolated in dogs and cats with the disease. Ultrasonography and cytology are helpful to confirm a presumptive diagnosis based on clinical signs and physical examination, and the preferred treatment is OHE. Aglepristone combined with antibiotics was used successfully for medical treatment of a golden hamster and a guinea pig.[163,164]

CLINICS CARE POINTS

Pearls:

- Be aware of potential life-threatening complications such as peritonitis or sepsis that may develop rapidly in any patient with pyometra and the uterus still in site. Additionally, focus on patients with significant comorbidities that may not provide as clear signs of illness or respond as promptly to treatment as expected.

- Use available predictive markers, clinical and laboratory, and diagnostic imaging techniques as tools for prognostication and treatment adjustments/response follow-up.

- Frequently reassess the patients to ensure identification of emerging complications early, and adjust treatments directly accordingly.

- Surgical ovariohysterectomy remains the safest and most efficient treatment for pyometra. Select patients for purely medical treatment carefully for best outcome.

Pitfalls:

- Insufficient or delayed identification and treatment of patients with organ dysfunctions due to dysregulated inflammation other complications.

- Not securing samples for culturing and sensitivity testing prior to initiating antimicrobial therapy in purely medical treatment protocols.

- Failure to follow the increasingly important antimicrobial stewardship recommendations to prevent inappropriate antimicrobial usage.

- Ovary-sparing surgical options for individuals with high risk for debilitating side effects of loss of reproductive hormones could be considered in uterine disorders without infection, but has not yet been evaluated for pyometra.

ACKNOWLEDGMENTS

The author is very grateful for the following experts' contributions: Dr Fredrik Södersten, DVM, PhD, Swedish University of Agricultural Sciences, performed histopathology examinations and provided the images in **Fig. 1**. Dr George Mantziaras, DVM, PhD, VetRepro, Athens, Greece, provided the ultrasonography Video 1 supplementary files and the stump pyometra ultrasonography image for **Fig. 12**. Associate Professor, Kerstin Hansson, DVM, PhD, Diplomate ECVDI, Swedish University of Agricultural Sciences and the University Animal Hospital, Swedish University of Agricultural Sciences provided the diagnostic imaging and text in **Fig. 3**, and together with Dr Chiara Mattei, Diplomate ECVDI, the radiography images in **Fig. 5**A and B.

DISCLOSURE

The author has nothing to disclose.

SUPPLEMENTARY DATA

Supplementary data related to this article can be found online at https://doi.org/10.1016/j.cvsm.2023.04.009.

REFERENCES

1. Egenvall A, Hagman R, Bonnett BN, et al. Breed risk of pyometra in insured dogs in Sweden. J Vet Intern Med 2001;15:530–8.
2. Hagman R, Strom Holst B, Moller L, et al. Incidence of pyometra in Swedish insured cats. Theriogenology 2014;82:114–20.
3. Dow C. The cystic hyperplasia-pyometra complex in the bitch. J Comp Pathol 1959;69:237–50.
4. Hagman R, Greko C. Antimicrobial resistance in Escherichia coli isolated from bitches with pyometra and from urine samples from other dogs. Vet Rec 2005; 157:193–6.
5. Sandholm M, Vasenius H, Kivisto AK. Pathogenesis of canine pyometra. J Am Vet Med Assoc 1975;167:1006–10.
6. Wadas B, Kuhn I, Lagerstedt AS, et al. Biochemical phenotypes of Escherichia coli in dogs: comparison of isolates isolated from bitches suffering from pyometra and urinary tract infection with isolates from faeces of healthy dogs. Vet Microbiol 1996;52:293–300.
7. Jitpean S, Hagman R, Strom Holst B, et al. Breed variations in the incidence of pyometra and mammary tumours in Swedish dogs. Reprod Domest Anim 2012; 47(Suppl 6):347–50.
8. Lansabakul N, Sirinarumitr K, Sirinarumitr T, et al. First report on clinical aspects, blood profiles, bacterial isolation, antimicrobial susceptibility, and histopathology in canine pyometra in Thailand. Vet World 2022;15:1804–13.
9. Davidson AP, Feldman EC, Nelson RW. Treatment of pyometra in cats, using prostaglandin F2 alpha: 21 cases (1982-1990). J Am Vet Med Assoc 1992;200:825–8.
10. Kenney KJ, Matthiesen DT, Brown NO, et al. Pyometra in cats: 183 cases (19791984). J Am Vet Med Assoc 1987;191:1130–2.
11. Arendt M, Ambrosen A, Fall T, et al. The ABCC4 gene is associated with pyometra in golden retriever dogs. Sci Rep 2021;11:16647.
12. Hagman R, Karlstam E, Persson S, et al. Plasma PGF 2 alpha metabolite levels in cats with uterine disease. Theriogenology 2009;72:1180–7.
13. Niskanen M, Thrusfield MV. Associations between age, parity, hormonal therapy and breed, and pyometra in Finnish dogs. Vet Rec 1998;143:493–8.
14. Von Berky AG, Townsend WL. The relationship between the prevalence of uterine lesions and the use of medroxyprogesterone acetate for canine population control. Aust Vet J 1993;70:249–50.
15. Hagman R, Lagerstedt AS, Hedhammar A, et al. A breed-matched case-control study of potential risk-factors for canine pyometra. Theriogenology 2011;75: 1251–7.
16. Cox JE. Progestagens in bitches: a review. J Small Anim Pract 1970;11:759–78.

17. England GC, Moxon R, Freeman SL. Delayed uterine fluid clearance and reduced uterine perfusion in bitches with endometrial hyperplasia and clinical management with postmating antibiotic. Theriogenology 2012;78:1611–7.

18. Santana CH, Santos DO, Trindade LM, et al. Association of pseudoplacentational endometrial hyperplasia and pyometra in dogs. J Comp Path 2020;180: 79–85.

19. Hollinshead F, Krekeler N. Pyometra in the queen: to spay or not to spay? J Feline Med Surg 2016;18:21–33.

20. Wijewardana V, Sugiura K, Wijesekera DP, et al. Effect of ovarian hormones on maturation of dendritic cells from peripheral blood monocytes in dogs. J Vet Med Sci 2015;77:771–5.

21. Rowson LE, Lamming GE, Fry RM. Influence of ovarian hormones on uterine infection. Nature 1953;171:749–50.

22. Hawk HW, Turner GD, Sykes JF. The effect of ovarian hormones on the uterine defense mechanism during the early stages of induced infection. Am J Vet Res 1960;21:644–8.

23. Chaffaux S, Thibier M. Peripheral plasma concentrations of progesterone in the bitch with pyometra. Ann Rech Vet 1978;9:587–92.

24. Prapaiwan N, Manee-In S, Olanratmanee E, et al. Expression of oxytocin, progesterone, and estrogen receptors in the reproductive tract of bitches with pyometra. Theriogenology 2017;89:131–9.

25. Ström Holst B, Larsson B, Rodriguez-Martinez H, et al. Prediction of the oocyte recovery rate in the bitch. J Vet Med A Physiol Pathol Clin Med 2001;48:587–92.

26. De Bosschere H, Ducatelle R, Vermeirsch H, et al. Cystic endometrial hyperplasia-pyometra complex in the bitch: should the two entities be disconnected? Theriogenology 2001;55:1509–19.

27. Moxon R, Whiteside H, England GCW. Prevalence of ultrasound-determined cystic endometrial hyperplasia and the relationship with age in dogs. Theriogenology 2016;86:976–80.

28. Reusche N, Beineke A, Urhausen C, et al. Proliferative and apoptotic changes in the healthy canine endometrium and in cystic endometrial hyperplasia. Theriogenology 2018;114:14.

29. Fransson BA, Karlstam E, Bergstrom A, et al. C-reactive protein in the differentiation of pyometra from cystic endometrial hyperplasia/mucometra in dogs. J Am Anim Hosp Assoc 2004;40:391–9.

30. Hagman R, Kindahl H, Fransson BA, et al. Differentiation between pyometra and cystic endometrial hyperplasia/mucometra in bitches by prostaglandin F2alpha metabolite analysis. Theriogenology 2006;66:198–206.

31. Schlafer DH, Gillford AT. Cystic endometrial hyperplasia, pseudo-placentational endometrial hyperplasia, and other cystic conditions of the canine and feline uterus. Theriogenology 2008;70:349–58.

32. Coggan JA, Melville PA, de Oliveira CM, et al. Microbiological and histopathological aspects of canine pyometra. Braz J Microbiol 2008;39:477–83.

33. Fransson B, Lagerstedt AS, Hellmen E, et al. Bacteriological findings, blood chemistry profile and plasma endotoxin levels in bitches with pyometra or other uterine diseases. Zentralbl Veterinarmed A 1997;44:417–26.

34. Hernandez JL, Besso JG, Rault DN, et al. Emphysematous pyometra in a dog. Vet Radiol Ultrasound 2003;44:196–8.

35. Børresen B. Pyometra in the dog. II.-A pathophysiological investigation. II. Anamnestic, clinical and reproductive aspects. Nord Vet Med 1979;31:251–7.

36. Vandeplassche M, Coryn M, De Schepper J. Pyometra in the bitch: cytological, bacterial, histological and endocrinological characteristics. Vlaams Diergeneeskd Tijdschr 1991;60:207–11.

37. Hardy RM, Osborne CA. Canine pyometra: pathophysiology, diagnosis and treatment of uterine and extra-genital lesions. J Am Anim Hosp Assoc 1974; 10:245–67.

38. Maddens B, Heiene R, Smets P, et al. Evaluation of kidney injury in dogs with pyometra based on proteinuria, renal histomorphology, and urinary biomarkers. J Vet Intern Med 2011;25:1075–83.

39. Jitpean S, Pettersson A, Höglund OV, et al. Increased concentrations of Serum amyloid A in dogs with sepsis caused by pyometra. BMC Vet Res 2014;10:273.

40. Borresen B, Naess B. Microbial immunological and toxicological aspects of canine pyometra. Acta Vet Scand 1977;18:569–71.

41. Grindlay M, Renton JP, Ramsay DH. O-groups of Escherichia coli associated with canine pyometra. Res Vet Sci 1973;14:75–7.

42. Zheng HH, Du CT, Zhang YZ, et al. A study on the correlation between intrauterine microbiota and uterine pyogenesis in dogs. Theriogenology 2023;196:97–105.

43. Wareth G, Melzer F, El-Diasty M, et al. Isolation of *Brucella abortus* from a Dog and a Cat Confirms their Biological Role in Re-emergence and Dissemination of Bovine Brucellosis on Dairy Farms. Transboundary Emerg Dis 2016;64:e27–30.

44. Watts JR, Wright PJ, Whithear KC. Uterine, cervical and vaginal microflora of the normal bitch throughout the reproductive cycle. J Small Anim Pract 1996;37: 54–60.

45. Nomura K, Yoshida K, Funahashi H, et al. The possibilities of uterine infection of Escherichia coli inoculated into the vagina and development of endometritis in bitches. Japanese Journal of Reproduction 1988;34:199–203.

46. Agostinho JM, de Souza A, Schocken-Iturrino RP, et al. Escherichia coli strains isolated from the uteri horn, mouth, and rectum of bitches suffering from pyometra: virulence factors, antimicrobial susceptibilities, and clonal relationships among strains. Int J Microbiol 2014;2014:979584.

47. Hagman R, Kuhn I. Escherichia coli strains isolated from the uterus and urinary bladder of bitches suffering from pyometra: comparison by restriction enzyme digestion and pulsed-field gel electrophoresis. Vet Microbiol 2002;84:143–53.

48. Xavier RGC, Santana CH, da Silva PHS, et al. Transmission of Escherichia coli Causing Pyometra between Two Female Dogs. Microorganisms 2022;10:2465.

49. Menard J, Goggs R, Mitchell P, et al. Effect of antimicrobial administration on fecal microbiota of critically ill dogs: dynamics of antimicrobial resistance over time. Anim Microbiome 2022;4:36.

50. Melo RT, Oliviera RP, Silva BF, et al. Phylogeny and Virulence Factors of Escherichia coli Isolated from Dogs with Pyometra. Vet Sci 2022;9:158.

51. Szczubial M, Kankofer M, Wawrykowski, et al. Activity of the glycosidases β-galactosidase, α-L-fucosidase, β-N-acetyl-hexosaaminidase, and sialidase in uterine tissues from female dogs in diestrus with and without pyometra. Therigenology 2021;177:133–9.

52. Mateus L, Henriques S, Merino C, et al. Virulence genotypes of Escherichia coli canine isolates from pyometra, cystitis and fecal origin. Vet Microbiol 2013;166: 590–4.

53. Siqueira AK, Ribeiro MG, Leite Dda S, et al. Virulence factors in Escherichia coli strains isolated from urinary tract infection and pyometra cases and from feces of healthy dogs. Res Vet Sci 2009;86:206–10.

54. Chen YM, Wright PJ, Lee CS, et al. Uropathogenic virulence factors in isolates of Escherichia coli from clinical cases of canine pyometra and feces of healthy bitches. Vet Microbiol 2003;94:57–69.

55. Lopes CE, De Carli S, Imperico Riboldi C, et al. Pet pyometra: Correlating Bacteria Pathogenicity to Endometrial histological changes. Pathogens 2021;10:833.

56. Fiamengo TE, Runcan EE, Premanandan C, et al. Evaluation of Biofilm Production by Escherichia coli Isolated From Clinical Cases of Canine Pyometra Topics in Companion Animal Medicine. Top Companion Anim Med 2020;39:100429.

57. Henriques S, Silva E, Silva MF, et al. Immunomodulation in the canine endometrium by uteropathogenic Escherichia coli. Vet Res 2016;47:114.

58. Hagman R, Rönnberg E, Pejler G. Canine bacterial uterine infection induces upregulation of proteolysis-related genes and downregulation of homeobox and zinc finger factors. PLoS One 2009;4:e8039.

59. Bukowska D, kempisty B, Zawirucha P, et al. Microarray analysis of inflammatory response-related gene expression in the uteri of dogs with pyometra. J Biol Regul Homeost Agents 2014;28:637–48.

60. Voorwalld FA, Marchi FA, Rios Villacis RA, et al. Molecular expression profile revelas potential biomarkers and therapeutic targets in canine endometrial lesions. PLoS One 2015;10:e0133894.

61. Pugliese M, La Maestra R, Passantino A, et al. Electrocardiographic Findings in Bitches Affected by Closed Cervix Pyometra. Vet Sci 2020;7:183.

62. Van Miert ASJ, Frens J. The reaction of different animal species to bacterial pyrogens. Zentralbl Veterinarmed A 1968;15:532–43.

63. McAnulty JF. Septic shock in the dog: a review. J Am Anim Hosp Assoc 1983;19: 827–36.

64. Okano S, Tagawa M, Takase K. Relationship of the blood endotoxin concentration and prognosis in dogs with pyometra. J Vet Med Sci 1998;60:1265–7.

65. Hagman R, Kindahl H, Lagerstedt AS. Pyometra in bitches induces elevated plasma endotoxin and prostaglandin F2alpha metabolite levels. Acta Vet Scand 2006;47:55–67.

66. Karlsson I, Wernersson S, Ambrosen A, et al. Increased concentrations of C-reactive protein but not high-mobility group box 1 in dogs with naturally occurring sepsis. Vet Immunol Immunopathol 2013;156:64–72.

67. Marretta SM, Matthiesen DT, Nichols R. Pyometra and its complications. Probl Vet Med 1989;1:50–62.

68. Wheaton LG, Johnson AL, Parker AJ, et al. Results and complications of surgical treatment of pyometra: a review of 80 cases. J Am Anim Hosp Assoc 1987; 25:563–8.

69. Singer M. The new sepsis consensus definitions (Sepsis-3): the good, the not-so-bad, and the actually-quite-pretty. Intensive Care Med 2016;42:2027–9.

70. Brady CA, Otto CM, Van Winkle TJ, et al. Severe sepsis in cats: 29 cases (19861998). J Am Vet Med Assoc 2000;217:531–5.

71. Jitpean S, Ambrosen A, Emanuelson U, et al. Closed cervix is associated with more severe illness in dogs with pyometra. BMC Vet Res 2017;13:11.

72. Jitpean S, Strom-Holst B, Emanuelson U, et al. Outcome of pyometra in female dogs and predictors of peritonitis and prolonged postoperative hospitalization in surgically treated cases. BMC Vet Res 2014;10:6.

73. Kondert L, Mayer J. Reproductive medicine in guinea pigs, chinchillas and degus. Vet Clin North Am Exot Anim Pract 2017;20:609–28.

74. Pailler S, Slater MR, Lesnikowski SM, et al. Findings and prognostic indicators of outcomes for queens with pyometra treated surgically in a nonspecialized hospital setting. J Am Vet Med Assoc 2022;260:S42–8.

75. Hagman R, Thorén E, Ström Holst B. A retrospective study of 92 female cats with pyometra. Abstract, 23rd European Veterinary Society for Small Animal Reproduction virtual congress, October 1-2 2021.

76. Talukdar D, Sarma K, Konwar B, et al. Clinico-pathological alterations of pyometra in cat. Indian J Anim Res 2022;B-4723:1–6.

77. Bjurstrom L. Aerobic bacteria occurring in the vagina of bitches with reproductive disorders. Acta Vet Scand 1993;34:29–34.

78. Nak D, Nak Y, Tuna B. Follow-up examinations after medical treatment of pyometra in cats with the progesterone-antagonist aglepristone. J Feline Med Surg 2009;11:499–502.

79. Garcia Mitacek MC, Stornelli MC, Tittarelli CM, et al. Cloprostenol treatment of feline open-cervix pyometra. J Feline Med Surg 2014;16:177–9.

80. Pugliese M, La maestro R, Passantino A, et al. Electrocardiographic findings in bitches affected by closed cervix pyometra. Vet Sci 2020;7:183.

81. Vilhena H, Figueiredo M, Céron JJ, et al. Acute phase proteins and antioxidant responses in queens with pyometra. Theriogenology 2018;115:30–7.

82. Mattei C, Fabbi M, Hansson K. Radiographic and ultrasonographic findings in a dog with emphysematous pyometra. Acta Vet Scand 2018;60:67.

83. Bigliardi E, Parmigiani E, Cavirani S, et al. Ultrasonography and cystic hyperplasia- pyometra complex in the bitch. Reprod Domest Anim 2004;39:136–40.

84. Asheim A. Renal function in dogs with pyometra. 8. Uterine infection and the pathogenesis of the renal dysfunction. Acta Pathol Microbiol Scand 1964;60:99–107.

85. Gasser B, Ramirez Uscategui RA, Maronezi MC, et al. Clinical and ultrasound variables for early diagnosis of septic acute kidney injury in bitches with pyometra. Sci Rep 2020;10:8994.

86. Heiene R, Kristiansen V, Teige, et al. Renal histomorphology in dogs with pyometra and control dogs, and long term clinical outcome with respect to signs of kidney disease. Acta Vet Scand 2007;49:13.

87. Pööpl AG, Valle SC, Mottin TS, et al. Pyometra-associated insulin resistance assessment by insulin binding assay and tyrosine kinase activity evaluation in canine muscle tissue. Domest Anim Endocrinol 2021;76:106626.

88. Dabrowski R, Kostro K, Lisiecka U, et al. Usefulness of C-reactive protein, serum amyloid A component, and haptoglobin determinations in bitches with pyometra for monitoring early post-ovariohysterectomy complications. Theriogenology 2009;72:471–6.

89. Dorsey TI, Rozanski EA, Sharp CR, et al. Evaluation of thromboelastography in bitches with pyometra. J Vet Diagn Invest 2018;30(1):165–8.

90. Becher-Deichsel A, Aurich JE, Schrammel N, et al. A surgical glove port technique for laparoscopic-assisted ovariohysterectomy for pyometra in the bitch. Theriogenology 2016;86:619–25.

91. Fieni F, Topie E, Gogny A. Medical treatment for pyometra in dogs. Reprod Domest Anim 2014;49(Suppl 2):28–32.

92. Fantoni D, Shih AC. Perioperative fluid therapy. Vet Clin North Am Small Anim Pract 2017;47:423–34.

93. Kirby R. An introduction to SIRS and the rule of 20. In: Kirby R, Linklater A, editors. Monitoring and intervention for the critically ill small animal. Ames (IA): Wiley Blackwell; 2017. p. 1–8.

94. DeClue A. Sepsis and the systemic inflammatory response syndrome. In: Ettinger SJ, Feldman EC, Cote E, editors. Textbook of veterinary internal medicine: diseases of the dogs and cat. 8th edition. St Louis (MO): Elsevier; 2016. p. 554–60.

95. Fernandes V, Cunha E, Nunes T, et al. Antimicrobial resistance of clinical and commensal Escherichia coli canine isolates: profile characterization and comparison of antimicrobial susceptibility results according to different guidelines. Vet Sci 2022;9:284.

96. Rocha MFG, Paiva DDQ, Amando BR, et al. Antimicrobial susceptibility and production of virulence factors by bacteria recovered from bitches with pyometra. Reprod Domest Anim 2022;57:1063–73.

97. Devey JJ. Surgical considerations in the emergent small animal patient. Vet Clin North Am Small Anim Pract 2013;43:899–914.

98. Larsson S, Jämtner M, Emanuelson U, et al. Perioperative antimicrobial usage in female dogs surgically treated for pyometra. Milan: Proceedings of the ISCFR-EVSSAR congress; 2022. p. 45.

99. Turkki OM, Sunesson KW, den Hertog E, et al. Postoperative complications and antibiotic use in dogs with pyometra: a retrospective review of 140 cases (2019). Acta Vet Scand 2023;65:11.

100. Liao PY, Chang SC, Chen KS, et al. Decreased postoperative C-reactive protein production in dogs with pyometra through the use of low-dose ketamine. J Vet Emerg Crit Care 2014;24:286–90.

101. Tobias KM, Wheaton LG. Surgical management of pyometra in dogs and cats. Semin Vet Med Surg (Small Anim) 1995;10:30–4.

102. Karnezi G, Tzimtzimmis E, Rafailidis V, et al. Body temperature fluctuation after ovariohysterectomy in dogs in luteal phase, inactive phase and pyometra: a clinical study of 77 cases. Top Companion Anim Med 2020;40:100440.

103. Bartoskova A, Vitasek R, Leva L, et al. Hysterectomy leads to fast improvement of hematological and immunological parameters in bitches with pyometra. J Small Anim Pract 2007;48:564–8.

104. Feldman EC, Nelson RW. Cystic endometrial hyperplasia/pyometra complex. In: Feldman EC, Nelson RW, editors. Endocrinology and reproduction. 3rd edition. St Louis (MO): Saunders; 2004. p. 852–67.

105. Fantoni DT, Auler Junior JO, Futema F, et al. Intravenous administration of hypertonic sodium chloride solution with dextran or isotonic sodium chloride solution for treatment of septic shock secondary to pyometra in dogs. J Am Vet Med Assoc 1999;215:1283–7.

106. Fransson BA, Lagerstedt AS, Bergstrom A, et al. C-reactive protein, tumor necrosis factor alpha, and interleukin-6 in dogs with pyometra and SIRS. J Vet Emerg Crit Care 2007;17:373–81.

107. Fieni F. Clinical evaluation of the use of aglepristone, with or without cloprostenol, to treat cystic endometrial hyperplasia-pyometra complex in bitches. Theriogenology 2006;66:1550–6.

108. England GC, Freeman SL, Russo M. Treatment of spontaneous pyometra in 22 bitches with a combination of cabergoline and cloprostenol. Vet Rec 2007;160:293–6.

109. Verstegen J, Dhaliwal G, Verstegen-Onclin K. Mucometra, cystic endometrial hyperplasia, and pyometra in the bitch: advances in treatment and assessment of future reproductive success. Theriogenology 2008;70:364–74.

110. Jurka P, Max A, Hawrynska K, et al. Age-related pregnancy results and further examination of bitches after aglepristone treatment of pyometra. Reprod Domest Anim 2010;45:525–9.

111. Ros L, Holst BS, Hagman R. A retrospective study of bitches with pyometra, medically treated with aglepristone. Theriogenology 2014;82:1281–6.

112. Trasch K, Wehrend A, Bostedt H. Follow-up examinations of bitches after conservative treatment of pyometra with the antigestagen aglepristone. J Vet Med A Physiol Pathol Clin Med 2003;50:375–9.

113. Gurbulak K, Pancarci M, Ekici H, et al. Use of aglepristone and aglepristone + intrauterine antibiotic for the treatment of pyometra in bitches. Acta Vet Hung 2005;53:249–55.

114. Contri A, Gloria A, Carluccio A, et al. Effectiveness of a modified administration protocol for the medical treatment of canine pyometra. Vet Res Commun 2015; 39:1–5.

115. Melandri M, Veronesi MC, Pisu MC, et al. Fertility outcome after medically treated pyometra in dogs. J Vet Sci 2019;20:e39.

116. Gobello C, Castex G, Klima L, et al. A study of two protocols combining aglepristone and cloprostenol to treat open cervix pyometra in the bitch. Theriogenology 2003;60:901–8.

117. Da Rosa Filho RR, Brito MM, Faustino TG, et al. Prostaglandin and antigestagen in pyometra bitches: vascular and stereological effect. Reprod fertil 2021;2: 95–105.

118. Corrada Y, Arias D, Rodriguez R, et al. Combination dopamine agonist and prostaglandin agonist treatment of cystic endometrial hyperplasia-pyometra complex in the bitch. Theriogenology 2006;66:1557–9.

119. Attard S, Bucci R, Parrillo S, et al. Effectiveness of a modified administration protocol for the medical treatment of feline pyometra. Vet Sci 2022;9:517.

120. Lopate C. Pyometra, cystic endometrial hyperplasia (hydrometra, mucometra, hematometra). In: Greco DS, Davidson AP, editors. Blackwell's five-minute veterinary consult clinical companion, small animal endocrinology and reproduction. Hoboken (NJ): Wiley-Blackwell; 2017. p. 53–62.

121. Davidson A. Female and male infertility and subfertility. In: Nelson RW, Couto CG, editors. Small animal internal medicine. 5th edition. St Louis (MO): Elsevier; 2014. p. 951–65.

122. Greer M. Canine reproduction and neonatology - a practical guide for veterinarians, veterinary staff and breeders. Jackson (WY): Teton Newmedia; 2015.

123. BSAVA small animal formulary. 8th edition. Gloucester (United Kingdom): British Small Animal Veterinary Association; 2014.

124. Jena B, Rao KS, Reddy KCS, et al. Comparative efficacy or various therapeutic protocols in the treatment of pyometra in bitches. Vet Med 2013;58:271–6.

125. Arnold S, Hubler M, Casal M, et al. Use of low dose prostaglandin for the treatment of canine pyometra. J Small Anim Pract 1988;29:303–8.

126. Sridevi P, Balasubramanian S, Devanathan T, et al. Low dose prostaglandin F2 alpha therapy in treatment of canine pyometra. Indian Vet J 2000;77:889–90.

127. Gogny A, Fieni F. Aglepristone: a review on its clinical use in animals. Theriogenology 2016;85:555–66.

128. Lagerstedt A-S, Obel N, Stavenborn M. Uterine drainage in the bitch for treatment of pyometra refractory to prostaglandin F2α. J Small Anim Pract 1987; 28:215–22.

129. Martini G, Bucci R, Parrillo S, et al. Treatment of a recurrent pyometra by surgical uterine drainage in a Main Coon cat. Vet Sci 2023;10:60.

130. Gabor G, Siver L, Szenci O. Intravaginal prostaglandin F2 alpha for the treatment of metritis and pyometra in the bitch. Acta Vet Hung 1999;47:103–8.

131. De Cramer KG. Surgical uterine drainage and lavage as treatment for canine pyometra. J S Afr Vet Assoc 2010;81:172–7.

132. Pailler S, Slater MR, Lesnikowski SM, et al. Findings and prognostic indicators of outcomes for bitches with pyometra treated surgically in a nonspecialized setting. J Am Vet Med Assoc 2022;260:S49–56.

133. Ahn S, Bae H, Kim J, et al. Comparison of clinical and inflammatory parameters in dogs with pyometra before and after ovariohysterectomy. Can J Vet Res 2021; 85:271–8.

134. Yazlik MO, Mutluer I, Yildirim M, et al. The evaluation of SIRS status with hematobiochemical indices in bitches affected from pyometra and the usefulness of these indices as a potential diagnostic tool. Theriogenology 2022;193:120–7.

135. Conti-Patara A, de Araujo Caldeira J, de Mattos-Junior E, et al. Changes in tissue perfusion parameters in dogs with severe sepsis/septic shock in response to goal-directed hemodynamic optimization at admission to ICU and the relation to outcome. J Vet Emerg Crit Care 2012;22:409–18.

136. Donati P, Londono LA, Tunes M, et al. Retrospective evaluation of the use of quick sepsis-related organ failure assessment (qSOFA) as predictor of mortality and length of hospitalization in dogs with pyometra (2013-2019): 52 cases. J Vet Emerg Crit Care 2022;32:223–8.

137. Kuplulu S, Vural MR, Demirel A, et al. The comparative evaluation of serum biochemical, haematological, bacteriological and clinical findings of dead and recovered bitches with pyometra in the postoperative process. Acta Veterinaria-Beograd 2009;59:193–204.

138. Hagman R. Diagnostic and prognostic markers for uterine diseases in dogs. Reprod Domest Anim 2014;49(Suppl 2):16–20.

139. Kuleš J, Horvatić A, Guillemin N, et al. The plasma proteome and the acute phase protein response in canine pyometra. J Proteomics 2020;223:103817.

140. Franco-Martinez L, Horvatic GA, Gelamanovic A, et al. Changes in the Salivary Proteome Associated With Canine Pyometra. Front Vet Sci 2020;7:277.

141. Tecles F, Escribano D, Contreras-Aguilar MD, et al. Evaluation of adenosine deaminase in saliva and serum, and salivary α-amylase, in canine pyometra at diagnosis and after ovariohysterectomy. Vet J 2018;236:102–10.

142. Dabrowski R, Wdowiak A, Contreras-Aguilar MD, et al. Serum and salivary adiponectin dynamics in septic and non-septic systemic inflammation in a canine model. Vet Immunol Immunopathol 2020;219:109961.

143. Zheng HH, Du CT, Zhang YZ, et al. Identification of Canine Pyometra-Associated Metabolites Using Untargeted Metabolomics. Int J Mol Sci 2022 Nov 16;23(22):14161.

144. Kutzler MA. Gonad-Sparing Surgical Sterilization in Dogs. Front Vet Sci 2020 Jun 12;7:342.

145. Kutzler MA. Understanding the effects of sustained supraphysiologic concentrations of luteinizing hormone in gonadectomized dogs: What we know and what we still need to learn. Theriogenology 2023 Jan 15;196:270–4. Epub 2022 Nov 9. PMID: 36459946.

146. Hart BL, Hart LA, Thigpen AP, et al. Assisting Decision-Making on Age of Neutering for 35 Breeds of Dogs: Associated Joint Disorders, Cancers, and Urinary Incontinence. Front Vet Sci 2020 Jul 7;7:388.

147. Hart BL, Hart LA, Thigpen AP, et al. Assisting Decision-Making on Age of Neutering for Mixed Breed Dogs of Five Weight Categories: Associated Joint Disorders and Cancers. Front Vet Sci 2020 Jul 31;7:472.

148. Sasidharan JK, Patra MK, Khan JA, et al. Differential expression of inflammatory cytokines, prostaglandin synthases and secretory leukocyte protease inhibitor in the endometrium and circulation in different graded CEH-pyometra in bitch. Theriogenology 2022;197:139–49.

149. Mir F, Fontaine E, Albaric O, et al. Findings in uterine biopsies obtained by laparotomy from bitches with unexplained infertility or pregnancy loss: an observational study. Theriogenology 2013;79:312–22.

150. Christensen BW, Schlafer DH, Agnew DW, et al. Diagnostic value of transcervical endometrial biopsies in domestic dogs compared with full-thickness uterine sections. Reprod Domest Anim 2012;47(Suppl 6):342–6.

151. Artl S, Wehrend A, Reichler IM. Kastration der Hundin - neue und alte Erkenntnisse zu Vor- und nachteilen. Tierärztliche Praxis Kleintiere 2017;45:253–63.

152. Waters DJ, Kengeri S, Maras AH, et al. Life course analysis of the impact of mammary cancer and pyometra on age-anchored life expectancy in female Rottweilers: Implications for envisioning ovary conservation as a strategy to promote healthy longevity in pet dogs. Vet J 2017;224:25–37.

153. Goericke-Pesch S, Wehrend A, Georgiev P. Suppression of fertility in adult cats. Reprod Domest Anim 2014 Jun;49(Suppl 2):33–40.

154. Kutzler MA. Estrus Suppression in Dogs. Vet Clin North Am Small Anim Pract 2018 Jul;48(4):595–603.

155. Ball RL, Birchard SJ, May LR, et al. Ovarian remnant syndrome in dogs and cats: 21 cases (2000-2007). J Am Vet Med Assoc 2010;236:548–53.

156. Demirel MA, Acar D. Ovarian remnant syndrome and uterine stump pyometra in three queens. J Feline Med Surg 2012;14:913–8.

157. Sterman A, Mankin K, Barton C. Stump Pyometra Secondary to Human Topical Estrogen Hormone Exposure in a Spayed Female Chihuahua. J Am Anim Hosp Asoc 2019;55:e55604.

158. Ehrhardt CM, Odunayo A, Pascutti K, et al. Stump pyometra in a spayed female dog secondary to tamoxifen. Vet Med Sci 2023;9:47–52.

159. Ivaldi F, Ogdon C, Khan FA. A rare case of vulvar discharge associated with exogenous oestrogen exposure in a spayed Weimaraner bitch. Vet Med Sci 2022;8:1872–6.

160. Martorell J. Reproductive disorders in pet rodents. Vet Clin North Am Exot Anim Pract 2017;20:589–608.

161. Mancinelli E, Lord B. Urogenital system and reproductive disease. Glouchester (United Kingdom): BSAVA; 2016.

162. Heap RB. Prostaglandins in pyometrial fluid from the cow, bitch and ferret. Br J Pharmacol 1975;55:515–8.

163. Engelhardt AB. Behandlung des Endometritis/Pyometrakomplexes eines Meerschweinchens - ein Fallbericht. Der Prakt Tierarzt 2006;87:14–6.

164. Pisu MC, Andolfatto A, Veronesi MC. Pyometra in a six-month-old nulliparous golden hamster (Mesocricetus auratus) treated with aglepristone. Vet Q 2012; 32:179–81.

Moving?

Make sure your subscription moves with you!

To notify us of your new address, find your **Clinics Account Number** (located on your mailing label above your name), and contact customer service at:

Email: journalscustomerservice-usa@elsevier.com

800-654-2452 (subscribers in the U.S. & Canada)
314-447-8871 (subscribers outside of the U.S. & Canada)

Fax number: 314-447-8029

Elsevier Health Sciences Division
Subscription Customer Service
3251 Riverport Lane
Maryland Heights, MO 63043

*To ensure uninterrupted delivery of your subscription, please notify us at least 4 weeks in advance of move.

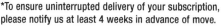

Printed and bound by CPI Group (UK) Ltd, Croydon, CR0 4YY

03/10/2024

01040471-0010